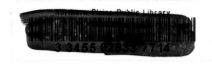

PRAC
STRAT

D0686328

GERIATRIC
MENTAL
HEALTH

CASES AND APPROACHES

PRACTICAL STRATEGIES IN

GERIATRIC MENTAL HEALTH

CASES AND APPROACHES

Edited by

Laura B. Dunn, M.D.
Erin L. Cassidy-Eagle, Ph.D.

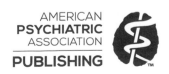
AMERICAN
PSYCHIATRIC
ASSOCIATION
PUBLISHING

Copyright © 2020 American Psychiatric Association Publishing

ALL RIGHTS RESERVED

First Edition

Manufactured in the United States of America on acid-free paper

23 22 21 20 19   5 4 3 2 1

American Psychiatric Association Publishing
800 Maine Avenue SW
Suite 900
Washington, DC 20024-2812
www.appi.org

Library of Congress Cataloging-in-Publication Data
Names: Dunn, Laura B., editor. | Cassidy-Eagle, Erin L., editor. | American
   Psychiatric Association, issuing body.
Title: Practical strategies in geriatric mental health cases and approaches /
   edited by Laura B. Dunn, Erin L. Cassidy-Eagle.
Description: First edition. | Washington, D.C. : American Psychiatric
   Association Publishing, [2019] | Includes bibliographical references and
   index. |
Identifiers: LCCN 2019015077 (print) | LCCN 2019016616 (ebook) | ISBN
   9781615372577 () | ISBN 9781615371488 (alk. paper)
Subjects: | MESH: Mental Disorders | Aged | Geriatric Psychiatry--methods |
   Case Reports
Classification: LCC RC451.4.A5 (ebook) | LCC RC451.4.A5 (print) | NLM WT
   150 | DDC 618.97/689--dc23
LC record available at https://lccn.loc.gov/2019015077

British Library Cataloguing in Publication Data
A CIP record is available from the British Library.

Contents

1 Late-Life Depression I

Dolores Gallagher-Thompson, Ph.D., ABPP
Ann Choryan Bilbrey, Ph.D.
Erin L. Cassidy-Eagle, Ph.D., CBSM, DBSM
Larry W. Thompson, Ph.D., ABPP

2 Late-Life Depression II

Aazaz U. Haq, M.D.
Christopher O'Connell, M.D.

3 Working With Depressed Caregivers: Behavioral Activation

Ann Choryan Bilbrey, Ph.D.
Erin L. Cassidy-Eagle, Ph.D., CBSM, DBSM
Dolores Gallagher-Thompson, Ph.D., ABPP

4 Diagnosis and Treatment of Generalized Anxiety Disorder

Marla Kokesh, M.D.
Daniel D. Sewell, M.D.

Contributors

Awais Aftab, M.D.
Geriatric Psychiatry Fellow, University of California–San Diego

Duane Allen, M.D.
Chief Resident, Eskenazi Health, Department of Medicine, Indiana University School of Medicine, Indianapolis

Ann Choryan Bilbrey, Ph.D.
Associate Director, Optimal Aging Center, Sunnyvale, California

Mary (Molly) E. Camp, M.D.
Assistant Professor of Psychiatry, University of Texas Southwestern Medical Center, Dallas, Texas

Erin L. Cassidy-Eagle, Ph.D., CBSM, DBSM
Clinical Associate Professor, Department of Psychiatry and Behavioral Sciences, Stanford University School of Medicine, Stanford, California

Cathy I. Cheng, M.D., FACP
Adjunct Clinical Assistant Professor, Department of Psychiatry and Behavioral Sciences, Stanford University, Stanford, California

Laura Clayton, LCSW
Senior Specialist, Collective Health, San Francisco, California

R. Ryan Darby, M.D.
Board Certified in Neurology by the American Board of Psychiatry and Neurology; Assistant Professor of Neurology, Vanderbilt University; Director of the Frontotemporal Dementia Clinic, Vanderbilt University Medical Center, Nashville, Tennessee

Beth D. Darnall, Ph.D.
Clinical Professor, Department of Anesthesiology, Perioperative and Pain Medicine, and Psychiatry and Behavioral Sciences (by courtesy), Stanford University School of Medicine, Stanford, California

Laura B. Dunn, M.D.
Professor of Psychiatry and Behavioral Sciences, Department of Psychiatry and Behavioral Sciences, Stanford University, Stanford, California

J. Kaci Fairchild, Ph.D., ABPP
Co-Associate Director, Sierra Pacific MIRECC at VA Palo Alto Health Care System, Palo Alto, California

Dolores Gallagher-Thompson, Ph.D., ABPP
Board Certified in Clinical and Geropsychology by the American Board of Professional Psychology; Professor Emerita, Department of Psychiatry and Behavioral Sciences, Stanford University School of Medicine; and Visiting Professor, Betty Irene Moore School of Nursing, University of California, Davis

Aazaz U. Haq, M.D.
Staff Psychiatrist, Veterans Administration Palo Alto; Assistant Professor of Psychiatry (Affiliated), Stanford University, Stanford, California

Elizabeth Hathaway, M.D.
Psychiatry Resident, Department of Psychiatry, Indiana University School of Medicine, Indianapolis

Alana Iglewicz, M.D.
Associate Clinical Professor, University of California, San Diego Department of Psychiatry

Kevin K. Johnson, M.D.
Clinical Faculty Instructor, Department of Psychiatry, SUNY Upstate Medical University, Syracuse, New York

Michael Kelly, M.D.
Senior Psychiatrist, Coalinga State Hospital, Coalinga, California; and Program Director, Forensic Psychiatry Fellowship, San Mateo County Behavioral Health and Recovery Services, San Mateo, California

Babar Khan, M.D., M.S.
Research Scientist, Indiana University Center of Aging Research, Regenstrief Institute; Associate Professor of Medicine, Division of Pulmonary, Critical Care, Sleep and Occupational Medicine, Department of Medicine, Indiana University School of Medicine; and Director of the Critical Care Recovery Center, Sandra Eskenazi Center for Brain Care Innovation, Eskenazi Hospital, Indianapolis, Indiana

Daniel Kim, M.D.
Clinical Assistant Professor, Department of Psychiatry and Behavioral Sciences, Stanford University, Stanford, California

Marla Kokesh, M.D.
Clinical Assistant Professor, University of California, San Diego

Clete A. Kushida, M.D., Ph.D.
Professor, Department of Psychiatry and Behavioral Sciences, Stanford University, Stanford, California

Sheila Lahijani, M.D.
Clinical Assistant Professor, Department of Psychiatry and Behavioral Sciences, Stanford University School of Medicine, Stanford, California

Peter Louras, M.S.
Pacific Graduate School of Psychology, Palo Alto University, Palo Alto, California

Ajita Mathur, M.D.
Psychiatrist, Department of Psychiatry, Einstein Healthcare Network, Philadelphia, Pennsylvania

Monica Mathys, Pharm.D.
Associate Professor of Pharmacy Practice, Texas Tech Health Sciences Center School of Pharmacy; and Clinical Pharmacy Specialist–Mental Health, Veterans Administration North Texas Healthcare System, Dallas

Leah McGowan, J.D.
Attorney, Robin, Ferguson and Kempton, LLP, Menlo Park, California

Christopher O'Connell, M.D.
Staff Psychiatrist, Veterans Administration St. Louis Health Care System, Missouri

Oxana Palesh, Ph.D., M.P.H.
Assistant Professor, Department of Psychiatry and Behavioral Sciences, Stanford University, Stanford, California

Kathryn Phillipps, M.S.
Pacific Graduate School of Psychology–Stanford PsyD Consortium, Palo Alto University, Palo Alto, California

Iuliana Predescu, M.D.
Staff Psychiatrist, University of Pittsburgh Medical Center (UPMC), Altoona, Pennsylvania

Karen Reimers, M.D., FRCPC
Adjunct Assistant Professor, Department of Psychiatry, University of Minnesota, Minneapolis

Patricia Serrano, M.D.
Geriatric Psychiatry Fellow, Department of Geriatric Psychiatry, Indiana University School of Medicine, Indianapolis

Daniel D. Sewell, M.D.
Professor of Clinical Psychiatry, University of California, San Diego

Kelli M. Smith, M.D.
Resident Physician, Department of Psychiatry and Behavioral Sciences, Stanford University, Stanford, California

Barbara R. Sommer, M.D.
Associate Professor Emerita, Department of Psychiatry and Behavioral Sciences, Stanford University School of Medicine, Stanford, California

Warren Taylor, M.D., MHSc
Board Certified in Psychiatry and Geriatric Psychiatry by the American Board of Psychiatry and Neurology; James G Blakemore Professor of Psychiatry, Department of Psychiatry and Behavioral Sciences, Vanderbilt University Medical Center, Nashville, Tennessee

Nishina A. Thomas, M.D.
Geriatric Psychiatry Fellow, Department of Psychiatry and Behavioral Sciences, Stanford University, Stanford, California

Larry W. Thompson, Ph.D., ABPP
Board Certified in Geropsychology by the American Board of Professional Psychology; Professor Emeritus, Division of Endocrinology, Gerontology and Metabolism, Stanford University School of Medicine, Stanford, California

Eveleigh Wagner, M.D.
Resident PGY-4, Department of Psychiatry and Behavioral Sciences, Vanderbilt University Medical Center, Nashville, Tennessee

Sophia Wang, M.D.
Assistant Professor of Clinical Psychiatry, Department of Psychiatry, Indiana University School of Medicine; and Implementation Scientist, Center of Health Innovation and Implementation Science, Center for Translational Science and Innovation, Indianapolis, Indiana

Ilse R. Wiechers, M.D., M.P.P., M.H.S.
Assistant Clinical Professor, Office of Mental Health and Suicide Prevention, Department of Veterans Affairs; and Assistant Clinical Professor, Department of Psychiatry, Yale University School of Medicine, New Haven, Connecticut

Tonita E. Wroolie, Ph.D., ABPP
Clinical Associate Professor, Department of Psychiatry and Behavioral Sciences, Stanford University School of Medicine, Stanford, California

Preface

As geriatric mental health specialists, we frequently field requests from colleagues along the lines of "Can you help me with this patient?" or "What would you think about implementing if you were seeing this patient?" Such calls have become more frequent as primary providers increasingly struggle to find geriatric mental health specialists with openings for new patients.

Whether the patient in question is a depressed older adult who has not responded to one or more trials of antidepressants and is now losing weight and rarely leaving home, or a patient with dementia whose behavior has becoming increasingly difficult for caregivers, older adults frequently present complex diagnostic and treatment challenges. Comorbid medical conditions frequently complicate the psychiatric presentation. Most patients are already taking numerous medications. Cognitive changes confuse the picture. Family members, who are often also caregivers, have questions and fears—and their own medical and mental health conditions. The so-called patient is not only a patient but also a family system.

The "chief complaint" often masks an underlying or latent problem or set of problems. "Depression" may turn out to be primarily due to cognitive impairment, or vice versa. In geriatric mental health, then, we are detectives trying to gather as many clues as possible to help us crack these complex cases.

And the cases keep coming. Older adults (those age 65 and older) are the fastest growing segment of the U.S. population. All of the baby boomers will be over age 65 years by 2030, meaning that one-fifth of the population will be older adults. As this population expands, the number of older adults with mental illness is expected to double.

Yet there are not enough geriatric mental health specialists to meet the needs of these patients, and there likely will never be enough of us. We cannot train enough specialists to meet the demographic demand.

Therefore, our motivation for compiling this book was to try to disseminate practical information and tools for working with older adults. We wanted to collect in one volume as many clinical pearls as possible, and we wanted the book to be accessible not only to physicians and mental health practitioners but also to a broader audience of care and service providers for older adults. Our hope is that we can help other providers see the patients through our eyes as they work diligently to improve their patients' health and mental health.

Another part of our motivation for putting this book together was our own fascination with the "detective work" of geriatric mental health. We hope that other providers, similarly intrigued, will enjoy the format of this book, where we organized each chapter around a chief complaint, followed by a case vignette that fleshes out the presentation. In older adults, the chief complaint, more often than not, will only lead us to part of the diagnostic and treatment picture. The chief complaint can also be misleading if the full range of possibilities is not considered. A patient complaining of depression may have cognitive impairment; a patient complaining of memory problems may also have depression; a patient exhibiting agitation may be in pain; a patient complaining of pain may also be depressed. Chasing down every lead, exploring every alley, is a crucial part of taking care of our older patients. It is also immensely rewarding and a continual source of renewed learning.

Indeed, as the chapter drafts started to roll in from our wonderful group of authors, we noticed that we ourselves were gaining new clinical knowledge—and better yet, practical advice—from our colleagues. For example, we learned about treatment agreements for anxiety and somatization (Chapter 4), about providing exercise prescriptions for older adults (Chapter 18), and about helpful and not-so-helpful things to say to grieving patients (Chapter 24). We gained a whole new perspective from our team's social worker, giving us renewed appreciation for the importance of social work in helping improve patients' and families' lives. We learned a new word, "kinesiophobia" (fear of movement; Chapter 6). We learned how to take a concise social history (Chapter 9).

We hope you too find some pearls in this book for your own work with older patients and their families. The collected knowledge gives us great hope that we as professionals can better meet the needs of this equally inspiring and vulnerable population.

Laura B. Dunn, M.D.
Erin L. Cassidy-Eagle, Ph.D.

Acknowledgments

We are extremely grateful not only to all of the authors who contributed to this book but also to the many patients who have taught us innumerable lessons about working compassionately and effectively with older adults.

We also want to thank our amazing families (Jim, Leah, and Tara; John, Ava, and Ellen) for their support and patience during the many hours spent working on this project.

Late-Life Depression I

"I Can't Keep Up With My Grandkids"

Dolores Gallagher-Thompson, Ph.D., ABPP
Ann Choryan Bilbrey, Ph.D.
Erin L. Cassidy-Eagle, Ph.D., CBSM, DBSM
Larry W. Thompson, Ph.D., ABPP

CHAPTER 1

Clinical Presentation

Chief Complaint

"I can't keep up with my grandkids."

Vignette

Mr. H is a 78-year-old married white man who enjoyed relatively good physical health (he has type 2 diabetes that is well controlled with medication) and a successful career in business until his retirement at age 73. He began to teach English as a second language (ESL) and was active at his church and with his family: his wife of 54 years, three middle-age children, and five grandchildren. Mr. H started showing mood changes about 2 years ago after several surgeries for various cardiovascular events that resulted in some functional impairment. He says he is unable to "keep up" with his grandchildren and often feels "winded" with little exertion, which resulted in his dropping the ESL program. Along with this fatigue, Mr. H has become more inactive in general and socially withdrawn. He reports that his mood is "down,"

1

and his wife agrees, saying he has become irritable and less able to help her at home and in her daily struggle with the chronic pain of fibromyalgia. Mr. H's primary care physician noted the fatigue and blue mood and inquired about it at a routine office visit.

Discussion

Differential Diagnosis of Depressive Symptoms

Depressive symptoms are common among older adults who experience multiple losses, including declines in physical health and cognitive abilities, deaths of close friends and family members (loss of social supports), financial setbacks, and a host of other biological and psychosocial changes (Aziz and Steffens 2013; Gallagher-Thompson et al. 2017). Detection and correct diagnosis of depression may be difficult in older adults for a variety of reasons; for example, neurological disorders or other medical conditions that often affect the elderly can mimic depression, and older adults tend to endorse a lack of emotions rather than depressed mood (Kotbi et al. 2010) or endorse feelings of irritability and fearfulness rather than sadness (Alexopoulos 2005; Blazer 2003; Haigh et al. 2018). Given this complex situation, it is not surprising that depression is common in later life.

It is estimated that major depressive disorder affects 1%–4% of older adults, while estimates for dysthymia and minor depression are higher, at 4%–13% (Gum et al. 2009; Steffens et al. 2009). In a population-based study of older adults administered the Cambridge Examination for Mental Disorders of the Elderly—Revised, mild depression or dysthymia was the most common depressive disorder (16.4%), with 7.5% experiencing moderate depression and 1.1% experiencing severe depression, while 5.6% endorsed subthreshold depressive symptoms (Forlani et al. 2014). The authors also found that depression decreased as age increased after age 81, although rates of suicide increased—particularly among white males.

Assessment Tools in Common Use

Patient Health Questionnaire

The Patient Health Questionnaire (PHQ-9; Spitzer et al. 1999) is the most widely used self-report screening tool in use today. It is available in multiple languages and is freely downloadable from the website www.phqscreeners.com, which includes a detailed scoring and instruction manual as well as other versions (shorter); the website also includes the Generalized Anxiety Disorder (GAD)–7 measure, which is a separate brief screen for anxiety (Spitzer et al. 2006). Although these measures were not developed specifically for use with older adults, they do the job in terms of getting a quick assessment of presence or absence of symptoms and their severity.

Geriatric Depression Scale

Another very useful screening measure for depression is the Geriatric Depression Scale (GDS; Sheikh and Yesavage 1986), which is also available in short and long forms and in multiple languages. All can be downloaded at no cost from a Stanford University website (web.stanford.edu/~yesavage/GDS.html). The 15-item version and clear scoring instructions can be found online as well (https://consultgeri.org/try-this/general-assessment/issue-4.pdf). The GDS is preferred to the PHQ-9 when there is possible cognitive impairment present because its response format is a simple Yes/No for each item, whereas the PHQ-9 requires more judgment because its response format uses a frequency rating (from "not at all" to "nearly every day") on a four-point scale. However, the PHQ-9 contains a suicide item that may be very relevant depending on the situation, and its responses were mapped onto existing psychiatric diagnostic criteria; thus, it is considered a more sensitive measure of both presence and severity of depressive symptoms.

In addition, screening for depression (as well as cognitive function, substance misuse, social isolation, and so forth) is an integral part of the Medicare Annual Wellness Visit. This annual wellness visit is described at www.medicareinteractive.org and more fully in a document called "Annual Wellness Visit" that is available online from www.cms.gov (Centers for Medicare and Medicaid Services and Medicare Learning Network 2018). We recommend clinicians become familiar with this visit so they can encourage their clients to take advantage of these screenings, which can give valuable information for subsequent treatment planning.

Decision Making for Treatment

A number of algorithms have been developed to assist practitioners in selecting appropriate treatments (Kotbi et al. 2010; Tufts Health Plan 2005). Although not necessarily focused on older adults, they provide thoughtful starting points for decision making. Kotbi and colleagues' algorithm published in 2010 illustrates choices for unipolar depression with and without psychotic features (Kotbi et al. 2010). The Tufts Health Plan algorithm is often used to guide decision making in primary care settings (Tufts Health Plan 2005). Based on our review of these algorithms and several others, we constructed our own algorithm that illustrates our collective thinking on this topic (see Figure 1–1).

Pharmacological and Cognitive-Behavioral Treatments

Late-life depression is commonly treated with pharmacotherapy or psychotherapy—most often cognitive-behavioral therapy (CBT), which has the most empirical support—or a combination of both (Castillo et al. 2013; Khouzam 2012; Substance Abuse and Mental Health Services Administration 2011), although acute episodes are known to respond favorably to electroconvulsive therapy (ECT) (Gautam et al. 2017). Late-life depression is typically treated first with antidepressant medication. However, this treatment can be mitigated by a number of factors, such as the differences in medication response between older adults and younger adults, with older adults often taking longer to respond and experiencing more side effects and more discomfort from these medications than younger adults. For more detailed discussion of this and related issues, it is strongly recommended that the interested reader consult the authoritative chapter by Blazer and Steffens (2015) on assessment and treatment of late-life depressive disorders.

For excellent review papers on treatment of late-life depression that cover a wide range of interventions, including indicators for ECT and transcranial magnetic stimulation (as well as discussion of some interventions that are not considered evidence based, such as acupuncture), see Frank 2014, Gautam et al. 2017, Khouzam 2012, Tedeschini et al. 2011, and Substance Abuse and Mental Health Services Administration 2011. Finally, there is a very thorough article on medication management for major depression in older adults written by a group of pharmacists (Castillo et al. 2013) that reviews not only commonly used antidepressants but also atypical medications that can be used. It should be noted that several influential professional organizations, such as the American Psychiatric Association and the American Psychological Association, have published practice guidelines on this topic (American Psychiatric Association 2010; Areán 2015).

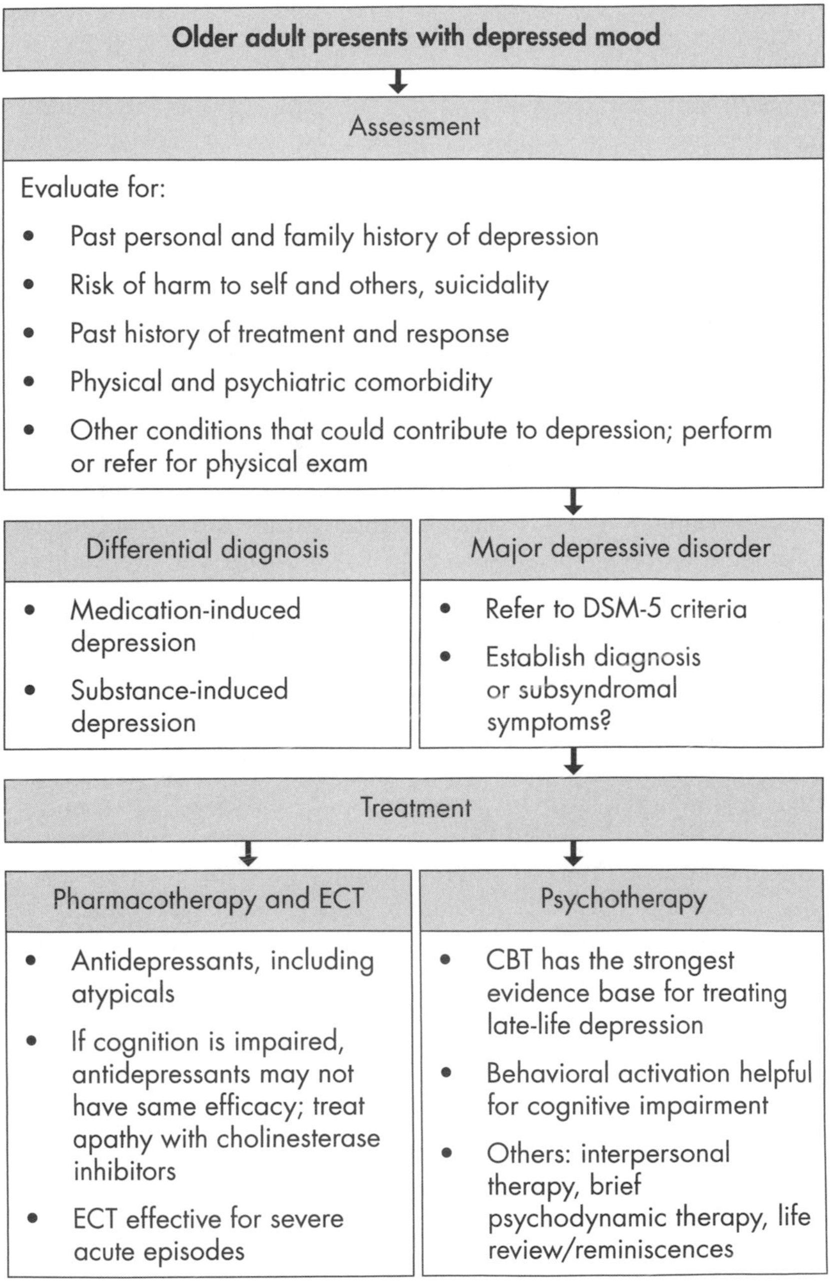

Older adult presents with depressed mood

↓

Assessment

Evaluate for:

- Past personal and family history of depression
- Risk of harm to self and others, suicidality
- Past history of treatment and response
- Physical and psychiatric comorbidity
- Other conditions that could contribute to depression; perform or refer for physical exam

↓

Differential diagnosis	Major depressive disorder
• Medication-induced depression • Substance-induced depression	• Refer to DSM-5 criteria • Establish diagnosis or subsyndromal symptoms?

↓

Treatment

↓ ↓

Pharmacotherapy and ECT	Psychotherapy
• Antidepressants, including atypicals • If cognition is impaired, antidepressants may not have same efficacy; treat apathy with cholinesterase inhibitors • ECT effective for severe acute episodes	• CBT has the strongest evidence base for treating late-life depression • Behavioral activation helpful for cognitive impairment • Others: interpersonal therapy, brief psychodynamic therapy, life review/reminiscences

FIGURE 1–1. Assessment and treatment for older adults presenting with depressed mood.

Note. CBT=cognitive-behavioral therapy; ECT=electroconsvulsive therapy.

Psychotherapeutic Interventions

Psychotherapy with older adults differs from work with younger people in that it considers increased physical comorbidities; lifetime experience of coping with stress; age-specific lifespan development factors, such as cohort effects; and social support systems (Laidlaw et al. 2003, in press). Of the various forms of psychotherapy available, the one with the strongest empirical support is CBT, which is described and listed as an evidence-based practice for treatment of depression in older adults in the Substance Abuse and Mental Health Services Administration (2011) evidence-based practices kit.

CBT is an effective treatment for depression in adults when used alone or in conjunction with medication (for review, see Driessen and Hollon 2010). A number of studies over the past 10–30 years have likewise demonstrated its efficacy with older adults (Areán and Cook 2002; Areán et al. 1993; Cuijpers et al. 2009; Laidlaw et al. 2003; Marquett et al. 2013; Thompson et al. 1987). One of the earliest studies of CBT with an older adult population compared CBT, behavior therapy, and brief dynamic therapy in 91 older adults who were followed for 1 year after treatment ended. Participants showed significant improvement over wait-list control subjects, and all three interventions continued to demonstrate positive outcomes during the 1-year follow-up period (Thompson et al. 1987). The efficacy of CBT has also been shown to be long-lasting; people who respond to CBT tend not to relapse up to 2 years after treatment (Gallagher-Thompson et al. 1990). CBT has also been evaluated for efficacy with family caregivers. A study by Gallagher-Thompson and Steffen (1994) found that longer-term caregivers of older adults with dementia were more responsive to CBT, possibly because CBT is suited to the more structured problem solving that caregivers need to perform when supporting their loved one with cognitive decline. Further discussion of this topic is found in Chapter 3, "Working With Depressed Caregivers."

However, for older adults with more severe symptoms who have been chronically depressed, it is likely that the combination of pharmacotherapy and psychotherapy will be most effective (see Thompson et al. 2001 for empirical support of this assertion). Also, whereas dysthymic disorder or subsyndromal depression can be effectively treated by psychotherapy alone, severe depression usually requires pharmacotherapy in combination with psychotherapy (for review, see Kotbi et al. 2010). Some studies show that older adults prefer nonmedical interventions and may need to limit use of psychiatric medications depending on other medications taken for their physical comorbidities (Kotbi et al.

2010; Kraus et al. 2007). Thus, in the final analysis, the choice is up to the individual as to which form of treatment (if any) he or she will comply with.

Cognitive-Behavioral Therapy

For a brief review of key components of how CBT is typically done with depressed older adults, the reader is referred to the article by Gallagher-Thompson et al. (2017). For a more detailed description, see our therapist manual and accompanying client workbook in the "Treatments That Work" series published by Oxford University Press: *Effective Treatment for Late-Life Depression: A Therapist Guide* (Gallagher-Thompson and Thompson 2010) and *Effective Treatment for Late-Life Depression: A Client Workbook* (Thompson et al. 2010). Used together, these books provide step-by-step guidance for therapists and include homework assignments, forms, and related resources. Our clinical research team has also published a comprehensive handbook on the use of CBT with older adults with a variety of presenting problems, including anxiety and substance use disorders, insomnia, chronic pain, serious mental illness, and suicide issues (Gallagher-Thompson et al. 2008).

Here we describe what we regard as the four key skills that need to be incorporated into all successful CBT work: goal setting, behavioral activation, cognitive reframing (with these three skills usually done in that order), and maintenance of gains and preparing for the future (i.e., developing "action plans" to help the client when adverse situations occur again).

1. **Goal setting** is done in an early session to help focus therapy and to clarify what can be accomplished in the time frame available. Often CBT is time limited (based on insurance concerns, health limitations, and the like), typically 10–20 individual sessions of at least 50 minutes each. Most older adults are not familiar with this form of therapy and do not understand that it is problem oriented and focused in the here and now, with little review of childhood experiences—except in cases in which long-term schema change work is necessary. Typically, goals involve such concrete, measurable targets as becoming more active with other people; reengaging with estranged adult children; seeking part-time or volunteer work; or adapting better to physical health and functional limitations. Setting goals helps structure session time well and reduce time spent on tangential information and discussion.
2. **Behavioral activation** is a brief, effective, empirically validated, first-line treatment for depression of mild to moderate severity. At

the core of behavioral activation are patient-specific activation strategies that focus on helping the depressed individual to a) decrease avoidance and depression-fueling behaviors (e.g., physical inactivity, social isolation, time spent ruminating) and b) increase the number and types of pleasant activities and engagement strategies (e.g., exercising, spending time with family and friends, attending and engaging in community-based activities). The technique often involves enlisting the patient in monitoring his or her activities and scheduling agreed-on "target behaviors" (e.g., having coffee with a friend once a week; going for a walk outside for 15 minutes three times a week). The target behaviors are tailored to the patient's individual interests, relationships, and values. The clinician works closely with the patient to educate, inspire, and document a personalized activity plan, taking into account the patient's baseline level of activity and personal interests. Several books and articles are available that discuss the various elements of behavioral activation and how it can be used with different groups, such as older adults (Kanter et al. 2010; Lejuez et al. 2001; Martell et al. 2013), and a more recent study illustrates its effectiveness with even one treatment session (Gum et al. 2016).

3. **Cognitive reframing** involves teaching clients how to understand and think about their current life situation differently. To do this effectively, clients need to learn how to identify unhelpful thinking patterns, such as all-or-none thinking, mind reading, and "would have/could have/should have" thinking, which are common ways that depressed persons think about themselves, their situation, and the future (Beck et al. 1979). They also need to see how negative thinking and negative mood states are related so that they are motivated to modify these thinking habits. This is not easy for older adults who may have thought certain ways for many years.

To assist older adults, therefore, we teach a variety of skills to challenge the negative thoughts, such as examining the evidence "for" and "against" particular beliefs; articulating what a friend might think in a similar situation; and thinking about the impact or consequences of maintaining specific negative thoughts. These skills enable the client to begin to think differently, which in turn leads to improved mood and everyday functioning. We use thought records to help clients see these relationships and generate appropriate alternative thoughts that are more adaptive and more associated with neutral or positive mood states. These thought records are worked on collaboratively with the therapist until clients are able to complete them on their own. Of course, such forms need to be tailored to the individual client—for example, some have Parkinson's disease or another disorder that prevents them from writing clearly. For such clients, recording the information on their phones and playing it in session or calling it in at certain times of the week can be very helpful. Discussing alternative thoughts and how they lead to better mood (and, often, to more adaptive behaviors as well) is the essence of this component of CBT.

4. **Maintenance of gains** involves helping clients anticipate and prepare for challenges. We ask them to think ahead to a future situation likely to make them depressed again, write it out, and think about how specific skills learned in therapy could help them deal with that situation *without* becoming depressed again. For example, persons with multiple physical health problems may be fearful that "one more bad thing happening" will result in another bout of serious depression. They can be asked to think about how they have coped with prior health challenges (to set the stage for the "action plan") and then asked how they can use those skills plus their new CBT skills to help reduce the negative impact of future health declines. Clients often realize that they are more resilient than they thought in coping with adverse events and that they can use both behavioral activation (possibly in a modified format, depending on the severity of the health condition) and cognitive reframing to help them focus on what they can still do rather than what they cannot do.

We also include in the action plan a section on identifying early warning signs (how the person will know he or she is getting seriously depressed again) along with emergency phone numbers and contact information to use if a serious episode of depression occurs. We explain that depression is, by its nature, cyclical, so it is not shameful to have a new episode and need further professional assistance.

Vignette *(continued)*

Mr. H was assessed as having dysthymic disorder because of the duration of his symptoms. On the PHQ-9 he scored 21, which placed him in the moderately severe range in terms of intensity of symptoms. He was offered a selective serotonin reuptake inhibitor medication by his primary care physician, which helped improve his mood to some degree: readministration of the PHQ-9 showed a decrease to 14 after 3 months. On his next visit, Mr. H said he was interested in adding "talking therapy" following his wife's reading him an AARP magazine article on CBT for late-life depression. He was referred to a trained CBT provider for 12 sessions of individual therapy focused on questioning his unrealistically negative beliefs about himself and his capabilities; increasing his engagement in everyday positive activities (such as short outings with his grandchildren); and resumption of participation in church events with his wife. Mr. H willingly completed "home practice" assignments to record and challenge his negative thoughts and to keep track of daily activities. His compliance increased treatment effectiveness. At the conclusion of therapy his PHQ-9 score was 5 (nondepressed), and his wife reported that he was less irritable and more helpful around the house.

KEY POINTS

- Late-life depression is common. While symptoms may not reach a diagnosable level, they reduce quality of life and should be inquired about, and treatment choices offered.
- Self-report questionnaires such as the Patient Health Questionnaire–9 and Geriatric Depression Scale are helpful for finding out the person's level of distress. In addition, asking direct questions during the Medicare Annual Wellness Visit can help clarify possible causes and contributors and treatment options.
- Pharmacotherapy, electroconvulsive therapy, and various forms of psychotherapy can all be effective ways to treat late-life depression. Decisions about what form of treatment to begin with (and to continue after an acute episode is over) can be informed by a number of existing treatment algorithms, including one provided in this chapter (see Figure 1–1).
- Of the psychotherapies, cognitive-behavioral therapy (CBT) is most effective for both acute and chronic depression. Variants of CBT, such as psychoeducational programs, have also been found to be effective with specific kinds of problems.

Resources

AARP Program Division, 601 E Street, NW, Washington, DC 20049; (888) 687-2277; www.aarp.org

American Association for Geriatric Psychiatry, 6728 Old McLean Village Dr., McLean, VA 22101; (703) 556-9222; www.aagponline.org

American Geriatrics Society, 40 Fulton St., 18th Floor, New York, NY 10038; (212) 308-1414; www.americangeriatrics.org

American Psychiatric Association, 800 Maine Ave., SW, Suite 900, Washington, DC 20024; (888) 357-7924; www.psychiatry.org (provides a curated information on depression: www.psychiatry.org/patients-families/depression)

American Psychological Association, 750 First St., NE, Washington, DC 20002-4242; (800) 374-2721; www.apa.org (Help Center offers information related to psychological issues written for the nonmedical consumer: http://www.apa.org/helpcenter/index.aspx)

Depression and Bipolar Support Alliance, 55 E Jackson Blvd., Suite 490, Chicago, IL 60604; (800) 826-3632; www.dbsalliance.org

National Alliance on Mental Illness (NAMI), Colonial Place Three, 3803 N. Fairfax Dr., Suite 100, Arlington, VA 22203; (800) 950-6264; www.nami.org (website links family members and caregivers with additional support and information: www.nami.org/Find-Support/ Family-Members-and-Caregivers)

National Institute of Mental Health, 6001 Executive Blvd., Room 6200, MSC 9663, Bethesda, MD 20892-9663; (866) 615–6464; www.nimh.nih.gov (website provides up-to-date information about depression: www.nimh.nih.gov/health/topics/depression/ index.shtml)

Substance Abuse and Mental Health Services Administration, 5600 Fishers Lane, Rockville, MD 20857; (877) 726-4727 (provides a wide range of information for both consumers and medical providers, including apps: www.samhsa.gov; also available is "Treatment of Depression in Older Adults Evidence-Based Practices (EBP) Kit," which can be found at: www.dmh.ms.gov/pdf/SAMHSA%20Toolkit.pdf)

References

Alexopoulos G: Late-life mood disorders, in Comprehensive Textbook of Geriatric Psychiatry, 3rd Edition. Edited by Grossberg GT, Sadavoy J, Jarvik LF, et al. New York, WW Norton, 2005, pp 609–654

American Psychiatric Association: Treating Major Depressive Disorder: A Quick Reference Guide. Arlington, VA, American Psychiatric Association, 2010, pp 1–28

Areán PA: Treatment of Late-Life Depression, Anxiety, Trauma, and Substance Abuse. Washington, DC, American Psychological Association, 2015

Areán PA, Cook BL: Psychotherapy and combined psychotherapy/pharmaco-therapy for late life depression. Biol Psychiatry 52(3):293–303, 2002 12182934

Areán PA, Perri MG, Nezu AM, et al: Comparative effectiveness of social problem-solving therapy and reminiscence therapy as treatments for depression in older adults. J Consult Clin Psychol 61(6):1003–1010, 1993 8113478

Aziz R, Steffens DC: What are the causes of late-life depression? Psychiatr Clin North Am 36(4):497–516, 2013 24229653

Beck AT, Rush JA, Shaw BF, et al: Cognitive Therapy of Depression. New York, Guilford, 1979

Blazer DG: Depression in late life: review and commentary. J Gerontol A Biol Sci Med Sci 58(3):249–265, 2003 12634292

Blazer DG, Steffens DC: Depressive disorders, in The American Psychiatric Publishing Textbook of Geriatric Psychiatry, 5th Edition. Washington, DC, American Psychiatric Publishing, 2015, pp 283–308

Castillo S, Sorrentino E, Twum-Fening K: Depression in the elderly: a pharmacist's perspective. Formulary 48(12):388–394, 2013

Centers for Medicare and Medicaid Services, Medicare Learning Network: Annual Wellness Visit (ICN 905706). Baltimore, MD, Centers for Medicare and Medicaid Services, 2018. Available at: https://www.cms.gov/Outreach-and-Education/Medicare-Learning-Network-MLN/MLNProducts/downloads/AWV_chart_ICN905706.pdf. Accessed December 11, 2018.

Cuijpers P, van Straten A, Smit F, et al: Is psychotherapy for depression equally effective in younger and older adults? A meta-regression analysis. Int Psychogeriatr 21(1):16–24, 2009 19040783

Driessen E, Hollon SD: Cognitive behavioral therapy for mood disorders: efficacy, moderators and mediators. Psychiatr Clin North Am 33(3):537–555, 2010 20599132

Forlani C, Morri M, Ferrari B, et al: Prevalence and gender differences in late-life depression: a population-based study. Am J Geriatr Psychiatry 22(4):370–380, 2014 23567427

Frank C: Pharmacologic treatment of depression in the elderly. Can Fam Physician 60(2):121–126, 2014 24522673

Gallagher-Thompson D, Steffen AM: Comparative effects of cognitive-behavioral and brief psychodynamic psychotherapies for depressed family caregivers. J Consult Clin Psychol 62(3):543–549, 1994 8063980

Gallagher-Thompson D, Thompson LW: Effective Treatment for Late-Life Depression: A Therapist Guide. New York, Oxford University Press, 2010

Gallagher-Thompson D, Hanley-Peterson P, Thompson LW: Maintenance of gains versus relapse following brief psychotherapy for depression. J Consult Clin Psychol 58(3):371–374, 1990 2365900

Gallagher-Thompson D, Steffen A, Thompson LW (eds): Handbook of Behavioral and Cognitive Therapies With Older Adults. New York, Springer, 2008

Gallagher-Thompson D, Cassidy-Eagle E, Dunn LB: Cognitive-behavioral therapy for treatment of late-life depression. Today's Geriatric Medicine 10(1):22–26, 2017

Gautam S, Jain A, Gautam M, et al: Clinical practice guidelines for the management of depression. Indian J Psychiatry 59 (suppl 1):S34–S50, 2017 28216784

Gum AM, King-Kallimanis B, Kohn R: Prevalence of mood, anxiety, and substance-abuse disorders for older Americans in the national comorbidity survey-replication. Am J Geriatr Psychiatry 17(9):769–781, 2009 19700949

Gum AM, Schonfeld L, Tyler S, et al: One-visit behavioral intervention for older primary care patients with mild to moderate depressive symptoms. South Med J 109(8):442–447, 2016 27490649

Haigh EAP, Bogucki OE, Sigmon ST, et al: Depression among older adults: a 20-year update on five common myths and misconceptions. Am J Geriatr Psychiatry 26(1):107–122, 2018 28735658

Kanter JW, Manos RC, Bowe WM, et al: What is behavioral activation? A review of the empirical literature. Clin Psychol Rev 30(6):608–620, 2010 20677369

Khouzam HR: Depression in the elderly: how to treat. Consultant 52(4):267–278, 2012

Kotbi N, Mahgoub N, Odom A: Depression in older adults: how to treat its distinct clinical manifestations. Curr Psychiatr 9(8):39–46, 2010

Kraus CA, Kunik ME, Stanley MA: Use of cognitive behavioral therapy in late-life psychiatric disorders. Geriatrics 62(6):21–26, 2007 17547480

Laidlaw K, Thompson LW, Gallagher-Thompson D, et al: Cognitive Behaviour Therapy With Older People: A Case Conceptualization Approach. New York, John Wiley and Sons, 2003

Laidlaw K, Thompson LW, Gallagher-Thompson D: Cognitive Behaviour Therapy With Older People: A Case Conceptualization Approach, 2nd Edition. New York, John Wiley and Sons (in press)

Lejuez CW, Hopko DR, Hopko SD: A brief behavioral activation treatment for depression. Treatment manual. Behav Modif 25(2):255–286, 2001 11317637

Marquett RM, Thompson LW, Reiser RP, et al: Psychosocial predictors of treatment response to cognitive-behavior therapy for late-life depression: an exploratory study. Aging Ment Health 17(7):830–838, 2013 23631698

Martell CR, Dimidijian S, Herman-Dunn R: Behavioral Activation for Depression: A Clinician's Guide. New York, Guilford, 2013

Sheikh JI, Yesavage JA: Geriatric Depression Scale (GDS): recent evidence and development of a shorter version. Clinical Gerontologist: The Journal of Aging and Mental Health 5(1–2):165–173, 1986

Spitzer RL, Kroenke K, Williams JB: Validation and utility of a self-report version of PRIME-MD: the PHQ primary care study. Primary Care Evaluation of Mental Disorders. Patient Health Questionnaire. JAMA 282(18):1737–1744, 1999 10568646

Spitzer RL, Kroenke K, Williams JB, et al: A brief measure for assessing generalized anxiety disorder: the GAD-7. Arch Intern Med 166(10):1092–1097, 2006 16717171

Steffens DC, Fisher GG, Langa KM, et al: Prevalence of depression among older Americans: the Aging, Demographics and Memory Study. Int Psychogeriatr 21(5):879–888, 2009 19519984

Substance Abuse and Mental Health Services Administration: The Treatment of Depression in Older Adults: How to Use the Evidence-Based Practices KITs (HHS Publ No SMA-11-4631). Rockville, MD, Center for Mental Health Services, Substance Abuse and Mental Health Services Administration, U.S. Department of Health and Human Services, 2011. Available at: http://www.dmh.ms.gov/pdf/SAMHSA%20Toolkit.pdf. Accessed May 4, 2019.

Tedeschini E, Levkovitz Y, Iovieno N, et al: Efficacy of antidepressants for late-life depression: a meta-analysis and meta-regression of placebo-controlled randomized trials. J Clin Psychiatry 72(12):1660–1668, 2011 22244025

Thompson LW, Gallagher D, Breckenridge JS: Comparative effectiveness of psychotherapies for depressed elders. J Consult Clin Psychol 55(3):385–390, 1987 3597953

Thompson LW, Coon DW, Gallagher-Thompson D, et al: Comparison of desipramine and cognitive/behavioral therapy in the treatment of elderly outpatients with mild-to-moderate depression. Am J Geriatr Psychiatry 9(3):225–240, 2001 11481130

Thompson LW, Dick-Siskin L, Coon DW, et al: Effective Treatment for Late-Life Depression: A Client Workbook. New York, Oxford University Press, 2010
Tufts Health Plan: Clinical Guidelines for the Treatment of Depression in the Primary Care Setting. Watertown, MA, Tufts Health Plan, 2005. Available at: https://www.jpshealthnet.org/sites/default/files/ clinical_guidelines_for_the_treatment_of_depression_in_primary_care .pdf. Accessed April 6, 2018.

Late-Life Depression II

"My Guilt Is So Intense, I Think of Ending My Life Every Day to Get Relief"

Aazaz U. Haq, M.D.
Christopher O'Connell, M.D.

CHAPTER 2

Clinical Presentation

Chief Complaint

"My guilt is so intense, I think of ending my life every day to get relief."

Vignette

Mr. F is a 78-year-old Hispanic man who was admitted to the hospital's inpatient psychiatry unit after jumping off an overpass into oncoming traffic. Fortunately, he had avoided major physical injury. On the unit, he was initially guarded but then revealed delusions that he was being tortured nightly by a group of people who came and whipped him with a cat-o'-nine-tails. He expressed severe guilt over having molested many children as a young man and insisted that the only way for him to atone for his sins was to take his life.

Discussion

Depression in older adults is about as common as in younger populations, with clinically relevant depressive syndromes being present in 13.5% of individuals older than age 55 years, minor depression present in 9.8%, and strictly defined major depression present in 1.8% in community populations (Beekman et al. 1999). The prevalence of depression in individuals over age 65 years increases in settings with higher medical illness burden; 5%–10% of elders in primary care clinics, 11.5% of elders on inpatient medicine and surgical units, and 14.4% of nursing home residents have presentations that meet criteria for major depressive disorder (Aziz and Steffens 2013). Depression is not a normal part of aging, and misperceiving it as such leads to underdetection and undertreatment. Depression in late life is treatable, and proper identification and treatment of depressive syndromes can decrease suffering, improve functioning, improve the outcomes of comorbid medical conditions, and decrease caregiver stress. Because of the relative shortage of geriatric mental health providers, up to 80% of late-life depression is treated in primary care settings (Kessler et al. 2010). This chapter aims to help nongeriatric specialists familiarize themselves with common depression syndromes in older adults and their treatment.

Of all age groups, suicide rates are highest in older individuals, with major risk factors being depression, social isolation/loneliness, poor sleep quality, perceived poor health status, and prior suicide attempts (Turvey et al. 2002; Wiktorsson et al. 2010). One study of older individuals who had attempted suicide found that psychiatric illness, most commonly major depression, was present in 71%–97% of attempters (Conwell et al. 2011). A study of individuals older than 65 years who had attempted suicide found that depressive symptoms in many of these patients were undiagnosed and untreated and that these individuals had received treatment only for anxiety and insomnia (Osváth and Fekete 2001).

Vignette *(continued)*

Mr. F was diagnosed with psychotic depression and started on sertraline, which was titrated up to 100 mg daily, and risperidone, titrated up to 5 mg daily, over the course of the next 2 weeks. He developed restlessness and bradykinesia, and gradual cross-titration to venlafaxine and aripiprazole, up to 225 mg and 20 mg daily, respectively, was carried out, with minimal improvement in symptoms.

Diagnosis and Evaluation

While a thorough clinical interview is the gold standard for diagnosing late-life depression, several screening tools are available to increase detection in primary care settings. In the waiting room, the 30-question

Geriatric Depression Scale (GDS-30) can be administered, with a sensitivity and specificity of 84.2% and 79.3%, respectively (Mitchell et al. 2010). Fifteen-, five-, and four-item versions of the scale are also available (GDS-15, GDS-5, GDS-4). The Patient Health Questionnaire–2 (PHQ-2) is a two-question instrument that asks the patient to rate feelings of depression and anhedonia over the past 2 weeks on a scale of 0–3, with a sensitivity and specificity of 82.9% and 90.0%, respectively, at a cutoff score of 3 (Kroenke et al. 2003). The complete nine-question version of this screener (PHQ-9) has evidence for comparable performance to the PHQ-2 and GDS in terms of detecting late-life depression in primary care settings (Phelan et al. 2010). The Cornell Scale for Depression in Dementia can be used for depression screening in patients with dementia (major neurocognitive disorder) and requires interview of a caregiver who is sensitive to the patient's psychiatric symptoms (Alexopoulos et al. 1988).

Prior to formal diagnosis of depression, it is important to exclude other neuropsychiatric syndromes in which apathy or withdrawal is prominent. Apathy, characterized by a loss of volition and diminished motivation to engage in activities, social interactions, or productive behaviors, can be seen in frontal lobe lesions, hypoactive delirium, early stages of Alzheimer's disease, and with the use of certain medications. Failure to properly consider and rule out these conditions can often inaccurately lead to diagnoses of depression. Hypoactive delirium in an older patient is marked by acute onset of diffuse cognitive impairments, particularly deficits in attention, leading to withdrawal and disengagement. Bedside testing of attention, such as by asking the patient to say the months of the year backward or to tap every time the letter A is mentioned, often reveals gross deficits. Frontal lobe disease, either from a primary degenerative illness or from stroke, trauma, or a tumor, is often accompanied by significant apathy, along with loss of social graces, disinhibition, expressive language impairment, and/or executive dysfunction. Patients with Alzheimer's disease often present with apathy as a prominent feature in the disease's early stages and this can be confused with depression. Use of high dosages of opioid medications or benzodiazepines can often cause a diminished sensorium and withdrawal that can be mistaken for depression.

These apathy or withdrawal syndromes generally lack the depressive mood and emotionality that usually accompany a true depressive syndrome—that is to say, the *look* of depression may be there, but the *music* of depression is absent. Most people who are depressed typically complain of some emotional symptoms, such as sadness, hopelessness, demoralization, despair, feelings of worthlessness, and so on, even in milder depressive syndromes. Absence of emotionality in the presence of apathy should trigger consideration for the presence of another neuropsychiatric syndrome.

If a true depressive syndrome is suspected, the next step is to see if a certain subtype can be identified. Important subtypes to keep in mind are discussed in the following subsections.

Melancholia

Melancholia refers to an endogenous, severe depressive syndrome with psychomotor disturbances, cognitive abnormalities, and neurovegetative (sleep and appetite) disturbances (Parker and Paterson 2014; Taylor and Fink 2006). Melancholia has been recognized since the days of Hippocrates as a distinct and serious condition that can have an impact on individuals of all ages. Patients with melancholia have pervasive and unremitting feelings of apprehension, dread, and gloom that affect all cognitive processes, leading to withdrawal, hopelessness, slowness in thinking, feelings of failure and worthlessness, and suicidal thoughts. Psychomotor disturbances are common, with retardation (i.e., slowness, reluctance to participate in daily activities, prolonged inactivity) and/or undirected agitation (i.e., hand wringing, pacing, restlessness) being present in almost all melancholic patients. These patients sleep poorly, often waking early in the morning and being unable to fall back asleep. Their appetite diminishes, and they need to be encouraged to eat. Weight loss is common.

Depression in older adults is more likely to be of the melancholic subtype. A Dutch study of 359 people age 60 years and older with depression found that 38.4% fell in the severe, melancholic subclass (Veltman et al. 2017). Psychotic depression, depression in bipolar disorder, depression with anxious distress, and abnormal bereavement can all be conceptualized as subtypes of melancholia and are best treated as such (Taylor and Fink 2006). Melancholic older patients are more likely to require hospitalization and to benefit from biological treatments, such as medications and electroconvulsive therapy (ECT). Psychotherapy is less likely to be effective.

Psychotic Depression

Psychotic features in the presence of depression indicate a severe illness and should raise concerns. The psychosis is often "mood congruent" and contains depressive and nihilistic themes, such as auditory hallucinations telling the patient that he or she is a failure and will be going to jail any day now, or delusions that the patient's family has abandoned him or her or that the patient's insides are rotting (Taylor and Fink 2006). The psychosis tends to have a pervasive character and colors all aspects of the patient's mental life and functioning. These individuals are at high risk of suicide and should be hospitalized. ECT generally brings about almost complete remission and should be considered early. If ECT is not available or not an option for other reasons, adequately dosed antidepressants and antipsychotics should be used concurrently (Andreescu and Reynolds 2011).

Vascular Depression

Vascular depression refers to a depressive syndrome in older adults that is hypothesized to be secondary to the effects of microvascular changes in the brain, presumably due to disruption of the frontal-subcortical-limbic networks responsible for mood regulation (Alexopoulos et al. 1997). Compared with elderly individuals with non–vascular depression, those with vascular depression are more likely to have an absence of a personal and family history of depression, higher medical comorbidity, more significant cognitive and functional impairment, lower response rates to treatment, higher residual symptoms, greater motivational problems, and more relapses (Aizenstein et al. 2016). This formulation remains controversial, however, because the causative role of the vascular lesions in the generation of the depressive syndrome has not been proven (Aizenstein et al. 2016).

Minor Depression

"Subsyndromal" or "subclinical" depressive symptoms, while not meeting full DSM criteria for an episode of major depression or melancholia, can still cause suffering, diminish occupational and social functioning, increase physical disability, and worsen the outcome of general medical conditions (Lyness et al. 2006). This less severe variant of depression is more prevalent than its more severe counterparts, with up to 27% of people above age 60 years demonstrating some depressive symptoms (Kessler et al. 1997). Strictly defined, *minor depression* refers to depression in which five of the nine criteria for a major depressive episode are *not* met (see Table 2–1) but the patient still has depressed mood or loss of interest in activities and meets three or fewer of the remaining criteria. Multiple types of psychotherapies, including interpersonal therapy, reminiscence therapy, cognitive-behavioral therapy (CBT), and problem-solving therapy, can be beneficial for minor depression, particularly when used in combination with antidepressant medications. Minor depression is different from persistent depressive disorder (dys-

TABLE 2–1.   Criterion A for major depressive episode

A. Five (or more) of the following symptoms have been present during the same 2-week period and represent a change from previous functioning; at least one of the symptoms is either (1) depressed mood or (2) loss of interest or pleasure.

1. Depressed mood most of the day, nearly every day, as indicated by either subjective report (e.g., feels sad, empty, hopeless) or observation made by others (e.g., appears tearful).

2. Markedly diminished interest or pleasure in all, or almost all, activities most of the day, nearly every day (as indicated by either subjective account or observation).

3. Significant weight loss when not dieting or weight gain (e.g., a change of more than 5% of body weight in a month), or decrease or increase in appetite nearly every day.

4. Insomnia or hypersomnia nearly every day.

5. Psychomotor agitation or retardation nearly every day (observable by others, not merely subjective feelings of restlessness or being slowed down).

6. Fatigue or loss of energy nearly every day.

7. Feelings of worthlessness or excessive or inappropriate guilt (which may be delusional) nearly every day (not merely self-reproach or guilt about being sick).

8. Diminished ability to think or concentrate, or indecisiveness, nearly every day (either by subjective account or as observed by others).

9. Recurrent thoughts of death (not just fear of dying), recurrent suicidal ideation without a specific plan, or a suicide attempt or a specific plan for committing suicide.

Source.   Adapted from the *Diagnostic and Statistical Manual of Mental Disorders,* 5th Edition. Arlington, VA, American Psychiatric Association, 2013, pp. 160–161. Used with permission. Copyright © 2013 American Psychiatric Association.

thymia), which refers to a chronic, low-grade depressive disorder that usually starts in early adulthood and may continue into late life.

Substance-Induced Depression

Several commonly used substances can precipitate depressive symptoms in older adults, either because of the direct neurophysiological effects of the substance or as a result of the deleterious effects of the substance on the patient's life. Alcohol is the most common substance of abuse in adults older than 65 years, with more than 978,000 elders in the United States having symptoms that met criteria for alcohol use disorder in 2014 (Center for Behavioral Health Statistics and Quality 2015). Comorbidity of alcohol use disorder and depression is common in late life; one study of 14,391 veterans over age 50 presenting for alcohol abuse treatment found that 21% had comorbid depression (Blow et al. 1992). There is evidence that cannabis use, particularly at heavy levels, is associated with the development of depressive disorders, although research specifically in older adults is lacking (Lev-Ran et al. 2014). Chronic use of opioids and benzodiazepines, both commonly prescribed classes of medications in older adults, is associated with cognitive impairment and functional decline in this age group and can be confused with a primary depressive syndrome. Use of any of these substances can contribute to treatment resistance, and the first step in treatment of depression needs to be cessation of substance use, with referral to formal substance abuse treatment if necessary. Targeting these individuals' depressive symptoms with medications or psychotherapy alone, without addressing the substance use, is likely to result in ineffective treatment and frustration for the patient and the provider.

Bereavement

Death of a loved one is one of the most common negative events of late life. Although most people are able to overcome their grief with time, grief can become prolonged or complicated in 10%–25% of cases (Hashim et al. 2013; Newson et al. 2011). Complicated grief is marked by 1) an inability to accept the death and 2) ongoing experiences of preoccupation with the deceased, along with distressing memories, intense yearning and searching, and difficulties with moving on (Prigerson et al. 1995). Risk factors for development of complicated grief include loss of a child or spouse, being age 75–85 years, lower education, lower socioeconomic function, and cognitive dysfunction (Newson et al. 2011). Complicated grief is a distinct syndrome from major depression, although clinical depression is present in a large percentage (92% in one sample; Kim and Jacobs 1991) of individuals with complicated grief. Symptoms of clinical depression in individuals with complicated grief should be actively sought and aggressively treated. It is a mistake to explain away clinical depression in a grieving individual as "understandable" and to forgo treatment.

Depression Secondary to a General Medical Condition

Certain general medical conditions have an increased prevalence of associated depressive symptoms. Endocrinopathies, such as hypothyroidism, hyperparathyroidism, Cushing's disease, Addison's disease, and low testosterone, are all associated with depression, as a direct consequence of either the hormone imbalance or its metabolic side effects. Patients with acute myocardial infarction, lupus erythematosus, Lyme disease, pancreatic carcinoma, and Crohn's disease are all at higher risk of depression. Many neurological conditions, such as stroke, traumatic brain injury, Parkinson's disease, Huntington's disease, and epilepsy, are also associated with an increased incidence of depression. These depressive syndromes represent more than just the demoralization that comes with having a chronic medical condition and are the consequences of the physiological aberrancies on the central nervous system by the primary disease process. Treatment strategies should include optimal management of the primary medical condition to the greatest extent possible, as well as the psychotherapeutic and medication treatments described later in this chapter.

Depression With Catatonic Features

Severe melancholia in older adults can sometimes present with features of a retarded catatonia, including stupor (nonresponsiveness to the environment despite being awake and alert); negativism (refusing to comply with all requests without a clear reason); catalepsy (rigidity of limbs and/or body in a fixed posture); verbigeration (repetition of nonsense words or phrases); and waxy flexibility (ability to be placed into different postures by the examiner). These patients are at risk for poor oral intake, dehydration, weight loss, development of pressure ulcers, and development of malignant catatonia. These patients often have the potential for almost complete remission of symptoms with early treatment with ECT. Misdiagnosis of these individuals as having "advanced dementia" and inappropriate treatment can lead to severe adverse consequences, including unnecessary "do not resuscitate" orders, consignment to long-term nursing home care, development of deep venous thromboses and pulmonary emboli, and death (Swartz and Galang 2001).

Depression in Major Neurocognitive Disorder

There are 10%–25% of individuals with major neurocognitive disorder (NCD) who meet diagnostic criteria for major depression (Nilsson et al. 2002), with depressive symptoms being more severe and more common in major vascular NCD compared with major NCD due to Alzheimer's disease (Ballard et al. 1996; Newman 1999). Alzheimer's disease patients who have anosognosia about their cognitive symptoms often also disavow any depressive symptoms that may be present, and clinicians should keep this in mind during assessments. Depression can significantly worsen prognosis in major NCD and precipitate decline in these individuals, and antidepressant treatment is often effective. Nonpharmacological treatments can include psychotherapy for people in the milder stages of NCD, increasing physical exercise, increasing participation in activities meaningful to the individual, and increasing social interactions.

Depressive Pseudodementia

Depression in older adults can often be accompanied by secondary cognitive deficits, particularly in executive functioning, working memory, and sustained attention (Korczyn and Halperin 2009). Treatment of depression can result in at least partial improvement of the cognitive deficits, although many of these individuals go on to develop major NCD in subsequent years (Sáez-Fonseca et al. 2007). Cognitive impairment secondary to depression is typically accompanied by a greater degree of emotional distress, bradyphrenia, and bradykinesia, whereas individuals with Alzheimer's disease typically have greater apathy, less emotionality, and less insight. It is important for clinicians to keep in mind that 81% of individuals who have Alzheimer's disease are over the age of 75 (Hebert et al. 2013), and it can prove useful to question every diagnosis of Alzheimer's disease in younger individuals to ensure that depression, or another reversible condition, is not the primary cause of the patient's cognitive impairments.

In older individuals with severe depression, impact on functioning should be assessed and mitigated to the greatest extent possible. Older adults often lack the functional reserve that younger adults often have, and even moderate depression can dramatically diminish their ability to provide for their needs. They may stop basic self-care activities, such as keeping clean or eating regularly. Days at a time may be spent in bed. Cooking, grocery shopping, or socializing may seem like impossible tasks and may be neglected. Hospitalization should strongly be considered if functioning is severely diminished. If these individuals are to remain at home, efforts should be made to find sources of support for them, such as family, friends, and/or social services, and close follow-up should be maintained.

Vignette *(continued)*

ECT was recommended, and Mr. F passively agreed to it. He was started on bilateral ECT treatments three times a week. After four treatments, he started to show improvement in his mood and less preoccupation with being tortured at night. By seven treatments, his depression and delusional beliefs were completely resolved. His reaction was one of surprise when his delusions were recounted to him, and he denied ever having molested any children in his life. He was continued on moderate doses of aripiprazole and venlafaxine and discharged back to his assisted living facility, where he remained well at 1-, 3-, and 6-month follow-up visits.

Treatment

Older depressed patients often respond well to treatment, and therapeutic nihilism should be actively avoided if the first and second treatment attempts do not bring about remission. Treatment resistance in late-life depression is estimated to occur at a rate of about 33%, which is comparable to younger patients with depression (Mulsant and Pollock 1998). Predictors of good treatment outcomes include younger age, absence of executive dysfunction, absence of comorbid anxiety, absence of physical illness, lower baseline depression severity, shorter episode duration, and early improvement (Tunvirachaisakul et al. 2018).

Psychotherapy

Mild to moderate varieties of depression in older adults can benefit from different types of psychotherapies, which are commonly recommended in conjunction with pharmacotherapy options. CBT can be used effectively in older adults, particularly when a few modifications are made, such as presenting the information slowly and presenting more complex materials in handouts (Thompson 1996). Bibliotherapy, which refers to the reading of certain literature for therapeutic benefit, can decrease depressive symptoms in properly selected older patients (Scogin et al. 1987). Life-review therapy, which consists of recounting key meaningful moments of the person's life with a therapist, has good evidence for treating depressive and anxiety symptoms and having positive effects on mental health and quality of life (Korte et al. 2012). Existential psychotherapy, based on the theories of existential philosophers, can help individuals confront issues such as the meaning of their existence and the human condition; this approach can help select older adults find greater meaning in life and can have a moderate effect on psychopathology (Vos et al. 2015).

Pharmacotherapy

Selective serotonin reuptake inhibitors (SSRIs) are the most common first-line treatment for depression in older adults. The SSRIs with the best evidence of efficacy and tolerability are sertraline, citalopram, and escitalopram (Allan and Ebmeier 2013). Serotonin-norepinephrine reuptake inhibitors, such as duloxetine, venlafaxine, and milnacipran, are also safe and well tolerated in older adults and can be tried if SSRIs prove ineffective. Mirtazapine can be used if the side effects of weight gain and sedation are desirable, and bupropion is thought to be slightly more activating. Tricyclic antidepressants (TCAs) are thought by some experts to be more effective for melancholia than SSRIs (Taylor and Fink 2006), although older adults may be more prone to experiencing anticholinergic side effects (i.e., constipation, dry mouth, urinary retention, confusion, blurry vision), orthostatic hypotension due to alpha blockade, and QT prolongation. If a TCA is to be used on a trial basis, nortriptyline and desipramine are often preferred because they confer the least anticholinergic effects. Combination therapy with a second antidepressant or augmentation with low-dose lithium or an atypical antipsychotic (e.g., aripiprazole, quetiapine) can be effective, although polypharmacy should be avoided whenever possible.

Hepatic metabolism and renal clearance of medications are reduced in older adults, so lower doses produce higher blood levels of drug than in younger people. "Start low and go slow—but don't stop" is a common guide. Medication trials often need to be longer in older adults than in younger patients. Drug-drug interactions are more common in older adults because they tend to be taking more medications, on average, than younger patients.

Electroconvulsive Therapy

ECT is considered the gold standard of treatment for late-life depression that is resistant to treatment with medications and psychotherapy, with remission rates between 50% and 90% (Gálvez et al. 2015). ECT should be considered first-line treatment for psychotic depression, catatonic depression, and severe melancholia with decreased oral intake, inanition, and/or suicidality, although it is equally effective and safe in milder depression. ECT is well tolerated in older adults. The most common side effect is anterograde and retrograde memory dysfunction surrounding the days of treatment, which improves over subsequent days. Modern ECT has several modifications in technique to minimize cognitive side effects, including dose titration to use the smallest energy dose needed to elicit a therapeutic seizure, use of ultrabrief pulse width, and unilateral electrode placement (McDonald 2016). In severe depression, cognitive dysfunction often actually improves with ECT, because the negative preoccupations and executive dysfunction of severe depression remit. ECT is often much better tolerated than many medications. After remission is achieved, maintenance treatment with either medications or periodic maintenance ECT treatments is needed to prevent relapse (Kellner et al. 2006).

Transcranial Magnetic Stimulation

Transcranial magnetic stimulation (TMS) has been increasingly used in younger individuals, although most TMS research trials have excluded adults older than 65 years. In five trials without control subjects with a mean sample age greater than 60, response rates to TMS varied between 18% and 58.5% (Sabesan et al. 2015). It is hypothesized that TMS may be less effective in older adults because of neuroanatomical changes common in this age group, including cortical atrophy, which increases the distance between the brain and the TMS stimulus, and white matter ischemic changes, which can disrupt cortical-subcortical circuits (McDonald 2016). Nevertheless, the data do not support a lower response rate to TMS in older adults, and increasing the stimulus dose can result in an equal response to TMS as to that in younger adults. TMS is well tolerated in older adults, with no significant effects on cognition and only occasional minor side effects, such as headache or dizziness (Gálvez et al. 2015).

Ketamine

Studies of ketamine for the treatment of late-life depression are limited to a total of seven case reports, with mixed results (Medeiros da Frota Ribeiro and Riva-Posse 2017). Ketamine has increasing evidence as a viable treatment for depression in younger people, although psychotomimetic and cognitive side effects can occur in a small percentage of people. More research is needed about the safety and efficacy of ketamine in older adults.

Exercise, Bright Light, and Family Support

Exercise has been shown to have a beneficial effect on late-life depression, particularly when it combines mixed aerobic and anaerobic efforts, is at moderate intensity, is group based, utilizes mixed supervised and unsupervised formats, and is used in people without other clinical comorbidities (Schuch et al. 2016). Bright light therapy has shown efficacy in regulating the circadian rhythm and improving the mood of older patients with major depressive disorder (Lieverse et al. 2011). Lastly, social isolation and loneliness are major contributors to depression in older adults, and increased support from family and others can be vital in helping to alleviate the suffering and improve functioning of depressed older adults.

KEY POINTS

- Depression is not an inevitable or natural part of aging.
- Depression in older adults is treatable, with many different psychotherapeutic, pharmacological, neuromodulation, and other treatment modalities available.
- Conditions that may mimic depressive symptoms, such as apathy secondary to Alzheimer's disease, frontal lobe injury, hypoactive delirium, or substance abuse, should be identified and treated.
- Severe forms of depression, such as melancholia, psychotic depression, and catatonic depression, typically require hospitalization and early consideration of electroconvulsive therapy.

Resources

Organizations

American Association for Geriatric Psychiatry: www.aagponline.org
International Psychogeriatric Association: www.ipa-online.org

Scales

Geriatric Depression Scale (GDS):
    https://web.stanford.edu/~yesavage/GDS.html
Patient Health Questionnaire–9 (PHQ-9): www.mdcalc.com/phq-9-
    patient-health-questionnaire-9#creator-insights

Patient Handouts

National Alliance on Mental Illness: "Depression in Older Persons" (Fact
    Sheet): www.ncoa.org/wp-content/uploads/Depression_Older_
    Persons_FactSheet_2009.pdf
World Health Organization: "Staying Positive and Preventing Depression as You Get Older": www.who.int/campaigns/world-health-
    day/2017/handouts-depression/older-age/en

Books for Patients

Fink M: Electroconvulsive Therapy: A Guide for Professionals and Their Patients. New York, Oxford University Press, 2010

Moak GS: Beat Depression to Stay Healthier and Live Longer: A Guide for Older Adults and Their Families. Lanham, MD, Rowman and Littlefield, 2016

References

Aizenstein HJ, Baskys A, Boldrini M, et al: Vascular depression consensus report: a critical update. BMC Med 14(1):161, 2016 27806704

Alexopoulos GS, Abrams RC, Young RC, et al: Cornell Scale for Depression in Dementia. Biol Psychiatry 23(3):271–284, 1988 3337862

Alexopoulos GS, Meyers BS, Young RC, et al: "Vascular depression" hypothesis. Arch Gen Psychiatry 54(10):915–922, 1997 9337771

Allan CL, Ebmeier KP: Review of treatment of late life depression. Adv Psychiatr Treat 19(4):302–309, 2013

Andreescu C, Reynolds CF III: Late-life depression: evidence-based treatment and promising new directions for research and clinical practice. Psychiatr Clin North Am 34(2):335–355, vii–iii, 2011 21536162

Aziz R, Steffens DC: What are the causes of late-life depression? Psychiatr Clin North Am 36(4):497–516, 2013 24229653

Ballard C, Bannister C, Solis M, et al: The prevalence, associations and symptoms of depression amongst dementia sufferers. J Affect Disord 36(3–4):135–144, 1996 8821316

Beekman AT, Copeland JR, Prince MJ: Review of community prevalence of depression in later life. Br J Psychiatry 174:307–311, 1999 10533549

Blow FC, Cook CA, Booth BM, et al: Age-related psychiatric comorbidities and level of functioning in alcoholic veterans seeking outpatient treatment. Hosp Community Psychiatry 43(10):990–995, 1992 1328023

Center for Behavioral Health Statistics and Quality: Behavioral Health Trends in the United States: Results from the 2014 National Survey on Drug Use and Health (HHS Publ No SMA 15-4927, NSDUH Series H-50). Rockville, MD, Substance Abuse and Mental Health Services Administration, 2015. Available at: https://www.samhsa.gov/data/sites/default/files/NSDUH-FRR1-2014/NSDUH-FRR1-2014.pdf. Accessed August 17, 2018.

Conwell Y, Van Orden K, Caine ED: Suicide in older adults. Psychiatr Clin North Am 34(2):451–468, ix, 2011 21536168

Gálvez V, Ho KA, Alonzo A, et al: Neuromodulation therapies for geriatric depression. Curr Psychiatry Rep 17(7):59, 2015 25995098

Hashim SM, Eng TC, Tohit N, et al: Bereavement in the elderly: the role of primary care. Ment Health Fam Med 10(3):159–162, 2013 24427183

Hebert LE, Weuve J, Scherr PA, et al: Alzheimer disease in the United States (2010–2050) estimated using the 2010 census. Neurology 80(19):1778–1783, 2013 23390181

Kellner CH, Knapp RG, Petrides G, et al: Continuation electroconvulsive therapy vs. pharmacotherapy for relapse prevention in major depression: a multisite study from the Consortium for Research in Electroconvulsive Therapy (CORE). Arch Gen Psychiatry 63(12):1337–1344, 2006 17146008

Kessler RC, Zhao S, Blazer DG, et al: Prevalence, correlates, and course of minor depression and major depression in the National Comorbidity Survey. J Affect Disord 45(1–2):19–30, 1997 9268772

Kessler RC, Birnbaum H, Bromet E, et al: Age differences in major depression: results from the National Comorbidity Survey Replication (NCS-R). Psychol Med 40(2):225–237, 2010 19531277

Kim K, Jacobs S: Pathologic grief and its relationship to other psychiatric disorders. J Affect Disord 21(4):257–263, 1991 1829747

Korczyn AD, Halperin I: Depression and dementia. J Neurol Sci 283(1–2):139–142, 2009 19345960

Korte J, Bohlmeijer ET, Cappeliez P, et al: Life review therapy for older adults with moderate depressive symptomatology: a pragmatic randomized controlled trial. Psychol Med 42(6):1163–1173, 2012 21995889

Kroenke K, Spitzer RL, Williams JBW: The Patient Health Questionnaire-2: validity of a two-item depression screener. Med Care 41(11):1284–1292, 2003 14583691

Lev-Ran S, Roerecke M, Le Foll B, et al: The association between cannabis use and depression: a systematic review and meta-analysis of longitudinal studies. Psychol Med 44(4):797–810, 2014 23795762

Lieverse R, Van Someren EJW, Nielen MMA, et al: Bright light treatment in elderly patients with nonseasonal major depressive disorder: a randomized placebo-controlled trial. Arch Gen Psychiatry 68(1):61–70, 2011 21199966

Lyness JM, Heo M, Datto CJ, et al: Outcomes of minor and subsyndromal depression among elderly patients in primary care settings. Ann Intern Med 144(7):496–504, 2006 16585663

McDonald WM: Neuromodulation treatments for geriatric mood and cognitive disorders. Am J Geriatr Psychiatry 24(12):1130–1141, 2016 27889282

Medeiros da Frota Ribeiro C, Riva-Posse P: Use of ketamine in elderly patients with treatment-resistant depression. Curr Psychiatry Rep 19(12):107, 2017 29138992

Mitchell AJ, Bird V, Rizzo M, et al: Which version of the geriatric depression scale is most useful in medical settings and nursing homes? Diagnostic validity meta-analysis. Am J Geriatr Psychiatry 18(12):1066–1077, 2010 21155144

Mulsant BH, Pollock BG: Treatment-resistant depression in late life. J Geriatr Psychiatry Neurol 11(4):186–193, 1998 10230997

Newman SC: The prevalence of depression in Alzheimer's disease and vascular dementia in a population sample. J Affect Disord 52(1–3):169–176, 1999 10357030

Newson RS, Boelen PA, Hek K, et al: The prevalence and characteristics of complicated grief in older adults. J Affect Disord 132(1–2):231–238, 2011 21397336

Nilsson FM, Kessing LV, Sørensen TM, et al: Enduring increased risk of developing depression and mania in patients with dementia. J Neurol Neurosurg Psychiatry 73(1):40–44, 2002 12082043

Osváth P, Fekete S: [Suicidal behavior in the elderly. Review of results at the Pécs Center of the WHO/EURO Multicenter Study on Suicide]. Orv Hetil 142(22):1161–1164, 2001 11424590

Parker G, Paterson A: Melancholia: definition and management. Curr Opin Psychiatry 27(1):1–6, 2014 24270479

Phelan E, Williams B, Meeker K, et al: A study of the diagnostic accuracy of the PHQ-9 in primary care elderly. BMC Fam Pract 11:63, 2010 20807445

Prigerson HG, Frank E, Kasl SV, et al: Complicated grief and bereavement-related depression as distinct disorders: preliminary empirical validation in elderly bereaved spouses. Am J Psychiatry 152(1):22–30, 1995 7802116

Sabesan P, Lankappa S, Khalifa N, et al: Transcranial magnetic stimulation for geriatric depression: promises and pitfalls. World J Psychiatry 5(2):170–181, 2015 26110119

Sáez-Fonseca JA, Lee L, Walker Z: Long-term outcome of depressive pseudodementia in the elderly. J Affect Disord 101(1–3):123–129, 2007 17184844

Schuch FB, Vancampfort D, Rosenbaum S, et al: Exercise for depression in older adults: a meta-analysis of randomized controlled trials adjusting for publication bias. Rev Bras Psiquiatr 38(3):247–254, 2016 27611903

Scogin F, Hamblin D, Beutler L: Bibliotherapy for depressed older adults: a self-help alternative. Gerontologist 27(3):383–387, 1987 2886403

Swartz C, Galang RL: Adverse outcome with delay in identification of catatonia in elderly patients. Am J Geriatr Psychiatry 9(1):78–80, 2001 11156756

Taylor MA, Fink M: Melancholia: The Diagnosis, Pathophysiology and Treatment of Depressive Illness. Cambridge, UK, Cambridge University Press, 2006

Thompson LW: Cognitive-behavioral therapy and treatment for late-life depression. J Clin Psychiatry 57 (suppl 5):29–37, 1996 8647790

Tunvirachaisakul C, Gould RL, Coulson MC, et al: Predictors of treatment outcome in depression in later life: a systematic review and meta-analysis. J Affect Disord 227:164–182, 2018 29100149

Turvey CL, Conwell Y, Jones MP, et al: Risk factors for late-life suicide: a prospective, community-based study. Am J Geriatr Psychiatry 10(4):398–406, 2002 12095899

Veltman EM, Lamers F, Comijs HC, et al: Depressive subtypes in an elderly cohort identified using latent class analysis. J Affect Disord 218:123–130, 2017 28472702

Vos J, Craig M, Cooper M: Existential therapies: a meta-analysis of their effects on psychological outcomes. J Consult Clin Psychol 83(1):115–128, 2015 25045907

Wiktorsson S, Runeson B, Skoog I, et al: Attempted suicide in the elderly: characteristics of suicide attempters 70 years and older and a general population comparison group. Am J Geriatr Psychiatry 18(1):57–67, 2010 20094019

Working With Depressed Caregivers: Behavioral Activation

"I Can't Find the Energy or Time to Leave the House"

Ann Choryan Bilbrey, Ph.D.
Erin L. Cassidy-Eagle, Ph.D., CBSM, DBSM
Dolores Gallagher-Thompson, Ph.D., ABPP

CHAPTER 3

Clinical Presentation

Chief Complaint

"I can't find the energy or time to leave the house."

Vignette

Ms. E is a 72-year-old married woman. Her 81-year-old husband of 54 years was diagnosed with Alzheimer's disease 3 years ago and has recently progressed into the moderate stage, requiring a notable increase in care. Ms. E reports feeling overwhelmed, noting feelings of sadness, markedly diminished interest in most activities, trouble falling asleep, guilt, fatigue, and impaired concentration. She reports that while she has been experiencing these feelings intermittently since her husband's diagnosis, they have intensified and become sustained over the past 4 weeks. Ms. E has adequate social support because their son lives close by and her church community has offered assistance; however, she rarely accepts the offers of assistance, stating, "I can't find the energy or time to leave the house." Before her husband's diagnosis, Ms. E was active in many local charity organizations, attended multiple lectures and talks at the local university, and participated in yoga and other routine exercise groups. She has discontinued attendance in all of the mentioned activities, citing the caregiving demand. The couple still maintains a subscription to the opera, and a failed attempt at attendance 1 month ago precipitated her visit to primary care. Ms. E noted that she finally realized that her husband "would never get better" and that she was "losing the love of her life."

Discussion

Depression and Caregivers: Unique Concerns

Family caregivers of persons with dementia may present in primary care with a variety of complaints, including depression, as a result of the increased stress and burden they experience during the caregiving experience. These patients can be difficult to treat because they can perceive the caregiving experience as restrictive, allowing little time for necessary self-care. Depression occurs in 30%–40% of family caregivers, and the risk of depression increases with the progression of the care recipient's dementia (Alzheimer's Association 2018). There are a number of risk factors in the development of depression in family caregivers, primarily the frequency of the care recipient's behavior problems, the feeling of role captivity or of being an unwilling or involuntary caregiver, and caregiver overload with fatigue and burnout (Alspaugh et al. 1999). The quantity and intensity of caregiving can also be a risk factor for depression in caregivers (Covinsky et al. 2003). Chronicity of risk can be best predicted by the caregivers' subjective experience of role captivity, which is difficult to change with typical treatment such as respite (Zarit et al. 1986). A number of caregivers even continue to be at risk following the care recipient's institutionalization, which would be expected to relieve the stress and burden of the caregiving (Gaugler et al. 2010). A meta-analysis comparing caregivers with noncaregivers showed that caregivers have more stress and depressive symptoms and report lower levels of subjective well-being, physical health, and self-efficacy (Pinquart and Sörensen 2003). In particular, depression in caregivers is associated with a variety of negative health outcomes, most notably cardiovascular disease (Mausbach et al. 2007). Early identification of caregivers with depression is vital in preserving their health and maintaining well-being.

Caregiver Assessment Tools

A variety of assessment measures are available to the primary care team to assist in the evaluation of the mental health of the caregiver. Assessments of stress, burden, and depression, along with basic information about caregivers and the care they provide, can all contribute to obtaining a clear picture of the caregiver's mental health status. A basic caregiver interview assesses information about the care recipient—when was the care recipient diagnosed, where is he or she in the progression of the dementia, and what is his or her relationship to the caregiver. It is also important to assess the support the caregiver has—who is involved in the care, including treatment team members, family, and community members and services. The caregiver interview should also ask about the consequences of caregiving and any unique or challenging caregiving circumstances the caregiver may be experiencing. Should the screening tools indicate depression, it is important to gather information on the caregiver's mental health history. Does he or she have a history of depression? If so, how long ago? How many previous episodes? How was it treated, and was the treatment successful? Family Caregiver Alliance's toolkit "Caregivers Count Too!" (www.caregiver.org/caregivers-count-too-section-3-nuts-bolts-caregiver-assessment) contains detailed information on such assessments.

Depression: Nonspecific for Caregivers

Center for Epidemiologic Studies Depression Scale Revised. The Center for Epidemiologic Studies Depression Scale Revised (CESD-R-10; Kohout et al. 1993) is a 10-item self-report measure that assesses for the presence of depressive symptoms during the past week. Items are scored on a four-point Likert scale (0–3), with higher total scores reflecting greater depressive symptoms, and a total score over 10 suggesting depression. This measure has been validated for use with older adults (Irwin et al. 1999). A copy of the measure and instructions on how to score it can be found elsewhere (www.brandeis.edu/roybal/docs/CESD-10_website_PDF.pdf).

Geriatric Depression Scale (Short Form). The Geriatric Depression Scale (Short Form) (GDS; Sheikh and Yesavage 1986) is a 15-item self-report measure designed to be used with older adults, with yes/no answers asking for confirmation or denial of feelings occurring in the past week. A score greater than 5 is suggestive of depression requiring a more comprehensive interview, and scores greater than 10 indicate depression. A copy of the measure in multiple languages with scoring instructions is available online (web.stanford.edu/~yesavage/GDS.html).

Depression and Burden: Specific for Caregivers

The Caregiver Self-Assessment Questionnaire (CSAQ; Epstein-Lubow et al. 2010) is an 18-item assessment designed by the American Medical Association to measure stress in caregivers. Further research established that this measure detects depression as well. Items elicit primarily yes/no answers to assess stress and health over the past week, with two items asking for ratings on a scale of 1 to 10. A copy of the measure in multiple languages and instructions on how to score it can be found online (www.healthinaging.org/tools-and-tips/caregiver-self-assessment-questionnaire).

Stress

Perceived Stress Scale.   The Perceived Stress Scale–4 (PSS-4; Cohen et al. 1983) consists of four items asking about stressful feelings and thoughts occurring over the past month. The items are scored on a five-point Likert scale (0=never to 4=very often), with reverse coding on items two and three. The higher the score, the higher the perceived stress. A copy of the measure and scoring instructions can be found online (www.psy.cmu.edu/~scohen/PSS4.html).

Caregiver Depression Treatment

Behavioral Activation

Behavioral activation has been shown to be an effective brief treatment for depressed mood in family caregivers (Au et al. 2015; Moore et al. 2013). It is a relatively simple intervention, is easy to understand for the busy caregiver, and is not dependent on learning complex skills. Behavioral activation can be a great start to cognitive-behavioral therapy or can be an intervention by itself.

Behavioral activation is an evidenced-based, structured, brief psychosocial approach applicable for reducing both depression and anxiety symptoms. It is the first-line behavioral treatment for mild to moderately depressed older adults and has been successfully implemented by a range of clinicians, including mental health professionals, nurses, and primary care physicians for depressed older adults (Dimidjian et al.

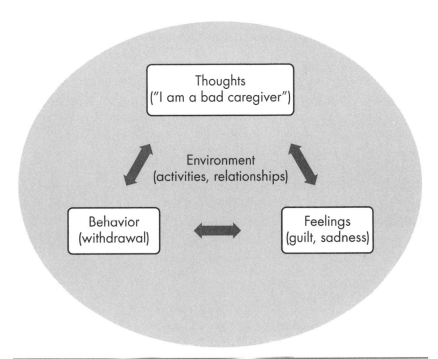

FIGURE 3–1.   Cognitive-behavioral model of depression.

2011) and their caregivers (Au et al. 2015). Behavioral activation has three goals: increase adaptive activities, reduce behaviors that maintain or worsen depression, and increase problem-solving skills that prevent a rewarding life. An individual who feels sad, tired, or worthless (feeling and thoughts) may withdraw from activities (behavior), leading to less social interaction, a loss of friendships, physical inactivity, and so forth, which then reinforces the depressive feelings and thoughts. This pattern in turn strengthens the withdrawal (Figure 3–1).

In essence, behavioral activation works on the premise that when patients feel bad, they do less. Acknowledging the research that social and physical activities tend to be potent mood boosters, the treatment focus is to increase the number of daily activities to four consciously and deliberately chosen pleasant events. Behavioral activation requires a person to change his or her approach to dealing with outside activities. Usually a person will wait to be motivated before doing an activity; however, in behavioral activation he or she is asked to act according to a plan rather than on the basis of feelings and thoughts. The treatment team helps the patient to choose activities that will make a difference in how he or she feels, assists with working out plans to carry them out, and monitors progress over time. Typically, the treatment requires four meetings, preferably in person; however, after the first meeting, follow-up can be done over the phone.

First meeting. In the first meeting with the depressed caregiver, it is important to prepare the caregiver for the behavioral activation. The first step is to educate about the benefits of taking action and help the caregiver to identify enjoyable activities. After talking about the theory and explaining the model, the clinician should note that behavioral activation is a systematic approach for accomplishing the addition of more pleasant activities and requires commitment from the caregiver to do things outside of the meetings. The clinician should point out that although being a caregiver is time-consuming, it is important to make the time to do enjoyable activities, because if all activities are limited to caregiving responsibilities, feelings of being burned out, frustrated, and even resentful can occur.

Once understanding and commitment has been secured, the next step is to identify what activities the caregiver enjoys doing. The clinician should ask about how the caregiver is currently spending his or her time. The clinician can then identify potential positive activities that the caregiver enjoyed doing in the past but is not currently doing. Can the activity noted still be done now? If not, how could it be modified to become more doable now? The clinician and caregiver then use this information to generate a list of 5–10 pleasurable activities. The list should start with pleasant activities that the caregiver is already doing. Then the clinician and caregiver can brainstorm other activities the caregiver is willing to try. It is important to write the activities down in the Pleasant Activities Log (PAL) (Figure 3–2). Ask the caregiver for a confidence rating—how confident is the caregiver that he or she can do the assignment? If the caregiver says 60%–70%, then the assignment can be modified until the caregiver's confidence level improves.

If caregivers experience difficulty identifying enjoyable activities, the California Older Person's Pleasant Events Schedule (COPPES) can be used to assist them (Rider et al. 2004). Most depressed people do not feel like doing things they used to enjoy, especially activities with other people. This common feeling is but one that leads to withdrawal, which reinforces the depression. It is important for the treatment team to design assignments that are manageable. The team should start small so that successful experiences occur. The caregiver's energy level and capacity to change should be matched to what he or she is being asked to do. Once 5–10 pleasant activities have been written down in the PAL, the clinician should ask the caregiver to commit to doing one or two a

PAL: Pleasant Activities Log – Mark each box to show which pleasant activities you've done and what your mood was

Name:	Day 1	Day 2	Day 3	Day 4	Day 5	Day 6	Day 7
1.							
2.							
3.							
4.							
5.							
6.							
7.							
8.							
9.							
10.							
Total # of activities done each day							
Overall Mood Score* for each day							

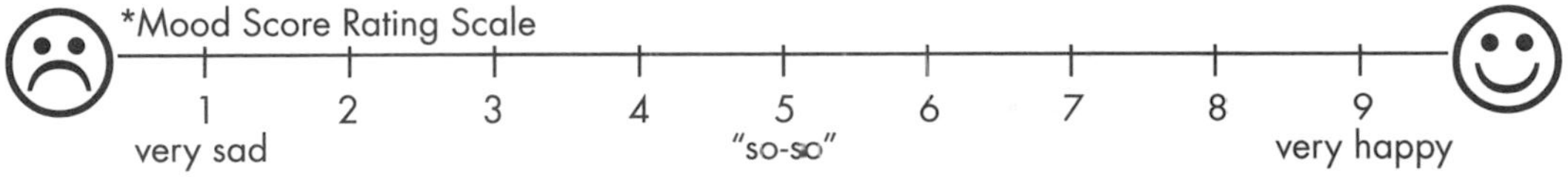

*Mood Score Rating Scale

```
  1    2    3    4    5    6    7    8    9
very sad        "so-so"              very happy
```

FIGURE 3–2. Pleasant Activities Log.

day until the clinician and caregiver next speak the following week, and to record his or her mood at the end of the day no matter how many activities have been completed.

The following are questions to ask in the follow-up meeting:

- What kinds of activities seem to give pleasure?
- Can these pleasurable activities be repeated on another day?
- Are ratings higher when other people are involved? If so, can social contact be increased?
- Are there activities that the caregiver has stopped doing? Is he or she interested in starting them again?
- Are there other activities the caregiver may be interested in doing?
- Is he or she willing to try something new?

Second through fourth meetings.   At the beginning of each meeting, the clinician should review the completed PAL with the patient. If the PAL was not completed, the clinician and caregiver should discuss reasons for and problem-solve any barriers together. The PAL should be reviewed each week. During the review of the PAL, the clinician should look for patterns between days with activity and mood. On the basis of the experience of the caregiver, the list of pleasant activities can be modified or added to depending on changing needs and observations about what works and what does not work. By the third meeting, the clinician should note if there has been an increase in pleasant activities. There should be three to four activities occurring each day, with mood ratings at 6 or higher. Are these activities planned, or are they just happening? The pleasant activities do not need to be huge—they can be something as small as taking a moment to enjoy a cookie and tea—but they need to be consciously chosen and deliberately done for the caregiver to experience a sense of control in his or her life. Many caregivers report a loss of control over the direction of their day-to-day life because it is absorbed by the needs and demands of their caregiving. After they consciously choose an activity they enjoy, deliberately schedule that activity into their day, and then actually do that activity, they report a sense of regaining some control over their lives, which has a positive effect on their mood. During the last meeting, the clinician should reinforce the progress the caregiver has made by attributing the success to the caregiver's efforts. The clinician should also stress that the caregiver can continue these gains, with mood management as the key to reducing depression, and that he or she now has the skills to maintain those gains himself or herself.

Vignette (continued)

At the start of treatment, Ms. E reported little to no pleasant activities in her day. Brainstorming was difficult because she could not spontaneously generate any activities to list. The COPPES was used to successfully prompt five activities. The first week, Ms. E completed one activity each day. The treatment team was able to note a slight trend toward a higher mood when Ms. E interacted socially, so her list was modified for the following week to include more social engagements. During week two, Ms. E struggled to balance her caregiving responsibilities with the need to have some time for herself. The team worked with Ms. E to role-play how to ask for assistance from her son and friends from her church. By week three, Ms. E was doing at least three scheduled pleasant activities, with a corresponding increase in mood. As her mood improved, Ms. E did need occasional reminders that the activities could be small in scope, because she liked to fill her schedule with difficult-to-accomplish grand plans. During the last meeting, the team and Ms. E brainstormed various plans to ensure Ms. E's continued improved mood despite the uncertainty of caregiving demands.

Behavioral activation strategies have been found to be effective in reducing symptoms of depression as well as increasing the frequency of healthy activity levels. Given the connection of mental health to physical health, brief and effective strategies are crucial to have in every clinician's toolbox.

KEY POINTS

- Early identification and treatment of caregivers with depression is vital in preserving health and maintaining well-being.
- Assessments of stress, burden, and depression, along with basic information about caregivers and the care they provide, can all contribute to obtaining a clear picture of the caregiver's mental health status.
- Behavioral activation has been shown to be an effective brief treatment for depressed mood in family caregivers because it is easy to understand for the busy caregiver and is not dependent on learning complex skills.
- Behavioral activation has three goals: increase adaptive activities, reduce behaviors that maintain or worsen depression, and increase problem-solving skills that prevent a rewarding life.

Resources

Online Resources

American Psychiatric Association provides a curated information on depression: www.psychiatry.org/patients-families/depression

American Psychological Association Help Center offers information related to psychological issues written for the nonmedical consumer: www.apa.org/helpcenter/index.aspx

National Alliance for Caregiving partners with other caregiving associations and groups to provide additional resources to help family caregivers address and cope with the challenges of caring for a loved one: www.caregiving.org/resources/general-caregiving

National Alliance on Mental Illness links family members and caregivers with additional support and information: www.nami.org/Find-Support/Family-Members-and-Caregivers

National Institute of Mental Health provides up-to-date information about depression: www.nimh.nih.gov/health/topics/depression/index.shtml

Video Illustrations With a Primary Care Provider

Online resources, including a video modeling the use of behavioral activation by a primary care physician with an older depressed woman, can be helpful for the established practitioner looking to expand their skill set.

Cassidy-Eagle E: "Behavioral Activation in a Primary Care Setting With Nancy Morioka-Douglas, MD, MPH." YouTube video, running time 11:06, July 29, 2018. Available at: www.youtube.com/watch?v=Vjq4Yap4gCo

Stanford Geriatric Education Center: Home (YouTube channel), 2011. Available at: www.youtube.com/user/StanfordGEC

Books, Articles, and Manuals for Providers

Kanter JW, Manos RC, Bowe WM, et al: What is behavioral activation? A review of the empirical literature. Clin Psychol Rev 30(6):608–620, 2010

Lejuez CW, Hopko DR, Hopko SD: A brief behavioral activation treatment for depression: treatment manual. Behav Modif 25(2):255–286, 2001

Martell CR, Dimidijian S, Herman-Dunn R: Behavioral Activation for Depression: A Clinician's Guide. New York, Guilford, 2013

References

Alspaugh MEL, Stephens MAP, Townsend AL, et al: Longitudinal patterns of risk for depression in dementia caregivers: objective and subjective primary stress as predictors. Psychol Aging 14(1):34–43, 1999 10224630

Alzheimer's Association: 2018 Alzheimer's disease facts and figures. Alzheimers Dement 14(3):367–429, 2018

Au A, Gallagher-Thompson D, Wong MK, et al: Behavioral activation for dementia caregivers: scheduling pleasant events and enhancing communications. Clin Interv Aging 10:611–619, 2015 25848237

Cohen S, Kamarck T, Mermelstein R: A global measure of perceived stress. J Health Soc Behav 24(4):385–396, 1983 6668417

Covinsky KE, Newcomer R, Fox P, et al: Patient and caregiver characteristics associated with depression in caregivers of patients with dementia. J Gen Intern Med 18(12):1006–1014, 2003 14687259

Dimidjian S, Barrera M Jr, Martell C, et al: The origins and current status of behavioral activation treatments for depression. Annu Rev Clin Psychol 7:1–38, 2011 21275642

Epstein-Lubow G, Gaudiano BA, Hinckley M, et al: Evidence for the validity of the American Medical Association's caregiver self-assessment questionnaire as a screening measure for depression. J Am Geriatr Soc 58(2):387–388, 2010 20370867

Gaugler JE, Mittelman MS, Hepburn K, et al: Clinically significant changes in burden and depression among dementia caregivers following nursing home admission. BMC Med 8(1):85, 2010 21167022

Irwin M, Artin KH, Oxman MN: Screening for depression in the older adult: criterion validity of the 10-item Center for Epidemiological Studies Depression Scale (CES-D). Arch Intern Med 159(15):1701–1704, 1999 10448771

Kohout FJ, Berkman LF, Evans DA, et al: Two shorter forms of the CES-D (Center for Epidemiological Studies Depression) depression symptoms index. J Aging Health 5(2):179–193, 1993 10125443

Mausbach BT, Patterson TL, Rabinowitz YG, et al: Depression and distress predict time to cardiovascular disease in dementia caregivers. Health Psychol 26(5):539–544, 2007 17845105

Moore RC, Chattillion EA, Ceglowski J, et al: A randomized clinical trial of behavioral activation (BA) therapy for improving psychological and physical health in dementia caregivers: results of the Pleasant Events Program (PEP). Behav Res Ther 51(10):623–632, 2013 23916631

Pinquart M, Sörensen S: Differences between caregivers and noncaregivers in psychological health and physical health: a meta-analysis. Psychol Aging 18(2):250–267, 2003 12825775

Rider KL, Gallagher-Thompson D, Thompson LW: California Older Person's Pleasant Events Schedule. Stanford, CA, Stanford Medicine Older Adult and Family Center, 2004. Available at: http://oafc.stanford.edu/coppes.html. Accessed April 6, 2018.

Sheikh JI, Yesavage JA: Geriatric Depression Scale (GDS): recent evidence and development of a shorter version. Clinical Gerontologist: The Journal of Aging and Mental Health 5(1–2):165–173, 1986

Zarit SH, Todd PA, Zarit JM: Subjective burden of husbands and wives as caregivers: a longitudinal study. Gerontologist 26(3):260–266, 1986 3721233

Diagnosis and Treatment of Generalized Anxiety Disorder

"Getting Old Is Not for Wimps!"

Marla Kokesh, M.D.
Daniel D. Sewell, M.D.

CHAPTER 4

If you ask what is the single most important key to longevity, I would have to say it is avoiding worry, stress and tension. And if you didn't ask me, I'd still have to say it.

George F. Burns

Clinical Presentation

Chief Complaint

"Getting old is not for wimps!"

Vignette

Ms. B is a 72-year-old retired, divorced woman who presented to a geriatric psychiatric clinic with a past medical history of type 2 diabetes mellitus, hypertension, hyperlipidemia, essential tremor, chronic insomnia, and worsening depression and anxiety. Her problems with anxiety began when she was in her teens. Her mother married a man who verbally terrorized the patient and her sister and physically abused their mother. Her emotionally traumatic childhood inspired her to seek psychotherapy in the past, but she reported no recent mental health care other than being prescribed medications by her primary care provider. During her initial visit, she reported that the increase in her problems with anxiety occurred after a number of major life stresses. Her sister (and only sibling) had recently been diagnosed with terminal cancer. She was involved in two recent minor motor vehicle accidents, which she attributed to her anxiety. She also acknowledged unhappiness about her loss of her autonomy and greater dependence on her grown children for help with finances and with transportation to appointments. Lastly, she had fallen several times recently. Although not resulting in loss of consciousness or serious injury, these falls contributed to her fear of losing her independence. She shared that she was "always a take-charge person" and that she was motivated to "grow old mindfully."

She acknowledged the following symptoms of anxiety and/or depression: irritability, hyperarousal, psychomotor restlessness, worry, ruminations, increased pessimism with a sense of impending doom, and exaggerated and inappropriate self-criticism. She seemed curiously unconcerned about her falls, however, and stated, "I just need to learn to fall better." She noted that her increased level of anxiety had worsened her essential tremor to the point of affecting her speech. She reported intentional weight loss for better management of her diabetes. She denied problems with depressed mood, low energy, anhedonia, or concentration, and she denied suicidal or homicidal ideation or intent or having a suicide plan. She explained that her problem with chronic insomnia, for which she was currently taking melatonin 3 mg nightly, had worsened. She described mild changes in memory not associated with changes in her instrumental activities of daily living or activities of daily living. She denied drug use but reported drinking one scotch every other night for several years. She denied a history of blackouts, citations for driving under the influence, or other alcohol-related problems. Ms. B had been prescribed nortriptyline by her local primary care provider, who later switched the medication to sertraline 50 mg daily, which worsened her essential tremor and agitation and decreased her sense of well-being. She elected to have pharmacogenomic testing, which revealed that she would likely be a poor responder to selective serotonin reuptake inhibitor (SSRIs), but nonetheless, she was continuing to take sertraline 50 mg po daily.

In addition to the medical history, the patient reported that she had noted a decrease in her sense of smell and that she had been evaluated by a neurologist, who determined that she did not have Parkinson's disease. She reported a family history of depression, dementia, essential tremor, and Parkinson's disease. She shared that she was living independently in a 55+ community, was divorced after a 27-year marriage, had two adult children, and was a retired executive director and lobbyist. Eight years ago, she moved to her current home and has been slow to find friends and a sense of community.

She scored in the severe range (37) on the Burns Anxiety Inventory (Burns 1993) and in the mild range (14) on the Beck Depression Inventory–II (Beck et al. 1996). Her Montreal Cognitive Assessment (MoCA; Nasreddine et al. 2005) score was 27/30, with mild deficits in recall and fluency. Her evaluation included a magnetic resonance imaging scan without contrast, which revealed only mild brain volume loss and white matter hyperintensities consistent with chronic small-vessel ischemia slightly increased for the patient's age. Her initial care included tapering her off the sertraline, initiating a trial of mirtazapine 7.5 mg nightly, and referring her to group psychotherapy.

Discussion

Team Commentary

Dr. Kokesh: One of the striking things about this patient is that her chief complaint did not at all suggest that her primary psychiatric challenge was anxiety.

Dr. Sewell: I agree. Just like in older adults with depression symptoms, older adults with anxiety may not be able to recognize symptoms of depression (Wetherell et al. 2009) or use precise terms to describe their underlying symptoms. I don't think we really know the reasons for this, but a number of theories exist including actual differences in the underlying physiological abnormalities responsible for these symptoms and cohort effects related to stigma and the cultural beliefs at the time these individuals were living through their formative years. Even though she had previously worked with a psychotherapist, this would not necessarily have helped her address internalized shame or stigma related to her psychiatric symptoms and may have influenced how she responded to the question about her chief complaint.

Dr. Kokesh: Do you think the toxic environment that her stepfather created may have played a role in her struggles with anxiety?

Dr. Sewell: Yes. Poor psychological support during childhood has been independently associated with incident generalized anxiety disorder (GAD) in later life (Zhang et al. 2015). The abuse that she witnessed and directly experienced in her youth shaped her sense of herself and the world and also influenced the coping strategies that she developed. I suspect that her becoming someone who "always takes charge" may have been, at least in part, a coping strategy that she began using in her childhood as a response to the chaos her stepfather created.

Dr. Kokesh: Like many geriatric patients who seek psychiatric care, there is certainly a richness to her presentation that makes caring for her somewhat more challenging than it might be in a younger patient with fewer medical comorbidities. From a medical point of view, her age, her vascular disease risk factors, and her report of mild changes in her memory mandated that an emerging cognitive illness be included in the differential diagnosis of her complaints. Her history of recent falls also adds to her complexity, and the etiology of the falls needs to be explored. Fear of falling is the most common specific fear among older adults (Bower et al. 2015). From a psychodynamic perspective, her experience of multiple losses and concerns about loss of autonomy are definitely two of the common challenges that occur in later life. She herself linked her losses to her recent struggles with anxiety.

Symptoms and Diagnostic Criteria

Anxiety helps contribute to our safety in everyday life by alerting us to potential danger. When anxiety occurs for no reason or becomes severe and enduring, however, it prevents a person from flourishing in the present moment where life is lived. Excessive worry represents a maladaptive focus on the future and often includes "what if" scenarios and a preoccupation with "what's going to happen?" Ruminations, on the other hand, anchor the person in the past with regrets, sorrows, and upsetting thoughts and feelings about past situations dominating the person's thoughts.

The first step in caring for a patient with painful and disruptive anxiety is to develop a differential diagnosis and then take the necessary steps to determine the most likely cause or causes. The causes of clinically significant anxiety can be separated into the following categories: medical, including various illnesses and medications; psychiatric; and situational. Sometimes a patient's anxiety may be due to more than one cause from the same category and/or causes from different categories (Tables 4–1 and 4–2).

A common dilemma for providers is determining whether a patient's level of worry reaches the point where it should be considered an anxiety disorder. As defined in DSM-5 (American Psychiatric Association 2013), the cardinal symptom of GAD is excessive and hard-to-control worry and anxiety about multiple problems or life events without relief. The DSM-5 criteria for GAD are included in Box 4–1.

Box 4–1.   Diagnostic Criteria for Generalized Anxiety Disorder

---

A. Excessive anxiety and worry (apprehensive expectation), occurring more days than not for at least 6 months, about a number of events or activities (such as work or school performance).
B. The individual finds it difficult to control the worry.

C. The anxiety and worry are associated with three (or more) of the following six symptoms (with at least some symptoms having been present for more days than not for the past 6 months):

Note: Only one item is required in children.

1. Restlessness or feeling keyed up or on edge.
2. Being easily fatigued.
3. Difficulty concentrating or mind going blank.
4. Irritability.
5. Muscle tension.
6. Sleep disturbance (difficulty falling or staying asleep, or restless, unsatisfying sleep).

D. The anxiety, worry, or physical symptoms cause clinically significant distress or impairment in social, occupational, or other important areas of functioning.

E. The disturbance is not attributable to the physiological effects of a substance (e.g., a drug of abuse, a medication) or another medical condition (e.g., hyperthyroidism).

F. The disturbance is not better explained by another mental disorder (e.g., anxiety or worry about having panic attacks in panic disorder, negative evaluation in social anxiety disorder [social phobia], contamination or other obsessions in obsessive-compulsive disorder, separation from attachment figures in separation anxiety disorder, reminders of traumatic events in posttraumatic stress disorder, gaining weight in anorexia nervosa, physical complaints in somatic symptom disorder, perceived appearance flaws in body dysmorphic disorder, having a serious illness in illness anxiety disorder, or the content of delusional beliefs in schizophrenia or delusional disorder).

Source. Reprinted from American Psychiatric Association: *Diagnostic and Statistical Manual of Mental Disorders,* 5th Edition. Arlington, VA, 2013, p. 222. Copyright © 2013 American Psychiatric Association. Used with permission.

Epidemiology and Presentation

Estimates of the prevalence of anxiety disorders in older adults have varied significantly. The clinical setting and methodological differences—including diagnostic criteria, which do not reflect age-related differences in symptom expression—contribute significantly to this variation. One review of epidemiological studies reported that the frequency of anxiety symptoms significant enough to impair function or require treatment was 15%–52% in community samples and 15%–56% in medical settings (Bryant et al. 2008).

The presentation of GAD in older adults, even with the physical symptoms of normal aging, does not differ significantly from that ob-

TABLE 4–1.   Illnesses and syndromes associated with anxiety

Disorder	References
Alcohol use disorder	Smith and Randall 2012
Alcohol withdrawal	Brady and Lydiard 1993
Allergic conditions	Sareen et al. 2006
Arthritic conditions	Sareen et al. 2006
Autoimmune diseases	Evers et al. 2002; Seguí et al. 2000
Cancer	Pitman et al. 2018
Cardiac disease	Ginzburg et al. 2002; Vilchinsky et al. 2017
Dementia	Seignourel et al. 2008
Endocrine conditions	
Diabetes	Bickett and Tapp 2016; Grigsby et al. 2002
Hyperparathyroidism	Locke et al. 2015
Hyperthyroidism	Locke et al. 2015
Gastrointestinal disorders	Härter et al. 2003; Sareen et al. 2006
Hypertension	Player and Peterson 2011
Major depressive disorder	Zhou et al. 2017
Migraine headaches	Sareen et al. 2006
Opiate withdrawal	Kosten and George 2002; Vernon et al. 2016
Respiratory diseases including asthma	Goodwin 2003; Sareen et al. 2006
Sedative-hypnotic withdrawal	Perry and Alexander 1986
Thyroid disease	Simon et al. 2002

served in younger adults, although in older adults worry predominates over symptoms reflecting sympathetic nervous system activity (Lenze and Wetherell 2011b). The most common GAD symptoms among older adults, in addition to worry and distress, appear to be restlessness, fatigue, and sleep disturbances, including insomnia with muscle tension (Wetherell et al. 2003). Laboratory and behavioral studies have found that older people also have a less intense physiological response to strong emotional states (Lawton et al. 1992; Neiss et al. 2009). Although an older person may not experience as strong an autonomic response as a younger person, they tend to attribute autonomic symptoms of anxiety, such as abdominal discomfort, palpitations, and tremor, to physical causes. The types of concerns older people report are related to stress-

TABLE 4–2. Common medications prescribed to older adults that include side effects of anxiety

Cognitive enhancers

    Donepezil

    Galantamine

    Memantine

    Rivastigmine

    Corticosteroids

    Cortisone

    Dexamethasone

    Prednisone

ADHD medications

    Amphetamine/dextromethamphetamine

    Methylphenidate (Ritalin)

Asthma medications

    Albuterol

    Salmeterol

    Theophylline

Medications with caffeine

    Aspirin, acetaminophen, and caffeine

    Aspirin and caffeine (Anacin)

    Ergotamine and caffeine (Cafergot)

Parkinson's disease medications

Selective serotonin reuptake inhibitors

Note.   ADHD=attention-deficit/hyperactivity disorder.
Source.   Adapted from WebMD: "What Meds Might Cause Anxiety?" (web page), 2017. WebMD medical reference reviewed by Smitha Bhandari, M.D., on June 20, 2017. Available at: www.webmd.com/anxiety-panic/anxiety-causing-meds. Accessed December 18, 2018.

ors, in particular loss (of identity with retirement and of independence), but also illness and disability, fears of being a burden on others, impending mortality, and reduced economic resources.

Somatic symptoms are a hallmark of anxiety disorder in older adults, and older adults frequently present with comorbid medical conditions. These disorders decrease quality of life and may increase the risk for other serious medical problems such as heart disease, depression, and dementia (Lenze and Wetherell 2011a). Cardiovascular disease, chronically painful conditions (e.g. arthritis, migraine), lung disease, gastrointestinal problems, and other medical conditions (Table 4–1) have been associated with anxiety symptoms and/or anxiety disorders in older adults (El-Gabalawy et al. 2011). Importantly, older adults with comorbid anxiety and physical illness rate their health as poorer than do those with anxiety or physical illness alone, indicating the importance of assessing for and treating anxiety in physically ill older adults.

Excessive anxiety is not a normal part of aging, and identification and treatment of anxiety can significantly improve health outcomes in older adults (El-Gabalawy et al. 2011). GAD is associated with increased stress and impairment relative to normal aging (Wetherell et al. 2003). An important question is whether anxiety increases the risk of developing dementia. Older adults with anxiety are more than two times as likely to develop dementia as those with low or no anxiety, independent of age, gender, and depression (Burton et al. 2013).

Treatment of Generalized Anxiety Disorder

A number of recent publications have provided algorithms for the assessment of anxiety disorders in older adults. Bower et al. (2015) published rules for managing anxiety in older adults (see Figure 4–1 for adaptation): 1) perform a comprehensive assessment; 2) provide psychoeducation; 3) avoid or clean up medications; 4) provide first-line medication treatment; 5) provide follow-up; and 6) consider augmentation.

Assessment

During step 1 (comprehensive assessment), keeping the DSM-5 criteria for GAD in mind as interview questions are formed and asked will help to determine if the diagnostic threshold for GAD is actually met. In addition, it is important to remember that patients living with GAD may have one or more comorbid psychiatric conditions. A significant proportion of patients with GAD may also have a somatization disorder and/or long-standing maladaptive patterns of viewing and responding to life events, such as maintaining an external locus of control. Awareness of these comorbid factors helps the clinician design a treatment plan with the highest likelihood of success and indicates that the treatment plan will likely need to include more than just the use of carefully selected psychiatric medication. Given that the single greatest risk fac-

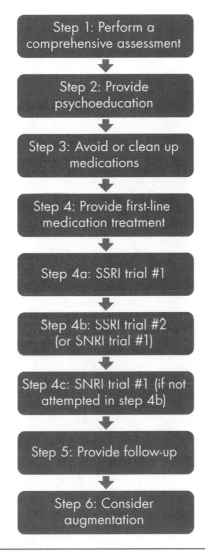

FIGURE 4–1. Algorithm for the assessment and management of anxiety in older adults.

Note. SNRI = serotonin-norepinephrine reuptake inhibitor; SSRI = selective serotonin reuptake inhibitor.
Source. Adapted from Bower et al. 2015.

tor of dementia is increasing age, and given the association between changes in cognition, including loss of short-term memory, and the development of anxiety, the initial assessment of an older adult with anxiety complaints should include some form of cognitive screening (e.g.,

MoCA). The use of rating scales for anxiety may be helpful in order to identify and quantify the patient's anxiety symptoms as well as to track changes over time. See Table 4–3 for a description of some anxiety assessment tools.

Psychoeducation

When psychoeducation is being provided (step 2), as Bower et al. (2015) emphasize, it is important to include family members or caretakers in discussions. Anxiety symptoms in an older adult inevitably impact the older adult's family and social support system in a variety of ways. Attempting to help older adults with anxiety, or even just being in the presence of an older adult with an anxiety problem, can trigger feelings such as annoyance, frustration, disappointment, or exhaustion. These feelings can worsen the situation for everyone—whether through avoidance of the anxious older adult or by saying things to the anxious older adult that evoke shame, pessimism, or worsened anxiety. Therefore, members of the patient's social support system may benefit from education and support delivered with a message of hope that things will likely improve. Including family members also allows the clinician to observe and help correct behaviors of family members that may be worsening the situation. In addition, inclusion of family members allows for these family members to become an active part of the treatment team—particularly helpful if a treatment agreement is one of the tools that is being employed. Treatment agreements are discussed in detail later in this chapter in the subsection titled as such.

Providing a patient with information about what is known about the neurobiology of anxiety may have therapeutic value. It is usually not necessary for the clinician to explain in great detail about the autonomic nervous system or to have all the neuroscience information memorized, but a simplified explanation will likely be well received. Here is an example of an explanation that might be appropriate and helpful:

> Our nervous system is composed of two opposing forces or systems, the sympathetic nervous system and the parasympathetic nervous system. The sympathetic nervous system (SNS) is responsible for protecting us from danger, both real and imagined. It produces the "fight, flight, or freeze response" to circumstances perceived as threatening, such as encountering a mother bear with cubs in the woods. In contrast, the parasympathetic nervous system (PNS) is about calm, relaxed, and vegetative states—digestion, immunology, reproduction, and so on. These two systems work in concert with each other, a dance of ebb and flow. The SNS speeds up our heart; the PNS slows it down. The PNS promotes digestion; the SNS inhibits it. When you get nervous about public speaking,

TABLE 4–3. Rating scales for anxiety

Scale	Number of questions	Scoring	Time to administer	Type of reporting	Source and cost
Beck Anxiety Inventory (Beck and Steer 1993)	21	Low: 0–21 Moderate: 22–35 Severe: ≥36	5–10 minutes	Self-report	The BAI was developed in 1990 and a revised manual was published in 1993 with some changes in scoring. The print manual costs $90.25; the digital manual costs $57.00. The print and digital manuals purchased together cost $90.25. The manuals are sold by Pearson and can be purchased online at www.pearsonassessments.com/professional-assessments/ordering/how-to-order.html.

TABLE 4–3. **Rating scales for anxiety** *(continued)*

Scale	Number of questions	Scoring	Time to administer	Type of reporting	Source and cost
Beck Depression Inventory IA (BDI-IA; Beck 1978) Beck Depression Inventory II (BDI-II; Beck et al. 1996)	21				The BDI-IA has 21 items and identifies symptoms and attitudes associated with depression; the respondent must recall the relevance of each statement based on the previous week including today. The BDI-II also consists of 21 items and was created to correspond with the updated DSM-IV criteria for depression. The BDI-IA and the BDI-II are copyrighted. The rights are held by Harcourt Assessment (Pearson Education) under contract from the author. A fee is required for the manual and record forms. This limits availability (Jackson-Koku 2016).

TABLE 4–3. Rating scales for anxiety (continued)

Scale	Number of questions	Scoring	Time to administer	Type of reporting	Source and cost
World Health Organization World Mental Health Composite International Diagnostic Interview (WHO WMH-CIDI; Robins et al. 1988)	Uses gateway questions that lead to other questions based on responses; total number is variable.	Establishes whether or not criteria for specific anxiety disorders, such as generalized anxiety disorder (GAD) and panic disorder, are met.	46 minutes (range 32–68 minutes)	Computer-based and clinician administered	To administer the WHO WMH-CIDI, you need to purchase a license (or licenses) for the Blaise software in which the WHO WMH-CIDI is programmed. Westat USA is the distributor of the Blaise system for North, Central, and South America. Contact: www.westat.com/capability/information-systems-software/blaise/blaise-licensing-ordering; blaise@westat.com
GAD-7 (Spitzer et al. 2006)	7	Mild: 5–9 Moderate: 10–14 Severe: >15	2–5 minutes	Self-report	No cost. The copyright is held by Pfizer Inc., but the questionnaire is free to use (Williams 2014).

TABLE 4–3. Rating scales for anxiety *(continued)*

Scale	Number of questions	Scoring	Time to administer	Type of reporting	Source and cost
Hamilton Rating Scale for Anxiety (HAM-A; Hamilton 1959)	14	Mild: 1–17 Moderate: 18–24 Severe: 25–30	10–15 minutes	Clinician administered	No cost. The HAM-A is in the public domain.
Hospital Anxiety and Depression Scale (HADS; Zigmond and Snaith 1983)	14; 7 for anxiety, 7 for depression	Normal: 0–7 Mild: 8–10 Moderate: 11–14 Severe: 15–21	2–5 minutes	Self-report	Use of the questionnaire is licensed by GL Assessment. A license agreement must be completed beforehand, and a user fee is required of all users (commercial and academic) (Bjelland et al. 2002). Please contact: GL Assessment Ltd. 1st Floor Vantage London Great West Road Brentford TW8 9AG London United Kingdom permissions@ gl-assessment.co.uk www.gl-assessment.co.uk

TABLE 4–3. Rating scales for anxiety *(continued)*

Scale	Number of questions	Scoring	Time to administer	Type of reporting	Source and cost
Penn State Worry Questionnaire (PSWQ; Meyer et al. 1990)	16	Total score range is 16–80; cutoff for GAD is 50	10–15 minutes	Self-report	No cost but copyrighted. The PSWQ can be obtained through the Measurement Instrument Database for the Social Sciences (MIDSS) at www.midss.org/content/penn-state-worry-questionnaire-pswq.
PROMIS Emotional Distress–Anxiety Short Form (PROMIS Health Organization and PROMIS Cooperative Group 2012)	29	Raw score × number of items on the short form divided by the number of items that were actually answered yields a T-score. The raw score can be rescaled into a standardized score with a mean of 50 and SD of 10.	Not reported	Self-report	No cost. To get a copy of this instrument, register with Assessment Center (www.assessmentcenter.net) and endorse the PROMIS terms and conditions of use (Pilkonis et al. 2011).

your mouth gets dry—the first sign that your SNS is in charge and shutting down digestion in preparation for a fight, flight, or freeze reaction that readies you to run hard and fast to get away by diverting blood (energy) from digestion and pumping blood to large muscle groups. After all, you do not need to digest your lunch when you are about to *be* lunch (real or imagined danger). Fortunately, most of us will rarely need to run away from a bear, but we may encounter conditions of psychological challenge (e.g., stressful circumstances, negative thoughts, worries) or physical challenge (e.g., a strange noise when alone in your house, physical assault, or threat) that are the modern-day equivalent of running from a bear. These challengers or "stressors" disrupt homeostatic balance and trigger the fight, flight, or freeze response, which is also referred to as "the stress response." It is a cascade of neural and endocrine changes designed to respond to and reestablish homeostasis.

Several books in the section "Resources" provide helpful explanations along these lines. It also may be helpful to tell patients something like the following:

> We have a dilemma in modern life because not all stress in bad. If your stress comes from real events that connect with an authentic medical crisis, the stress response is lifesaving. But if, instead, you are chronically assaulted with the psychological stress of modern life, which is more diffuse and chronic, your health suffers. Often, we get sick from activating this lifesaving stress response too often, for too long, and for purely psychological reasons.

See McGonigal (2015) for further discussion of the evolutionary role of stress.

Correcting Suboptimal Prescribing

The third step is to begin with a general review of all medications the patient is currently taking. If the patient has been taking medications included on the Beers List (American Geriatrics Society 2015 Beers Criteria Update Expert Panel 2015), serious consideration should be given to stopping the medication if possible and, if not, switching the patient to a medicine for the same indication that is believed to be a better choice for someone who is older. Making these changes, of course, requires coordination with the other clinicians working with the patient. In addition, any medication for which there is no clear indication, any medication prescribed for a problem that it did not improve, and any medication that is not appropriate for the treatment of an anxiety disorder that is chronic should be discontinued. These would include sedatives (e.g., benzodiazepines), anticholinergics, and antihistaminergic medications, all of which are generally not well tolerated by older adults. In the case of medications such as benzodiazepines or SSRIs, the discontinuation will need to be done in a stepwise fashion to avoid withdrawal symptoms that regrettably, often include anxiety and will likely be both uncomfortable and disconcerting to the anxious patient. Correcting suboptimal prescribing also should include a review of any over-the-counter (OTC) medications and complementary and alternative medicines (CAMs). Although a small number of studies suggest that certain CAMs, such as kava, may be helpful, scientific evidence also indicates that both OTC medication products and CAMs have the potential to make anxiety worse, such as caffeine-containing OTC products and St. John's wort (Ravindran and da Silva 2013; Saeed et al. 2007).

If completion of the first three steps in the algorithm (Figure 4–1) has not yielded satisfactory improvement in the patient's anxiety, then consideration of the use of pharmacological and nonpharmacological interventions is necessary.

Pharmacological Strategies

Avoidance of benzodiazepines (if possible). The benzodiazepines are a useful treatment for short term anxiety. They provide a rapid anxiolytic effect, but the risk to-benefit ratio in older adults is not favorable and becomes even more unfavorable with long-term use, especially with the recent research that identifies benzodiazepine medication use as a risk factor for dementia (Billioti de Gage et al. 2012). Using a very low dose of a "senior-friendly" benzodiazepine (Solai et al. 2001) may be appropriate for situational anxiety such as the initial phase of grieving. Benzodiazepine medication is not recommended for long-term use to treat anxiety problems because its use in this way increases the risk of 1) cognitive decline, 2) decreased respiratory drive, 3) substance use disorder, and 4) additive sedation (Benítez et al. 2008). In addition, the immediate relief often provided by the benzodiazepines with short-term or as-needed use is short-lived, does not address these maladaptive behaviors (e.g., avoidance) to improve quality of life in the long term, and in many cases reinforces maladaptive behaviors often associated with anxiety. Even if the only initial treatment in step four is medication, psychoeducation on the nature of anxiety disorders and the value of the person taking as much responsibility for his or her anxiety as possible remains an essential element of the treatment and may improve treatment adherence and compliance.

First-line medication treatment. If the patient agrees to start pharmacotherapy, SSRIs are first-line treatments, and some categorize serotonin-norepinephrine reuptake inhibitors (SNRIs) as first-line treatments as well. Abejuela and Osser (2016) published an algorithm specifically focused on selection of a medication for the treatment of GAD. In this algorithm, at least one, and possibly two, SSRI trials are recommended before a trial of duloxetine, an SNRI, is considered. These authors suggest that when a medication from either of these categories is being chosen, those options that are considered more likely to be successfully used with an older adult should be given careful consideration. For example, among the SSRIs, sertraline, citalopram, and escitalopram are generally considered to be the preferred options for older adults because of their relatively favorable side-effect profiles, relatively fewer potential drug-drug interactions, and intermediate half-lives (Solai et al. 2001). Lenze et al. (2009) found that escitalopram was superior to placebo in cumulative response. Among the SNRIs, venlafaxine extended release and duloxetine were found to be useful (Davidson et al. 2008; Katz et al. 2002).

When a medication is being introduced, it is important to start at a low dosage and then make relatively small increases separated by at least a few days—that is, "Start low and go slow." In older adults, it is better to start low and slow with a dosage that may be subtherapeutic but better tolerated. Once there is a therapeutic alliance and the patient has a sense of trust in the clinician, it is much easier to titrate upward as needed to a therapeutic dosage. Warning patients about potential side effects is one important way to build trust.

Frequent follow-up during the first month of treatment is necessary to encourage adherence and to monitor treatment response. Patients living with problematic levels of anxiety may be especially at risk for problematic side effects to medications. As a rule, they are concerned about the side-effect profile and have anticipatory anxiety with a tendency to catastrophize about any sensation they detect or experience in taking medications. Often these patients have an external locus of control and/or have spent years being hypervigilant about bodily sensations as well as being prone to interpret any new or unexpected bodily sensation as the harbinger of an emerging health threat, which paradoxically worsens the anxiety symptoms the new medication was intended to treat.

A patient starting an SSRI or SNRI benefits from warnings about common initial side effects and the knowledge that these are rarely serious and often transient. In addition, patients benefit from knowing that the maximum therapeutic effect may take at least 4–6 weeks to achieve, in stark contrast with the benzodiazepines, which are initially fast-acting (20–30 minutes). In addition, the use of anxiety self-report measures helps patients develop insight into their progress.

Follow-Up and Augmentation Strategies

Under the follow-up step, Bower et al. (2015) recommend slow titration of the psychotropic medication along with carefully checking for medication side effects and offering reassurance to improve compliance. During this phase of care, Bower and colleagues also list a number of potentially helpful nonpharmacological augmentation strategies, including relaxation therapy or cognitive-behavioral therapy (CBT) with a relaxation component. These authors also acknowledge that consulting an expert may be necessary if none of the initial interventions have been helpful.

Pharmacological augmentation.   In some cases, monotherapy may be unsuccessful in treating the anxiety symptoms. The patient may not tolerate the increase to a more therapeutic dosage, may not obtain a therapeutic response at the maximum recommended dosage, or may not be able to tolerate the side effects. When this occurs, it may be necessary to augment with a second medication or refer the patient to a geriatric psychiatrist who has more expertise.

Nonpharmacological augmentation.   There are a variety of psychotherapeutic and behavioral interventions in various stages of development and study that may prove helpful to older adults with problematic anxiety. The primary and simplest mechanism to break the cycle of anxiety is breath work. A person's breath is the cheapest, most neutral, and universally available intervention. Breath work is the foundation for mindfulness training. Mindfulness is a state of nonjudgmental awareness of present moment experience (Shapiro et al. 2006).

Wetherell et al. (2011, 2013) found that CBT maybe an effective augmentation strategy when added to SSRI medication. Combination therapy treatment may be introduced sequentially or simultaneously. The potential advantage for simultaneous introduction is that the SSRI can reduce the acute distress and somatic symptoms, while the CBT can address the underlying maladaptive behaviors of worry, improve coping skills, and review cognitive distortions. Patients overcome by anxiety have a heightened state of fear, and it can be nearly impossible to "talk them through the anxiety." The key is to regulate their body response first and then address the personal narrative or story that is layered on top: "I'm fearful of...." Assuring patients that their body is a source of safety when overcome by anxiety and has the capacity to override the anxious thought is a useful tool to address their maladaptive behaviors.

Energy follows attention. When the attention is on worry, anxiety, and the body's response to this fear, a break in the cycle is needed. In other words, attention must be captured to redirect it. A simple and easy mechanism is to direct the patient to "bring your attention to the back of the room; bring your attention to the front of the room; and now bring your attention to reading level." At this point the attention is in the here and now, and you can introduce an intervention to bring the energy from the head, where worry and ruminations reside, to the body, where a source of safety and assurance can be learned. This then provides an excellent time to do further interventions such as breath work, because the patient is less consumed with the worry and more receptive to a nonpharmacological intervention.

Treatment Agreements

A nonpharmacological approach that works especially well with patients who have the triad of GAD (i.e., frequently co-occurring presence of chronic disabling anxiety, somatization symptoms or a full disorder, and psychological developmental delays or arrests)—or some combination of these features—is to partner with the patient in the development of a written *treatment agreement*. Psychological delays or arrests are usually not difficult to recognize because they announce their presence via long-standing maladaptive patterns of coping such as all-or-none thinking, externalization of responsibility (i.e., an external locus of control), and splitting. Other comparable terms that are sometimes used to describe a treatment agreement include a *treatment memorandum of understanding*, a *treatment roadmap*, a *treatment outline*, or a *treatment guide*.

The theoretical underpinnings of these documents may include one or more of the following: behavior therapy, cognitive therapy, insight-oriented psychotherapy, and supportive psychotherapy. Some of the goals of a treatment agreement may include fostering accurate and realistic expectations for the patient, family members, and staff; avoiding pointless debates about the reality or etiology of symptoms (e.g., physical vs. psychological); increasing the patient's ownership of the recovery process; reducing splitting behaviors; and binding the negative countertransference that members of the treatment team often develop when caring for patients with these challenges. Characteristics of these patients that make them challenging to care for, and that can be a source of negative feelings in members of the treatment team, include the following: 1) they often improve slowly, requiring patience on the part of team members; 2) their myriad somatic concerns can be exhausting to listen to; and 3) their external locus of control often causes them to blame team members for their lack of improvement or slowness to improve.

The psychotherapeutic treatment agreement approach developed and refined at the University of California, San Diego, yields treatment agreements that consist of four main sections (see Table 4–4 for more details and Table 4–5 for a deidentified version of an actual treatment agreement). Although the elements of each of these sections usually cluster together within the agreement, this is not a requirement. Also, certain tasks listed as part of one section may also contribute helpfully to the goals and tasks of another section.

The goal of Section 1 is for the patient's primary concerns and goals to be recorded as specifically as possible using the patient's own words, along with their scope, severity, and history, and to help manage expectations regarding the anticipated rate of improvement in symptoms. Many older patients may have lived with uncomfortable anxiety symptoms for a long time and may have failed multiple treatment trials of various types. Alternatively, the past treatment received may have been suboptimal at best or inappropriate at worst (e.g., long-term use of a benzodiazepine medication). As a result, the patient may be skeptical about the ability of the treatment agreement approach to be helpful or may rather quickly sabotage or devalue the agreement.

To overcome any hesitation or resistance to the treatment agreement approach early in the process, patients may benefit from a homework assignment that requires them to list all of the previous clinicians who have attempted to help them with their anxiety. Often this list can be quite long. When the patient brings this list to the subsequent meeting, the clinician should carefully review the list. After doing so, the therapist should make a statement such as the following:

> I see that you have sought treatment from quite a few clinicians of various types and yet here you are still suffering and asking for my help. Some of the clinicians on your list I know well and consider to be very talented. Your list of past providers demonstrates to me that your symptoms must be quite serious if none of these clinicians were able to help resolve them. Your list also suggests to me that if you have never had your symptoms treated using a treatment agreement approach, then you don't have much to lose and it may be reasonable to have a new approach that you have never had before. In other words, everything else has not been successful, so why not try a new/different approach?

For the treatment agreement approach to be successful, it is essential for the patient to move toward an understanding that the nature and extent of the person's recovery are fundamentally up to the patient, and to obtain the patient's "buy in" or "ownership" of the treatment agreement. A number of specific techniques help to achieve these goals. Almost every statement in a treatment agreement is written using first-

TABLE 4–4. **Organization of a treatment agreement for patients with generalized anxiety disorder and/or somatization**

Section 1: Identifying the patient's primary concerns and goals

Use the patient's own words/direct quotes.

Record scope, severity, and history, and help manage expectations regarding the anticipated rate of improvement in symptoms.

Validate the reality of the patient's suffering without concern for underlying etiology or the degree to which medical versus psychological issues are responsible.

Help the patient manage expectations about the rate of improvement.

Consider adding the most complete list possible for all clinicians, past and present, who have had any role in helping the patient with assessment and treatment of the presenting complaints.

Section 2: Imparting important foundational concepts

List the possible various tools that may prove helpful.

Identify and describe other problems connected to the presenting problem.

Define various terms such as *splitting*.

Create a list of activities that the patient has historically found relaxing and rewarding.

Section 3: Assigning and reviewing homework

Record regular homework assignments:

Work with the patient to establish homework that the patient believes is a reasonable amount to accomplish before the due date.

Consider use of a behavioral contingency table to provide the patient with acknowledgment of success.

Include an "enforcement clause" if the patient does not complete the homework.

Remember: The most accessible and perhaps the most powerful tool a clinician has to inspire behavior change is the amount of face time given to a patient. Depending on the clinical setting, something like the following may be possible: if a patient completes a homework assignment successfully, then give the patient 30 minutes of face time. If the patient does not, then limit face time with the patient to 5 minutes.

TABLE 4–4. **Organization of a treatment agreement for patients with generalized anxiety disorder and/or somatization** *(continued)*

Section 4: Defining and expanding the current "treatment team"

Note: This is a different task from the similar, last task described in section 1 of this table. The purpose of this task is to make sure that the patient, members of the patient's family, and current members of the treating team know each other, that everyone is striving to be on the same page, and that everyone (patient, clinicians, and family members) has communicated and will likely continue to communicate with each other on an ongoing basis.

List the key clinicians currently working with the patient (both inpatient and outpatient).

List important members of the patient's social network.

Make sure that anyone listed is given up-to-date copies of the agreement. (These individuals should be considered active members of the patient's treatment team and should partner in the patient's care, including adhering to the treatment agreement.)

Consider a "signing ceremony" at times of transitions in care, such as from inpatient to outpatient.

person singular pronouns and verbs. For example, the first statement of a treatment agreement could be "I have agreed to meet with Dr. X on a regular and voluntary basis in order to receive evaluation and treatment of severe and persisting symptoms of anxiety and problematic patterns of interaction with my spouse." Another technique that often helps patients own the treatment agreement is to encourage the patient to find problems or mistakes with the agreement, big or small, and to respond quickly and positively to the patient's request for changes or improvements to the agreement. By doing this, the language in the agreement becomes more and more dominated by the patient's own thoughts and words. In addition, responding quickly and affirmatively helps the patient feel heard and respected, which may not happen very often outside the therapist's office, and helps strengthen the therapist's rapport with the patient.

Particularly for patients who have some degree of vulnerability to somatization, past negative experiences seeking help from a medical professional may have left these patients feeling disrespected, disbelieved, or devalued—the feelings that statements like "It's all in your head" often evoke. Because of these experiences, and especially if one of the presenting problems includes some form of physical pain, it may be helpful to include a statement early in the agreement, such as "I under-

TABLE 4–5. **A deidentified example of a treatment agreement**

Treatment Agreement for Jane Smith

Tuesday, August 6, 2019

Draft #6

1. I recently began working with Dr. X on a voluntary basis in order to receive evaluation and treatment for my complicated, distressing, and ongoing problems, which include chronic abdominal pain, chronic diarrhea, chronic burning pain, nausea, insomnia, anxiety, depressed mood, hopelessness, and overall diminished life quality.

2. I understand that Dr. X, Dr. Y, Dr. Z, and the other members of the treatment team in no way questioned the reality of my physical and emotional pain and suffering.

3. I acknowledge that despite repeatedly seeking care, I have been suffering from physical and associated psychological symptoms for a number of years. The seriousness of my symptoms is underscored by the fact that I have consulted with multiple clinicians and yet have not obtained satisfactory relief of my pain and suffering. The list of clinicians with whom I have previously consulted includes:

   a. Dr. A, my current psychiatrist.

   b. Dr. B, my current primary care physician.

   c. Dr. C, my gastroenterologist.

   d. Dr. D, my former psychotherapist.

   e. Dr. E, a neurologist.

   f. Dr. F, my cardiologist.

   g. Dr. G, my former primary care physician.

4. Because of the duration, severity, and complexity of my health problems, I understand that it may take some time for me to achieve the health and happiness that I desire and that it is unlikely that I will be completely recovered before my work with Dr. A comes to an end.

5. I understand that the primary goal of this therapy experience is to begin my journey down a path that will ultimately help me achieve the health and happiness I desire. I understand that the treatment program that I initiate with Dr. A will require me to make gradual, ongoing changes in my thoughts, habits, and behaviors and that the full benefit of this program will take months and possibly years. I understand that this treatment agreement will help guide this journey and that I will have access to a number of individuals who may be willing and able to help coach me on this journey. These individuals may include my son, my primary care physician, and the members of my mental health treatment team.

TABLE 4–5. **A deidentified example of a treatment agreement** *(continued)*

6. I understand that even if I am never completely free of physical and emotional symptoms, I will be able to live a rich, full, and meaningful life in spite of the physical and emotional symptoms.

7. I understand that my physical problems cause me stress, anxiety, and depression and that stress, anxiety, and depression make my physical problems worse. In order to achieve the best possible outcome, I will need ongoing treatment of my medical problems as well as treatment of depression and anxiety.

8. I understand that my work with Dr. A will include homework that will help me regain my health.

9. I understand that in order to achieve the highest degree of relief from my chronic abdominal pain, chronic diarrhea, chronic burning pain, nausea, insomnia, anxiety, depressed mood, hopelessness, and overall diminished life quality, every possible helpful tool will be considered. These tools will include but are *not* limited to:

    a. Medications.
    b. Exercise and stretching.
    c. Physical therapy.
    d. Deep breathing exercises.
    e. Mindfulness.
    f. Group therapy.
    g. Individual therapy.
    h. Cognitive-behavioral therapy.
    i. Art therapy.
    j. Horticultural therapy.
    k. Music.
    l. Volunteering.
    m. Other.

10. Below is a list of activities that historically I have generally found to be enjoyable, relaxing, rewarding, fulfilling, worthwhile, and/or engaging:

    a. Watching the television program *The Young and the Restless*.
    b. Listening to classical music/orchestral music.
    c. Listening to audio books.
    d. Going to Broadway stage performances at places like the Lawrence Welk Resort.
    e. Watching *Pink Panther* movies, especially the original ones with Peter Sellers.

TABLE 4–5.   A deidentified example of a treatment agreement *(continued)*

---

   f.   Being with and visiting with family members and children.

   g.   Socializing and talking with people of all ages.

   h.   Window shopping.

   i.   Listening to soothing, relaxing music.

   j.   Watching shows on public television.

   k.   Watching documentaries.

   l.   Learning new things.

   m.   Enjoying quiet and peaceful nights.

11. I acknowledge that there are aspects of my communication style that may unintentionally frustrate or annoy others and may even lead to others, including members of my family, limiting their time with me or avoiding me. One aspect of my interpersonal communication that I recognize could be improved is my conversational sensitivity. As a result, I have agreed to reflect on what it means to converse with others in a mutually respectful and courteous manner. I have agreed to be mindful of giving others the opportunity to speak without interrupting them. In order to help me improve in this area, if I interrupt a member of my clinical team or member of my family more than twice during a conversation, this person will immediately announce what has happened and promptly end the interaction.

12. Another aspect of my communication style that I am working to improve is my habit of "splitting." *Splitting* is a term used to describe a statement or other behavior that reveals that a person is having difficulty with holding opposing thoughts, feelings, or beliefs about someone or about himself or herself. In other words, positive and negative attributes of a person or event are not joined together into a cohesive set of beliefs.

13. Splitting represents a distorted way of thinking and is a coping mechanism used to protect the person from feeling hurt or rejected.

14. Someone who is vulnerable to splitting finds it difficult to recognize that good people sometimes do things imperfectly or make mistakes. The experience of splitting is very confusing and frustrating for people who split, their loved ones, and those who care for the person. For example, when a basically good person who is caring for me makes a mistake and because of that mistake is labeled publicly by me as "all bad," this person may feel unfairly judged and may no longer be as enthusiastic about caring for me. When other caregivers learn that I have unfairly judged one of their peers, then they may also lose their enthusiasm for helping me because they are anticipating that eventually they may do something that is less than perfect in my eyes and then they will also be publicly labeled by me in an unflattering way.

TABLE 4–5.   A deidentified example of a treatment agreement *(continued)*

15. Splitting is considered normal, natural, and expected in young children whose brains are not fully mature and, therefore, lack the sophistication required to see the world in terms that are other than black and white, all or none. In reality, most things in the world are not black and white but are actually varying shades of gray.

16. When a young person experiences painful psychological experiences, this sometimes interferes with psychological growth and results in this person no longer maturing at the same rate as his or her peers. This person may not achieve the level of maturity needed to avoid splitting.

17. In order to help me begin to be less prone to splitting, if I am observed to be splitting a member of my clinical team or a member of my family more than twice during a conversation, this person will immediately announce what has happened and promptly end the interaction.

18. My homework assignments to be completed by 4 P.M., Wednesday, 8/7/19:

    a. Read and critique draft #6 of my treatment agreement.

    b. Read another section in the booklet titled "Senior Behavioral Health Program Recovery Tools for Depressions and Anxiety."

Name of patient's spouse   Date

Name of patient's son   Date

Name of patient's geriatric psychiatrist   Date

Name of patient's primary care physician   Date

Note.   Although some items in the above treatment agreement could correctly be associated with more than one of the sections outlined in Table 4–4, one possible categorization by section is as follows: section 1: items 1–5; section 2: items 6–16; section 3: items 17–18; and section 4: signature section of agreement.

stand that my physical problems causes me stress and anxiety and that stress and anxiety make my physical problems worse. In order to achieve the best possible outcome, I will need ongoing treatment of my medical problems as well as treatment of depression and anxiety." Including a statement like this often helps to avoid pointless debates about the reality or etiology of symptoms (e.g., whether they are physical, psychological, or both).

The final important element of the first section of the treatment agreement is to help the patient manage expectations about the rate of improvement. By the time the patient arrives in the therapist's office, the years of suffering may have magnified the patient's hope for a rapid and complete response. This type of response, however, is only rarely possible. As a result, it is often helpful to include a statement that indicates that full recovery will likely take months, if not years. This level of transparency may inspire the patient to terminate and find another therapist, perhaps continuing a search for the elusive pill that will quickly resolve symptoms. If the patient does terminate, this is most likely a clear indication that for some reason a treatment agreement approach was not what the patient was seeking or, possibly, not what the patient was ready to try. Often a discussion of the time required for improvement triggers very strong emotions that may require an entire session to process. Acknowledging repeatedly that the therapist is aware of the pain the patient is experiencing and the understandable disappointment about the absence of a quick cure may help the patient recommit to the treatment agreement. If the therapist acknowledges an awareness of the many past treatment failures and then explains that a primary goal is not to mislead the patient or set the patient up for future disappointments when the recovery takes longer than expected, this also may help retain the patient in therapy.

Section 2 of the agreement consists of important foundational concepts such as a list of the possible various tools that may prove helpful, including medications; various forms of psychotherapy, including CBT; regular physical exercise; and maintaining a healthy diet that avoids foods and beverages that may increase anxiety (e.g., caffeinated beverages). This section may also include other problems connected to the presenting problem that need to be addressed, definitions of various terms such as *splitting,* and a list of activities that the patient has historically found relaxing and rewarding. This list helps serve as a source of potential activities that can be used to recognize successful completion of various tasks or the achievement of a therapeutic goal. The items on this list may also be helpful if the therapist elects to include a behavioral contingency table in the agreement.

The third section of the agreement contains the patient's homework assignment. These assignments are generally due at the time of the therapist's next anticipated contact with the patient. Keeping in mind a key principle from CBT, the clinician should work with the patient to make sure that the quantity of each homework assignment is reasonable for the time allotted. Many of the homework assignments will begin with the patient being asked to review and critique the most recent version of the agreement. Homework assignments often include CBT homework, such as being assigned certain pages to read and exercises to complete in a CBT workbook. If a patient is not able or willing to complete homework assignments, then this may require some statements of consequences. Generally, repeated failure to complete homework assignments, especially if care was taken to keep them a reasonable size, suggests that the patient is either not ready or not appropriate for this intervention. For patients receiving this treatment during an inpatient hospitalization setting, this may result in discharge, with a message such as "Your inability to complete your homework assignment for 2 days in a row suggests that the maximum benefit of this hospitalization has been obtained, and so you are being discharged. You are welcome to return when you are ready to resume the work we initiated." Depending on the patient's circumstances, including the number and acuity of symptoms and their impact on patient function, "return" may mean return to the hospital for readmission or return to the outpatient setting where members of the same group of clinicians previously caring for the patient can care for him or her as an outpatient.

The final section of the agreement is reserved for listing the patient's name, all of the members of the patient's treatment team, and key members of the patient's support network that the patient elects to include. These names are included for a variety of reasons. It is important that the patient understands that the success of the agreement, in part, hinges on everyone whose name is included having a copy of the agreement, being aware of its contents, and being willing to abide by what the agreement stipulates. If the agreement has been completed in an inpatient setting, then shortly before discharge, all included parties can be asked to sign the agreement, which is meant to be confirmation that this version of the agreement has been read, that the individual has had the opportunity to influence the content of the agreement, and that each signer agrees with its contents.

Treatment agreements generally need to be updated on a regular basis, so each update is assigned a number in chronological order. As drafts of the agreement accumulate, they serve as a concrete reminder of the effort that has been expended by the patient, the therapist, and others. In addition, the drafts help mark progress, and this can help mitigate feelings of restlessness or impatience in the therapist, as enduring changes in behavior take time. Changes to a draft of the agreement are sometimes placed in bold font to make them easier to identify. Lastly, copies of the agreement should be distributed to all clinicians caring for the patient and, with the patient's permission, to key members of the patient's support system. Widely disseminating the agreement helps keep everyone on the same page and helps to prevent splitting. Table 4–6 contains "Pointers" that may help ensure that the use of a treatment agreement is successful.

There are pitfalls to the treatment agreement approach. Perhaps the biggest is that the creation and use of a treatment agreement is time intensive. Other potential pitfalls include situations in which all staff are not aware of the details of the agreement; certain staff do not adhere to the agreement; the patient feels infantilized by the process; the agreement fosters hospital or other forms of dependency; goals or homework assignments are overly ambitious; or the patient or others believe that a "final draft" of the agreement must be created. Another potential pitfall is that members of the treatment team develop strongly negative countertransference toward the patient and begin "acting out" these negative feelings through avoidance or other unhelpful behaviors.

Lifestyle Modifications

Including lifestyle modifications in the treatment of anxiety can help improve a patient's health and quality of life, as well as empower the patient to engage in his or her own treatment plan. Such modifications are in addition to any psychopharmacological and psychotherapy interventions. Three lifestyle modifications to consider involve physical activity, sleep, and diet. Sleep is discussed in other chapters (see Chapter 7, "Primary Sleep Disorders," and Chapter 8, "Evaluation and Management of Insomnia"). Diet, albeit relevant, is beyond the scope of this chapter. Dietary modifications that may help reduce anxiety include reducing and/or avoiding consumption of caffeine, alcohol, and processed sugar. Additional helpful information about how diet has an impact on anxiety can be found in a number of places, including direct-to-consumer newsletters from well-respected health systems such as Harvard and Mayo Clinic, or a number of reputable books, including one by the certified dietitian, Trudy Scott (2011).

In general, aerobic exercise has been shown to be a powerful and cost-efficient treatment alternative for a variety of anxiety disorders (Salmon 2001). Several studies have indicated that aerobic exercise may be as effective in reducing generalized anxiety as CBT (McEntee and Haglin 1999). In the treatment of anxiety, exercise has been shown to alleviate anxious feelings. Exercising at 70%–90% of maximum heart rate

TABLE 4–6. **Pointers to consider when using a treatment agreement approach for generalized anxiety disorder**

1. Make plenty of copies of each draft of the agreement and widely distribute them to the patient, family members, and members of the treatment team.

2. Create the agreement using large type so that it can be easily read by all.

3. Listen carefully for the patient to disclose directly or indirectly what he or she finds rewarding or important and use this information.

4. Start slowly: the first draft of the agreement may be only one page.

5. Label and date each draft.

6. From draft to draft, put changes or edits in bold type.

7. Write the agreement so that the patient is not able to use nonadherence with the agreement to manipulate or control; for example, include a statement such as "Failure to complete my assigned homework 2 days in a row or 3 times total during the course of this hospital stay will be interpreted as a sign that the treatment is moving too fast and that I should be discharged and allowed to take a breather before additional work is attempted."

8. Consider putting in a few "outrageous" items or silly mistakes in order to confirm that the patient is reading the agreement. If the patient does not spontaneously mention these items, then this suggests that the patient may not be carefully reading the agreement. If the patient's commitment to the process is unclear, then this needs to be discussed openly with the patient. If the patient is not genuinely willing to commit to the process, then the patient may need to be informed that the maximum benefit of the therapy has been obtained and the patient will be discharged from care.

9. Partner with members of the patient's family or support system and keep them supplied with the latest version of the agreement.

10. Emphasize that the agreement will be useful even after discharge from the hospital.

11. Share the latest version of the agreement with all providers.

12. Remember that the most powerful tool available to you to inspire the patient to change is the provision or removal of your attention.

13. In any given encounter, if the patient engages in toxic thoughts or behaviors (e.g., verbalizing a cognitive distortion that serves to heighten anxiety), gently remind the patient that this has happened and ask him or her to stop the behavior. If the patient does it again, gently point this out, ask the patient to stop, and tell him or her that if it happens again, you will immediately end the interaction.

for 20 minutes three times a week has been shown to significantly reduce anxiety sensitivity (Smits et al. 2008).

Physicians should recommend that adults participate in at least 30 minutes of accumulated moderate-intensity physical activity (e.g., walking fast) on most days of the week. Key principles for physical activity are as follows (Meriwether et al. 2008): 1) the more activity the better; 2) accumulated time is more important than intensity; 3) activity can be accumulated in 10-minute increments; and 4) lifestyle activities (e.g., substituting walking or biking for short car rides, parking in the spot farthest from the door) are more likely to be sustained than are structured activities such as exercising at a gym. See Chapter 18, "Physical Activity," for further discussion about helping patients initiate and maintain physical activity.

Vignette *(continued)*

Ms. B responded well to mirtazapine at a low dosage (7.5 mg po nightly). Moreover, a strong therapeutic alliance was developed, facilitating not only her transition from the discontinuation of the SSRI, which was clearly part of the problem leading to the exacerbation of her anxiety disorder, but also the management of her hypervigilance to possible side effects and the reassurance needed to stay the course. She was referred to a senior psychotherapy group and attended once. She felt strongly that the group was "not for her," and a referral to a mindfulness group was successfully made. In the office, breathing techniques were practiced, and within minutes she was able to feel a change in her arousal state and a decrease in her symptoms. This small victory gave her confidence in her ability to be calm and manage her maladaptive behaviors that would have been lost with the introduction of a fast-acting benzodiazepine.

KEY POINTS

- Excessive anxiety is not a normal part of aging. Accurate identification and treatment of anxiety symptoms can significantly improve health outcomes and quality of life in older patients.
- The initial goals in caring for someone with problematic anxiety symptoms is to develop a differential diagnosis, then to take the necessary steps to determine the most likely cause or causes, and then treat these causes.
- When psychoeducation is being provided to an older adult with anxiety, it is important to include family members or caretakers.
- If an older adult with anxiety agrees to a medication trial, one of the selective serotonin reuptake inhibitors known to be better tolerated

by older patients, such as sertraline, citalopram, or escitalopram, is considered first-line treatment. Some experts consider the newer serotonin-norepinephrine reuptake inhibitors also to be first-line treatments.

- Benzodiazepine medications are not recommended for long-term use to treat anxiety in adults of any age.

Resources

Organizations and Other Online Resources

American Psychiatric Association, 800 Maine Ave., SW, Suite 900, Washington, DC 20024; (888) 357-7924; www.psychiatry.org

American Psychological Association, 750 First St., NE, Washington, DC 20002-4242; (800) 374-2721; www.apa.org

Anxiety and Depression Association of America, 8701 Georgia Ave., Suite 412, Silver Spring, MD 20910; (240) 485-1001; https://adaa.org

Anxiety.org (for complementary and alternative treatments for anxiety)

Centers for Disease Control and Prevention, Division of Mental Health, 1600 Clifton Rd., Atlanta, GA 30329-4027; (800) CDC-INFO (800-232-4636); www.cdc.gov/mentalhealth

National Alliance on Mental Illness (NAMI), Colonial Place Three, 3803 N. Fairfax Dr., Suite 100, Arlington, VA 22203; (800) 950-6264; www.nami.org

National Institute of Mental Health, 6001 Executive Blvd., Room 6200, MSC 9663, Bethesda, MD 20892-9663; (866) 615–6464; www.nimh.nih.gov

PsychologyTools: www.psychologytools.com; (for CBT-relevant free handouts)

Books

Burns DD: Ten Days to Self-Esteem. New York, Quill, 1993

Burns DD: Feeling Good: The New Mood Therapy. New York, HarperCollins, 2012

Greenberger D, Padesky CA: Mind Over Mood: Change How You Feel by Changing the Way You Think, 2nd Edition. New York, Guilford, 2016

Harris R: The Happiness Trap: How to Stop Struggling and Start Living. Boston, MA, Trumpeter Books, 2008

Kahn JP: Angst: Origins of Anxiety and Depression. New York, Oxford University Press, 2013

McGonigal K: The Upside of Stress: Why Stress Is Good for You, and How to Get Good at It. London, Avery, 2015

Sapolsky RM: Why Zebras Don't Get Ulcers. New York, Owl Book/ Henry Holt and Co, 2004

Scott T: The Antianxiety Food Solution: How the Foods You Eat Can Help You Calm Your Anxious Mind, Improve Your Mood, and End Cravings. Oakland, CA, New Harbinger, 2011

References

Abejuela HR, Osser DN: The Psychopharmacology Algorithm Project at the Harvard South Shore Program: an algorithm for generalized anxiety disorder. Harv Rev Psychiatry 24(4):243–256, 2016 27384395

American Geriatrics Society 2015 Beers Criteria Update Expert Panel: American Geriatrics Society 2015 updated Beers criteria for potentially inappropriate medication use in older adults. J Am Geriatr Soc 63(11):2227–2246, 2015 26446832

American Psychiatric Association: Diagnostic and Statistical Manual of Mental Disorders, 5th Edition. Arlington, VA, American Psychiatric Association, 2013

Beck AT, Steer RA: Beck Anxiety Inventory Manual. San Antonio, TX, Psychological Corporation, 1993

Beck AT, Steer RA, Brown GK: Beck Depression Inventory: Manual. San Antonio, TX, Psychological Corporation, 1996

Benítez CI, Smith K, Vasile RG, et al: Use of benzodiazepines and selective serotonin reuptake inhibitors in middle-aged and older adults with anxiety disorders: a longitudinal and prospective study. Am J Geriatr Psychiatry 16(1):5–13, 2008 18165458

Bickett A, Tapp H: Anxiety and diabetes: Innovative approaches to management in primary care. Exp Biol Med (Maywood) 241(15):1724–1731, 2016 27390262

Billioti de Gage S, Bégaud B, Bazin F, et al: Benzodiazepine use and risk of dementia: prospective population based study. BMJ 345:e6231, 2012

Bjelland I, Dahl AA, Haug TT, et al: The validity of the Hospital Anxiety and Depression Scale. An updated literature review. J Psychosom Res 52(2):69–77, 2002 11832252

Bower ES, Wetherell JL, Mon T, Lenze EJ: Treating anxiety disorders in older adults: current treatments and future directions. Harv Rev Psychiatry 23(5):329–342, 2015 26332216

Brady KT, Lydiard RB: The association of alcoholism and anxiety. Psychiatr Q 64(2):135–149, 1993 8316598

Bryant C, Jackson H, Ames D: The prevalence of anxiety in older adults: methodological issues and a review of the literature. J Affect Disord 109(3):233–250, 2008 18155775

Burns DD: Ten Days to Self-Esteem. New York, Quill, 1993

Burton C, Campbell P, Jordan K, et al: The association of anxiety and depression with future dementia diagnosis: a case-control study in primary care. Fam Pract 30(1):25–30, 2013 22915794

Davidson J, Baldwin DS, Stein DJ, et al: Effects of venlafaxine extended release on resilience in posttraumatic stress disorder: an item analysis of the Connor-Davidson Resilience Scale. Int Clin Psychopharmacol 23(5):299–303, 2008 18703940

El-Gabalawy R, Mackenzie CS, Shooshtari S, Sareen J: Comorbid physical health conditions and anxiety disorders: a population-based exploration of prevalence and health outcomes among older adults. Gen Hosp Psychiatry 33(6):556-564, 2011 21908055; Erratum in: Gen Hosp Psychiatry 35(3):325, 2013

Evers AW, Kraaimaat FW, Geenen R, et al: Longterm predictors of anxiety and depressed mood in early rheumatoid arthritis: a 3 and 5 year followup. J Rheumatol 29(11):2327–2336, 2002 12415588

Ginzburg K, Solomon Z, Bleich A: Repressive coping style, acute stress disorder, and posttraumatic stress disorder after myocardial infarction. Psychosom Med 64(5):748–757, 2002 12271105

Goodwin RD: Asthma and anxiety disorders. Adv Psychosom Med 24:51–71, 2003 14584347

Grigsby AB, Anderson RJ, Freedland KE, et al: Prevalence of anxiety in adults with diabetes: a systematic review. J Psychosom Res 53(6):1053–1060, 2002 12479986

Hamilton M: The assessment of anxiety states by rating. Br J Med Psychol 32(1):50–55, 1959 13638508

Härter MC, Conway KP, Merikangas KR: Associations between anxiety disorders and physical illness. Eur Arch Psychiatry Clin Neurosci 253(6):313–320, 2003 14714121

Jackson-Koku G: Beck Depression Inventory. Occup Med (Lond) 66(2):174–175, 2016 26892598

Katz IR, Reynolds CF III, Alexopoulos GS, Hackett D: Venlafaxine ER as a treatment for generalized anxiety disorder in older adults: pooled analysis of five randomized placebo-controlled clinical trials. J Am Geriatr Soc 50(1):18–25, 2002 12028242

Kosten TR, George TP: The neurobiology of opioid dependence: implications for treatment. Sci Pract Perspect 1(1):13–20, 2002 18567959

Lawton MP, Kleban MH, Dean J, et al: The factorial generality of brief positive and negative affect measures. J Gerontol 47(4):228–237, 1992 1624699

Lenze EJ, Wetherell JL: Anxiety disorders: new developments in old age. Am J Geriatr Psychiatry 19(4):301–304, 2011a 21427638

Lenze EJ, Wetherell JL: A lifespan view of anxiety disorders. Dialogues Clin Neurosci 13(4):381–399, 2011b 22275845

Lenze EJ, Rollman BL, Shear MK, et al: Escitalopram for older adults with generalized anxiety disorder: a randomized controlled trial. JAMA 301(3):295–303, 2009 19155456

Locke AB, Kirst N, Shultz CG: Diagnosis and management of generalized anxiety disorder and panic disorder in adults. Am Fam Physician 91(9):617–624, 2015 25955736

McEntee RJ, Haglin RP: Cognitive group therapy and aerobic exercise in the treatment of anxiety. Journal of College Student Psychotherapy 13:37–55, 1999

McGonigal K: The Upside of Stress. New York, Avery, 2015

Meriwether RA, Lee JA, Lafleur AS, et al: Physical activity counseling. Am Fam Physician 77(8):1129–1136, 2008 18481560

Meyer TJ, Miller ML, Metzger RL, Borkovec TD: Development and validation of the Penn State Worry Questionnaire. Behav Res Ther 28(6):487–495, 1990 2076086

Nasreddine ZS, Phillips NA, Bédirian V, et al: The Montreal Cognitive Assessment, MoCA: a brief screening tool for mild cognitive impairment. J Am Geriatr Soc 53(4):695–699, 2005 15817019

Neiss MB, Leigland LA, Carlson NE, et al: Age differences in perception and awareness of emotion. Neurobiol Aging 30(8):1305–1313, 2009 18155323

Perry PJ, Alexander B: Sedative/hypnotic dependence: patient stabilization, tolerance testing, and withdrawal. Drug Intell Clin Pharm 20(7–8):532–537, 1986 2874971

Pilkonis PA, Choi SW, Reise SP, et al: Item banks for measuring emotional distress from the Patient-Reported Outcomes Measurement Information System (PROMIS): depression, anxiety, and anger. Assessment 18(3):263–283, 2011 21697139

Pitman A, Suleman S, Hyde N, et al: Depression and anxiety in patients with cancer. BMJ 361:k1415, 2018 29695476

Player MS, Peterson LE: Anxiety disorders, hypertension, and cardiovascular risk: a review. Int J Psychiatry Med 41(4):365–377, 2011 22238841

PROMIS Health Organization and PROMIS Cooperative Group: LEVEL 2—Anxiety—Adult (PROMIS Emotional Distress—Anxiety—Short Form) 2012. Available at: http://www.psychiatry.org/practice/dsm/dsm5/online-assessment-measures. Accessed May 7, 2019.

Ravindran AV, da Silva TL: Herbal remedies and nutraceuticals as augmentation or adjunct for mood and anxiety disorders: evidence for benefit and risk, in Polypharmacy in Psychiatry Practice, Vol II. Edited by Ritsner M. New York, Springer Dordrecht, 2013

Robins LN, Wing J, Wittchen HU, et al: The Composite International Diagnostic Interview: An epidemiologic instrument suitable for use in conjunction with different diagnostic systems and in different cultures. Archives of General Psychiatry, 45(12):1069–1077, 1988

Saeed SA, Bloch RM, Antonacci DJ: Herbal and dietary supplements for treatment of anxiety disorders. Am Fam Physician 76(4):549–556, 2007 17853630

Salmon P: Effects of physical exercise on anxiety, depression, and sensitivity to stress: a unifying theory. Clin Psychol Rev 21(1):33–61, 2001 11148895

Sareen J, Jacobi F, Cox BJ, et al: Disability and poor quality of life associated with comorbid anxiety disorders and physical conditions. Arch Intern Med 166(19):2109–2116, 2006 17060541

Scott T: The Antianxiety Food Solution: How the Foods You Eat Can Help You Calm Your Anxious Mind, Improve Your Mood, and End Cravings. Oakland, CA, New Harbinger, 2011

Seguí J, Ramos-Casals M, García-Carrasco M, et al: Psychiatric and psychosocial disorders in patients with systemic lupus erythematosus: a longitudinal study of active and inactive stages of the disease. Lupus 9(8):584–588, 2000 11035432

Seignourel PJ, Kunik ME, Snow L, et al: Anxiety in dementia: a critical review. Clin Psychol Rev 28(7):1071–1082, 2008 18555569

Shapiro SL, Carlson LE, Astin JA, Freedman B: Mechanisms of mindfulness. J Clin Psychol 62(3):373–386, 2006

Simon NM, Blacker D, Korbly NB, et al: Hypothyroidism and hyperthyroidism in anxiety disorders revisited: new data and literature review. J Affect Disord 69(1–3):209–217, 2002 12103468

Smith JP, Randall CL: Anxiety and alcohol use disorders: comorbidity and treatment considerations. Alcohol Res 34(4):414–431, 2012 23584108

Smits JAJ, Berry AC, Rosenfield D, et al: Reducing anxiety sensitivity with exercise. Depress Anxiety 25(8):689–699, 2008 18729145

Solai LK, Mulsant BH, Pollock BG: Selective serotonin reuptake inhibitors for late-life depression: a comparative review. Drugs Aging 18(5):355–368, 2001 11392444

Spitzer RL, Kroenke K, Williams JB, et al: A brief measure for assessing generalized anxiety disorder: the GAD-7. Arch Intern Med 166(10):1092–1097, 2006 16717171

Vernon MK, Reinders S, Mannix S, et al: Psychometric evaluation of the 10-item Short Opiate Withdrawal Scale Gossop (SOWS-Gossop) in patients undergoing opioid detoxification. Addict Behav 60:109–116, 2016 27124502

Vilchinsky N, Ginzburg K, Fait K, Foa EB: Cardiac-disease-induced PTSD (CDI-PTSD): A systematic review. Clin Psychol Rev 55:92–106, 2017 28575815

Wetherell JL, Le Roux H, Gatz M: DSM-IV criteria for generalized anxiety disorder in older adults: distinguishing the worried from the well. Psychol Aging 18:622–627, 2003

Wetherell JL, Petkus AJ, McChesney K, et al: Older adults are less accurate than younger adults at identifying symptoms of anxiety and depression. J Nerv Ment Dis 197(8):623–626, 2009 19684501

Wetherell JL, Stoddard JA, White KS, et al: Augmenting antidepressant medication with modular CBT for geriatric generalized anxiety disorder: a pilot study. Int J Geriatr Psychiatry 26(8):869–875, 2011 20872925

Wetherell JL, Petkus AJ, White KS, et al: Antidepressant medication augmented with cognitive-behavioral therapy for generalized anxiety disorder in older adults. Am J Psychiatry 170(7):782–789, 2013 23680817

Williams N: The GAD-7 questionnaire. Occup Med (Chic Ill) 64(3):224, 2014

Zhang X, Norton J, Carrière I, et al: Risk factors for late-onset generalized anxiety disorder: results from a 12-year prospective cohort (the ESPRIT study). Transl Psychiatry 5:e536, 2015 25826111

Zhou Y, Cao Z, Yang M, et al: Comorbid generalized anxiety disorder and its association with quality of life in patients with major depressive disorder. Sci Rep 7:40511, 2017 28098176

Zigmond AS, Snaith RP: The hospital anxiety and depression scale. Acta Psychiatr Scand 67(6):361–370, 1983 6880820

Somatic Complaints and Anxiety

"I Wish the Doctor Would Figure Out What's Wrong With Me"

Sheila Lahijani, M.D.

CHAPTER 5

Clinical Presentation

Chief Complaint

"I wish the doctor would figure out what's wrong with me."

Vignette

Mr. A is a 72-year-old widowed man who visits with his primary care physician complaining of a headache. He has a history of type 2 diabetes mellitus, chronic renal insufficiency, and hypertension. He denies any associated symptoms of vision problems, fevers, chills, dizziness, lightheadedness, nausea, vomiting, or weight loss. Mr. A relates the onset of his headache as 2 weeks prior to presentation and characterizes the headache as being diffuse and throbbing in sensation. He describes the headache as persisting throughout the day without any identifiable triggers. Mr. A has not hit his head or had any traumatic brain injury. He has not had any recent colds or infections. He admits to some improvement in the headache while lying down and sleeping, taking acetaminophen, or drinking more water. He denies any sick contacts. He denies any deviation from his diet or nonadherence to his medications. His current medications include aspirin, glucophage, insulin, and lisinopril.

Mr. A has a history of headaches that started 2 years before this current episode. During that time his wife of 40 years passed away from cancer. He states he was very worried at the time about her and their children. He remembers feeling nervous each time she had a doctor's appointment and remembers having headaches then, too. The headaches were unrelenting at first and then eventually subsided with minimal interventions. Since then, Mr. A has continued his activities of going to the gym, spending time with his friends, reading, and visiting his children, who live out of state.

Mr. A reports that he had not experienced any further headache until recently, when he developed diffuse pain throughout his head. Mr. A does not use any alcohol, tobacco, or illicit substances. He drinks a cup of black tea every morning. With respect to stressors, he does cite some financial distress and also feeling isolated because he is now living alone. His son moved out of state recently for a new job. Since then, Mr. A. spends more time on his own and notes that he worries more about day-to-day tasks and the future. Mr. A states he has otherwise been in his usual state of health. When asked if he would like to discuss his worries, he initially declines but then becomes tearful. He describes feeling more lonely and isolated and having a harder time living by himself than he had thought he would.

Discussion

Interdisciplinary Team Commentary

Psychologist: Mr. A is resilient and possesses many strengths. He has continued to move forward with his life in spite of the loss of his wife. He knows when to seek medical care when he needs it. However, when it comes to addressing his psychological and emotional health, he has a harder time. I would want to know more about why this is so hard for him and to whom he reaches out to talk about such difficult issues. I am curious how he usually expresses himself and what defenses he employs in doing so. I would want to ask him more about his childhood and developmental history, occupational history, how he spends his time on a daily basis now since he does not work, and how he goes about planning his days. I would want to know more about how he sleeps and his eating habits. I wonder how he thinks about his future and what kinds of things he looks forward to doing. It appears important to him to be present for his children and manage his physical health. I wonder what may help him express himself and what reasons prevent him from doing so.

Psychiatrist: I agree. Perhaps there are reasons in his family life that made it difficult for him to express emotions and seek help, or perhaps that has been how he has managed hard times in the past through his work environment. It may be culturally more appropriate for him to express his distress or worry through somatic symptoms, such as a headache. Also of importance is how his headaches are associated with stress, given his experiences with his wife's illness and recently with his son moving out. Because he also has significant medical problems, the headaches may be associated with higher blood sugar or blood pressure. Maybe this would be a way to frame the importance of stress, anxiety, and headaches for him. He would also benefit from a diagnostic evaluation for anxiety and depression. He would benefit from knowing that these disorders are particularly prevalent in people who have other medical illness, such as diabetes. It may be important to talk with him once the reasoning is given about the use of anxiolytics or antidepressants. Management of the anxiety and somatic symptoms may contribute to better outcomes for his diabetes management as well.

Anxiety

Among older adults, anxiety symptoms and disorders are associated with increased disability, increased risk for cognitive impairment and dementia, worse quality of life, and increased health care utilization. Studies have shown persistence of anxiety over time, significantly increased risk for depression, and high relapse rates. Thus, the public health and personal impact of anxiety in older adults require clinical attention (Porensky et al. 2009). Given the association between anxiety and somatic complaints in older adults, approaching somatic complaints in older adults should involve a thoughtful evaluation of anxiety symptoms with the aim of improving quality of life, preventing disease progression, and reducing health care costs.

Anxiety symptoms are often a normal reaction to the surrounding environment. Anxiety disorders tend to begin in early adulthood and continue throughout a patient's lifetime, with periods of relapses and remissions. Prevalence estimates of anxiety disorders in late age range from 3.2% to 14.2% (Wolitzky-Taylor et al. 2010). Anxiety may increase in older adults as a result of isolation, loss of independence, illness, disability, and bereavement (Edmeads 1997).

An important consideration is whether the clinical manifestations and severity of anxiety change with age. In a review of anxiety in older adults, it was suggested that older adults experience and process emotions differently than younger adults, with older adults having less of a bias toward negative emotion and possibly less autonomic response to strong emotional states (Wolitzky-Taylor et al. 2010). This review also noted that the expressions of symptoms may differ in older adults. The reviewers suggest that certain clusters of symptoms or clinical anxiety-related presentations may be commonly observed among older adults but not delineated in DSM. Older adults may present with subclinical anxiety or symptoms of anxiety that cause distress and/or impairment but do not meet diagnostic criteria for an anxiety disorder.

Diagnosing anxiety in older adults is challenging because anxiety may manifest as somatic symptoms and be associated with several medical comorbidities. A recent cross-sectional multicenter survey (Canuto et al. 2018) using an adapted, age-specific World Health Organization Composite International Diagnostic Interview (WHO CIDI) demonstrated that the prevalence of anxiety disorders in community-dwelling adults ages 65–84 years was 17.2%. Agoraphobia, panic disorder, GAD, and specific phobias emerged as more frequent disorders. Age-related aspects of social context, such as retirement or loss of a partner, and subthreshold expression of anxiety in older adults may impair the sensitivity of assessment tools. Results of the cross-sectional survey suggest that anxiety disorders in older adults may be more prevalent than previously reported, and use of age-specific diagnostic tools is indicated.

There is no clear consensus among researchers and clinicians regarding the available anxiety measures used in older adults. In a systematic review (Therrien and Hunsley 2012), the Beck Anxiety Inventory, Penn State Worry Questionnaire, Geriatric Mental State Examination, Worry Scale, and Geriatric Anxiety Inventory showed psychometric properties and appropriateness for use in older adults. The authors (Therrien and Hunsley 2012) advocated for more research in the development and validation of anxiety measures for older adults given specific challenges, such as comorbid depressive symptoms and the coexistence of somatic symptoms.

Somatic Symptoms

According to Lipowski (1988), *somatization* is defined as a tendency to experience and express somatic distress in response to psychosocial stress and then seek medical attention for it. The concept of somatization comprises three essential components: the experiential, the cognitive, and the behavioral (Table 5–1). Anxiety disorders are commonly associated with somatic complaints, and patients with these disorders can present with chest pain, palpitations, dyspepsia, headache, dizziness, fainting, and dyspnea (Figure 5–1). The following factors can facilitate somatization in anxiety disorders: enhanced awareness of and

TABLE 5–1. **Components and characteristics of somatization**

Somatization component	Description	Examples
Experiential	Bodily perceptions Bodily dysfunctions Changes in appearance Distressing bodily sensations	Pain Dizziness Weakness Fatigue
Cognitive	Interpretation and attribution of perceptions Meaning of perceptions Decision-making perception surrounding the symptoms	I am sick I am unable to work I always will suffer I am not good at "x"
Behavioral	Actions and communications that stem from attributions of perceptions	Isolation Withdrawal Avoiding responsibility

Source. Lipowski 1988.

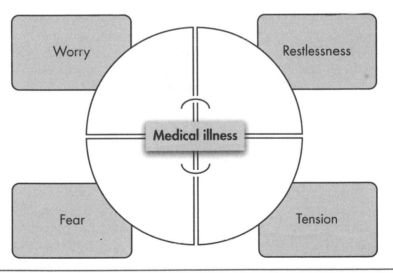

FIGURE 5–1. **Scheme of anxiety, somatic symptoms, and medical illness.**

selective attention to bodily sensations and danger-related information, increased sympathetic nervous system arousal, and a negative bias in appraising the individual's own health (Lipowski 1988).

Evidence suggests that somatization may be underestimated in research and clinical samples of older adults because of the method of diagnosis and the high symptom and disability thresholds required by DSM. Older adults may also experience difficulty in distinguishing somatic symptoms in the setting of medical comorbidities and a tendency to respond to somatic symptoms with a normalizing attribution and adaptation. Psychological distress, including anxiety and depression, may increase somatic symptom distress (Wijeratne 2011).

Somatization may result from a combination of cultural, familial, and personal factors, including biases against the expression of psychological distress (Katon and Walker 1998). Patients may fear being stigmatized by a psychiatric diagnosis, or they may be concerned about the physician's reaction to their nonsomatic complaints (Zajecka 1997). A study of primary care patients found that anxiety disorders were associated with a significantly higher rate of comorbid somatization disorder than that observed in the absence of anxiety disorders (Nisenson et al. 1998).

Consideration of somatization of anxiety in the primary care setting may help to identify patients who have an anxiety disorder. It has been estimated that as many as 53% of patients with symptoms that meet the criteria for a psychiatric disorder may receive an incorrect diagnosis in this setting (Ormel et al. 1991). Medical providers may therefore inappropriately attribute a patient's somatic symptom to an underlying medical disorder. Alternatively, when there is no evidence of a medical etiology, providers might not pursue any evaluation or treatment of a psychiatric cause.

The benefits of referring a patient to a mental health provider are multifold. Before doing so, however, the framing of the referral is key. Primary care providers may suggest such a consultation as a way of providing an expert evaluation of a patient's somatic complaints; this can foster the reassurance to the patient that his or her concerns are considered seriously and do warrant more of an assessment. The primary care provider also may feel more supported collaborating with a mental health provider who can elicit additional history and integrate those elements in the impression and recommendations. Furthermore, patients with high medical use, such as those who have both medical and psychiatric problems, benefit from the collaboration between their primary care provider and a psychiatric provider (Katon et al. 2007).

In addition to the presence of unexplained somatic complaints and the high rate of psychiatric comorbidities, anxiety itself may be a factor in provoking or maintaining medical conditions or diseases. Anxiety, without an intervention, may prolong or worsen a medical illness. Moreover, both anxiety and somatization can contribute to high health care costs and high health care utilization (Gelenberg 2000). Prompt recognition of anxiety presenting as a somatic complaint not only can ease patients' suffering but also can improve health care systems and reduce costs.

Cultural Issues

Understanding the relationship between somatic complaints and anxiety should take cultural contexts into account. Culture has effects on neural systems, psychological presentations, and interactional patterns throughout the lifespan. Culture influences the sources of distress, the illness experience, the interpretation of symptoms, mechanisms of coping, help seeking, and the social response to such distress. Clusters of symptoms may reflect the interactions of bodily processes and cognitive schemata based on ethnic beliefs. Furthermore, disturbances of mood in many cultures may be viewed less as psychological problems and more as social or moral problems (Kirmayer 2001).

The clinical presentation of anxiety is a function not only of a patient's cultural background but also of the health care system the patient finds himself or herself in and the diagnostic criteria used by providers. In a review of the literature, discordance was found between DSM criteria and local phenomenology of anxiety disorders in specific cultural contexts, particularly in panic disorder, social anxiety disorder, and GAD (Lewis-Fernández et al. 2010).

In a multicenter primary care study (Piccinelli and Simon 1997), the General Health Questionnaire and the CIDI—Primary Health Care Version were used to assess gender and cross-cultural differences in the association between somatic symptoms and emotional distress in subjects ages 15–65. The study concluded that there are no gender differences and that somatic symptoms and emotional distress are strongly associated in primary care patients.

In an effort to improve diagnosis and care to people of all backgrounds, DSM-5 (American Psychiatric Association 2013) incorporates criteria to reflect cross-cultural variations in presentations, provides more detailed and structured information about cultural concepts of distress, and includes a clinical interview tool to facilitate comprehensive assessments.

Treatment Strategies

Each presentation of a somatic complaint warrants a thorough evaluation of the etiology of symptoms and the relationship between the physical complaints and objective evaluation of those complaints. This may be challenging when there are medical comorbidities, particularly in the case of older adults. Valid and reliable diagnoses of somatic symptom disorders can be made based on comprehensive clinical evaluations, including interviews, physical examination, biomarkers, and careful evaluation of medical records (Schneider et al. 2003).

Validated instruments, such as the General Health Questionnaire (Kroenke et al. 2010) and the CIDI (Simms et al. 2012), may be used in the primary care setting to elicit somatic complaints and emotional distress. Additionally, the Patient Health Questionnaire–9 (PHQ-9) and PHQ-15 (Kroenke et al. 2010), as well as the GAD-7 scale (Spitzer et al. 2006), are brief, well-validated measures for detecting and monitoring depression, anxiety, and somatization. There are other scales that may be used in screening patients with somatic symptoms, mood symptoms, and health anxiety; these include the Whiteley 7 Index (Fink et al. 1999; Speckens et al. 1996), Health Anxiety Inventory (Salkovskis et al. 2002), Illness Attitude Scale and Somatosensory Amplification Scale (Speckens et al. 1996), and the somatization dimension of the Symptom Checklist–90—Revised and the Brief Symptom Inventory (Derogatis and Savitz 2000).

A "graduated care approach" suggested by Lenze et al. (2005) includes four major steps that proceed from history taking to initial recommendations and follow-up, to modification of treatment with persistence of somatic symptoms, and implementation of additional treatment such as psychotherapy, exercise, and complementary medicine. This approach places emphasis on taking a careful history to elucidate any medical basis for the somatic symptoms and thereafter pursuing a collaborative approach with the patient's primary care doctor to offer psychopharmacological and nonpsychopharmacological interventions as indicated.

Among the psychosocial treatments that may be tried are cognitive-behavioral therapy, supportive therapy, acceptance-based and mindfulness-based interventions, and relaxation training. Practical tips for talking with older adults about somatic symptoms and anxiety are presented in Table 5–2.

TABLE 5–2. **Tips on talking to older adults with somatic symptoms of anxiety**

Start off with a validating statement.	"It seems like this headache is really distressing to you."
Express a curiosity about how to handle it.	"I wonder how we can help you feel more comfortable right now."
Frame the intervention in an accommodating way.	"Treating both your headache and the distress it is causing you seems like the next best step."
Use sequential words to indicate a future plan.	"For right now, we can help you feel better, and then we can continue figuring out what's causing this."
Identify the intervention and define it skillfully.	"I am going to offer you a medicine to help calm your nerves and improve how you feel day to day."
Link the intervention with an additional corresponding plan for the present time.	"I think you may also benefit from talking to my colleague, who can support you further right now." "We know that physical activity can help treat pain and also the emotional discomfort caused by the pain."
Suggest a daily plan until the next appointment.	"I would like for you to create a schedule for yourself and arrange an appointment with me in 2 weeks." "It is very important for you to get regular, consistent sleep each night."
Specify the goal of the next visit.	"We will then assess how you are feeling and what further evaluation is needed then."

First-line medications for anxiety in older adults include the selective serotonin reuptake inhibitors and the serotonin-norepinephrine reuptake inhibitors. Clinical trials have demonstrated benefits with citalopram, escitalopram, paroxetine, sertraline, venlafaxine, and duloxetine. Although these medications are generally well tolerated among older adults, increased attention should be given to adverse effects in older adults, such as gait impairment and nongastrointestinal and gastrointestinal bleeding, relative to younger adults (Ramos and Stanley 2018).

Vignette *(continued)*

Mr. A is offered support by his primary care doctor and administered a GAD-7. Mr. A scores a 17. Mr. A is encouraged to consider a number of options at this time. He is advised to keep a headache log to identify what the triggers are, what helps, and what worsens his symptom. He is also encouraged to keep a sleep log while also monitoring his dietary intake and blood sugars.

Duloxetine is discussed as a medication that potentially can manage the pain caused by the headache and additionally help him feel less anxious. The medication is started using the controlled-release formulation at 20 mg daily as his creatinine clearance is monitored. Mr. A is also offered a referral to physical therapy to help him with physical reconditioning. In addition, his doctor refers him to the social worker in the clinic to help Mr. A identify community resources to increase his socialization.

Mr. A returns in 1 month endorsing an abatement of his headache after having had one other significant incident in the interim time. He shares his headache log and sleep log with his doctor. He describes feeling better physically and also admits he has made a few friends at a local community center. Mr. A talks about feeling less isolated and not experiencing as many worries for the future.

KEY POINTS

- Older adults may experience somatic distress in response to a psychosocial stressor.
- Anxiety in older adults may be secondary to isolation, loss of independence, illness, disability, and grief.
- Evaluating older adults' somatic symptoms using the biopsychosocial framework may reveal rich historical information.
- Framing interventions in a validating and future-oriented way can strengthen the therapeutic alliance and provide further reassurance to the older adult with anxiety.

Resources

Online Resources

American Association for Geriatric Psychiatry: www.aagponline.org

Anxiety and Depression Association of America: https://adaa.org/living-with-anxiety/older-adults

Mental Health America: www.mentalhealthamerica.net/anxiety-older-adults

Scales

Beck Anxiety Inventory (Beck and Steer 1993)
Brief Symptom Inventory (Derogatis and Savitz 2000)
Geriatric Mental State Examination (Copeland et al. 2002)
Health Anxiety Inventory (Salkovskis et al. 2002)
Illness Attitude Scale (Speckens et al. 1996)
Penn State Worry Questionnaire (Meyer et al. 1990)
Somatization Symptom Checklist–90–Revised (Derogatis and Savitz 2000)
Somatosensory Amplification Scale (Speckens et al. 1996)
Whiteley 7 Index (Fink et al. 1999; Speckens et al. 1996)
Worry Scale (Wisocki et al. 1986) and Geriatric Anxiety Inventory (Pachana et al. 2007)

Publications to Recommend to Patients

Craske MG, Barlow DH: Mastering Your Anxiety and Worry. New York, Oxford University Press, 2006
D'Arrigo T: Finesse required to treat anxiety in the elderly. ACP Internist: Mental Health (website), January 2013. Available at: American College of Physicians (ACP) Internist: https://acpinternist.org/archives/2013/01/elderly.htm
Friedman MB, Furst L, Gellis ZD, et al: Anxiety disorders in older adults. Social Work Today 13(4):10, 2013. Available at: http://www.socialworktoday.com/archive/070813p10.shtml.
Greenstein M, Holland J: Lighter As We Go: Virtues, Character Strengths, and Aging. New York, Oxford University Press, 2014
Kabat-Zinn J: Full Catastrophe Living. New York, Delacorte Press, 1990
Martins C: Mindfulness-Based Interventions for Older Adults: Evidence for Practice. London, Jessica Kingsley, 2014
Richmond L: Aging as a Spiritual Practice. New York, Avery, 2012
Yalom I: Staring at the Sun: Overcoming the Terror of Death. San Francisco, CA, Jossey-Bass, 2009

References

American Psychiatric Association: Diagnostic and Statistical Manual of Mental Disorders, 5th Edition. Arlington, VA, American Psychiatric Association, 2013
Beck AT, Steer RA: Beck Anxiety Inventory Manual. San Antonio, TX, Psychological Corporation, 1993
Canuto A, Weber K, Baertschi M, et al: Anxiety disorders in old age: psychiatric comorbidities, quality of life, and prevalence according to age, gender, and country. Am J Geriatr Psychiatry 26(2):174–185, 2018 29031568

Copeland JR, Prince M, Wilson KC, et al: The geriatric mental state examination in the 21st century. Int J Geriatr Psychiatry 17(8):729–732, 2002

Derogatis LR, Savitz KL: The SCL-90-R and Brief Symptom Inventory (BSI) in primary care, in Handbook of Psychological Assessment in Primary Care Settings. Edited by Maruish ME. Mahwah, NJ, Lawrence Erlbaum, 2000, pp 297–334

Edmeads J: Headaches in older people: How are they different in this age-group? Postgraduate Med 101(5):91–94, 98–100, 1997

Fink P, Ewald H, Jensen J, et al: Screening for somatization and hypochondriasis in primary care and neurological in-patients: a seven-item scale for hypochondriasis and somatization. J Psychosom Res 46(3):261–273, 1999 10193917

Gelenberg AJ: Psychiatric and somatic markers of anxiety: identification and pharmacologic treatment. Prim Care Companion J Clin Psychiatry 2(2):49–54, 2000 15014583

Katon WJ, Walker EA: Medically unexplained symptoms in primary care. J Clin Psychiatry 59 (suppl 20):15–21, 1998 9881537

Katon W, Lin EH, Kroenke K: The association of depression and anxiety with medical symptom burden in patients with chronic medical illness. Gen Hosp Psychiatry 29(2):147–155, 2007 17336664

Kirmayer LJ: Cultural variations in the clinical presentation of depression and anxiety: implications for diagnosis and treatment. J Clin Psychiatry 62 (suppl 13):22–28, discussion 29–30, 2001 11434415

Kroenke K, Spitzer RL, Williams JB, et al: The Patient Health Questionnaire somatic, anxiety, and depressive symptom scales: a systematic review. Gen Hosp Psychiatry 32(4):345–359, 2010 20633738

Lenze EJ, Karp JF, Mulsant BH, et al: Somatic symptoms in late-life anxiety: treatment issues. J Geriatr Psychiatry Neurol 18(2):89–96, 2005 15911937

Lewis-Fernández R, Hinton DE, Laria AJ, et al: Culture and the anxiety disorders: recommendations for DSM-V. Depress Anxiety 27(2):212–229, 2010 20037918

Lipowski ZJ: Somatization: the concept and its clinical application. Am J Psychiatry 145(11):1358–1368, 1988 3056044

Meyer TJ, Miller ML, Metzger RL, Borkovec TD: Development and validation of the Penn State Worry Questionnaire. Behav Res Ther 28(6):487–495, 1990 2076086

Nisenson LG, Pepper CM, Schwenk TL, et al: The nature and prevalence of anxiety disorders in primary care. Gen Hosp Psychiatry 20(1):21–28, 1998 9506251

Ormel J, Koeter MWJ, van den Brink W, et al: Recognition, management, and course of anxiety and depression in general practice. Arch Gen Psychiatry 48(8):700–706, 1991 1883252

Pachana NA, Byrne GJ, Siddle H, et al: Development and validation of the Geriatric Anxiety Inventory. Int Psychogeriatr 19(1):103–114, 2007

Piccinelli M, Simon G: Gender and cross-cultural differences in somatic symptoms associated with emotional distress. An international study in primary care. Psychol Med 27(2):433–444, 1997 9089835

Porensky EK, Dew MA, Karp JF, et al: The burden of late-life generalized anxiety disorder: effects on disability, health-related quality of life, and health-care utilization. Am J Geriatr Psychiatry 17(6):473–482, 2009 19472438

Ramos K, Stanley MA: Anxiety Disorders in Late Life. Psychiatr Clin North Am 41(1):55–64, 2018 29412848

Salkovskis PM, Rimes KA, Warwick HMC, et al: The Health Anxiety Inventory: development and validation of scales for the measurement of health anxiety and hypochondriasis. Psychol Med 32(5):843–853, 2002 12171378

Schneider G, Wachter M, Driesch G, et al: Subjective body complaints as an indicator of somatization in elderly patients. Psychosomatics 44(2):91–99, 2003 12618530

Simms LJ, Prisciandaro JJ, Krueger RF, Goldberg DP: The structure of depression, anxiety and somatic symptoms in primary care. Psychol Med 42(1):15–28, 2012

Speckens AE, Spinhoven P, Sloekers PP, et al: A validation study of the Whitely Index, the Illness Attitude Scales, and the Somatosensory Amplification Scale in general medical and general practice patients. J Psychosom Res 40(1):95–104, 1996 8730649

Spitzer RL, Kroenke K, Williams JB, et al: A brief measure for assessing generalized anxiety disorder: the GAD-7. Arch Intern Med 166(10):1092–1097, 2006 16717171

Therrien Z, Hunsley J: Assessment of anxiety in older adults: a systematic review of commonly used measures. Aging Ment Health 16(1):1–16, 2012 21838650

Wijeratne C. Somatization in older people. Psychiatr Clin North Am 34(3):661–671, 2011 21889685

Wisocki PA, Handen B, Morse CK: The Worry Scale as a measure of anxiety among homebound and community active elderly. Behavior Therapist 5:91–95, 1986

Wolitzky-Taylor KB, Castriotta N, Lenze EJ, et al: Anxiety disorders in older adults: a comprehensive review. Depress Anxiety 27(2):190–211, 2010 20099273

Zajecka J: Importance of establishing the diagnosis of persistent anxiety. J Clin Psychiatry 58 (suppl 3):9–13, discussion 14–15, 1997 9133488

Pain and Psychological Factors

"I Need More Pain Medication, Not Less!"

Beth D. Darnall, Ph.D.

CHAPTER 6

Clinical Presentation

Chief Complaint

"I need more pain medication, not less!"

Vignette

Ms. L is 71-year-old woman who lives alone. Her daughter be-came concerned when she was finding that her mother was slur-ring her words during their monthly phone calls. Ms. L has been taking Vicodin for the past year. Her doctor prescribed the pain medication after she fell and injured her hip. As an aside, Ms. L has had chronic low back pain for many years, but she has never sought treatment for it. Ms. L finds that the Vicodin takes the edge off her pain, and she also finds it helps her think less about the death of her husband, which happened 2 years ago. Her daughter is concerned and brings Ms. L in for an evaluation. You learn that Ms. L has been drinking two generous-sized martinis nightly for the past few years. She is largely sedentary. Her sleep is poor; she tosses and turns, awakens in pain, and ruminates on it. At some point in the early morning, she is able to fall back asleep, but she then must remain in bed until almost noon because of exhaustion.

Ms. L rarely leaves her home anymore. She feels comforted being in bed and prefers to just watch television or read. When she moves she hurts and the pain scares her, so she has avoided most of her regular activities since she fell. In fact, the fall itself had a tremendous impact on her. She was alone when she fell and found she could not to get up. She cried out for help, but no one was there to help her, and her neighbors could not hear her. Eventually she was able to crawl to a phone and call for help. Since then she has felt extremely vulnerable. She worries about falling again and imagines how awful that would be. Somehow, being in pain reminds her that she is all alone. She feels anxious a lot and finds that taking her pain medication helps lessen her anxiety, and so does her nightly martini or two. Her primary care doctor is dismayed that a year has passed and there is no real progress with her hip pain or her life. Her hip imaging is negative. She encouraged Ms. L to begin moving more and maybe join a gentle yoga class at the senior center. Ms. L says she will be happy to move more once her pain is better controlled. Ms. L believes that the solution is for her doctor to give her more pain medication, not less.

Discussion

Pain and Psychological Factors

Pain is a highly individual experience. Two people can experience the same stimulus or injury, and one may recover while the other goes on to develop severe, life-altering chronic pain. In aggregate, while the vast majority of pain has a medical basis, psychological and behavioral factors are key determinants for the development of chronic pain and its trajectory (Table 6–1).

Ms. L has chronic pain, and she is noted to have several risk factors that associate strongly with chronic pain and place her at risk for poor outcomes. She is known to have experienced physical and psychological trauma after she fell and was injured, and she potentially was also traumatized after her husband's death. Her workup should include assessment for the following symptoms and differential diagnoses.

Chronic Pain: Differential Diagnosis

Major depression (or complicated grief).   Major depression frequently co-occurs with chronic pain. Depression can impede engagement in treatment, activation, and the behavioral change that is essential for recovery from chronic pain. Multiple factors common to pain and depres-

TABLE 6–1. Factors associated with chronic pain

History of psychological trauma	Substance use disorder
History of abuse	Sleep disorder
Pain-related anxiety/fear of pain/ pain catastrophizing	Age
	Race
Lower socioeconomic status	Poor nutritional status
Female sex	Sedentary or low activity levels
Smoking	Mental disorders (depression, anxiety, posttraumatic stress disorder)
Anger	Perceptions of injustice

sion can serve to maintain lack of exercise, social isolation, feelings of helplessness, loss of identity, and a sense of worthlessness, as the quality of the patient's life deteriorates within the context of pain. A lower threshold for addressing depressive symptoms should be considered in individuals who have chronic pain, simply because the effects of those depressive symptoms have a negative impact on pain. Evidence based treatment may include cognitive-behavioral therapy (CBT) for pain or a variant of CBT, acceptance and commitment therapy. When possible, the patient should be referred to pain-related CBT versus general CBT unless the primary presenting condition is preexisting organic major depression. Good screening tools for level of depressive symptoms include the Center for Epidemiologic Studies Depression Scale, the Patient Health Questionnaire–9, and PROMIS Depression (Amtmann et al. 2014; Helmes and Nielson 1998). In Ms. L's case, in addition to screening for depression, she should be assessed for extended bereavement or complicated grief related to her husband's death (see Chapter 24, "Practical Strategies for Approaching Grief"). If either is present, the clinician should consider referral to a grief specialist. Finally, it is common for individuals with chronic pain to report some cognitive effects, such as poor memory, slowed cognition, or a sense of mental "fogginess"; these could be attributable to the distracting effects of pain itself, to co-occurring depression, to sleep disturbance and related fatigue, or to medication side effects.

Posttraumatic stress disorder or other specified or unspecified anxiety disorder. If the patient discloses a history of trauma or if the treatment team suspects it, the clinician should consider administering the Posttraumatic Stress Disorder Checklist–Civilian (Weathers et al. 1994). Additionally, if the patient endorses anxiety or panic attacks, psychological treatment is warranted. Posttraumatic stress disorder (PTSD) and chronic pain are mutually maintaining, and it is difficult to reduce pain when PTSD is untreated (Sharp and Harvey 2001). Similarly, anxiety disorders represent difficulties in the ability to self-regulate, which is an essential skill for pain management. Ms. L was demonstrating symptoms of anxiety related to her fall that require further workup to determine their severity and a proper treatment plan.

Sleep disturbance.   Poor sleep is a major contributor to next-day pain and fatigue. There is a bidirectional relationship between pain and sleep disturbance. However, contrary to what is commonly believed, sleep disturbance has a greater impact on pain intensity than pain does on sleep, thereby underscoring the importance of treating any medical and behavioral sleep issues. Improvements in pain are often experienced once sleep problems have been effectively addressed.

While it is clear that Ms. L has sleep disturbance, it is unclear whether she has an underlying medical condition contributing to or maintaining the problem. The clinician may consider referral to a sleep medicine specialist to rule out an obstructive or central sleep apnea. Ms. L is at increased risk for sleep apnea because she is taking opioids (Dimsdale et al. 2007; Guilleminault et al. 2010). This condition can resolve when the opioids are discontinued (Davis et al. 2012). Ms. L is also drinking alcohol at night, and alcohol metabolizes into a stimulant, thereby contributing to nighttime awakening and disrupted sleep (Thakkar et al. 2015). Alcohol cessation is indicated, particularly given that she should not consume alcohol when taking opioids. Alcohol and opioids are both central nervous system depressants, thereby placing her at risk for accidental overdose and death.

Finally, Ms. L should be evaluated for general sleep hygiene. It is unclear whether she is engaging in behaviors that are serving to maintain and worsen her sleep problems, such as watching television late at night or eating late. Her sedentary habits and sleep patterns are contributing factors that should be assessed and addressed, likely with a health or pain psychologist. Finally, her reported nighttime rumination on pain suggests that she is probably engaging in pain catastrophizing (discussed in a later subsection) and can certainly benefit from acquiring self-regulatory skills that will help her calm her nervous system and disengage from negative thought patterns that serve to amplify the experience of pain. Ms. L may be an excellent candidate for CBT for insomnia (see Chapter 8, "Evaluation and Management of Insomnia").

Alcohol use disorder.   Ms. L should be evaluated for alcohol use disorder. For instance, was her fall related to her alcohol use? Any negative impacts related to alcohol use should be fully assessed. Most likely her prescribing physician cautioned her against consuming alcohol in combination with opioids. As such, she may be violating an opioid agreement that was likely established with her doctor at the outset of her opioid prescription, or at a minimum, she may be knowingly placing herself at risk. The clinician should consider referring Ms. L to a substance disorder specialist or addictionologist for full evaluation. At a minimum, the risks of combining alcohol and opioids should be reviewed with her.

Opioid use disorder.   Ms. L should be evaluated for potential opioid use disorder. Her alcohol use is one red flag. Is she taking her medications as prescribed? The clinician should assess whether she has prescriptions from more than one prescriber, has lost prescriptions in the past, has reported medications stolen, has engaged in doctor shopping for opioids, or has visited an emergency department for opioid medication. The state prescription drug monitoring database is an excellent resource to help identify individuals with opioid use disorder so they may be referred to an addictionologist and harm reduction strategies can be implemented.

Additional Factors to Consider

Deconditioning.   Deconditioning is a common consequence of fear avoidance behaviors. Ms. L is exhibiting fear avoidance by minimizing movement and activity out of fear her pain will worsen; she is also in bed much of the day and sedentary. Over time, deconditioning results, and this muscular atrophy and weakness places patients at risk for worsening existing pain as well as for developing new pain problems. Deconditioning is often created and maintained by psychological factors, such as fear avoidance, anxiety, or depression. Barriers to movement and exercise should be assessed, and referral to a pain psychologist or skilled chronic pain physical therapist can elucidate psychobehavioral barriers and help the team develop a plan for rehabilitation.

Social network/social isolation.   Social isolation is a predictor for pain and depression. Older adults who are socially isolated may have a more difficult time with self-care related to pain and health. Lack of social support may contribute to increased utilization of medical care (Sterling et al. 2018). Patients with chronic pain should be assessed for frequency of social contact and social support. Older adults may be encouraged to join a free chronic pain support group (the American Chronic Pain Association website has helpful information; see "Resources" later in this chapter), local senior center classes, church or other spiritual services, or warm water senior aqua therapy through the Arthritis Foundation. Clinicians who work within a larger organization may connect the individual with social services or a geropsychologist who can better determine needs, any barriers (e.g., travel), and local options.

Thinking Beyond Diagnoses: Reducing Pain and Suffering

Chronic pain erodes the health and quality of life for up to one-third of the U.S. population (Institute of Medicine Committee on Advancing Pain Research, Care, and Education 2011) and is a source of untold suffering for patients, their families, and caregivers. The incidence of chronic pain is greater than the incidence rates for heart disease, cancer, and diabetes combined. To one degree or another, the high prevalence of pain in older adulthood is due to a convergence of factors—for example, increasing longevity (more years spent in older adulthood), the obesity epidemic, reduced activity, and emergence of painful age-related health conditions such as osteoarthritis, degenerative bone disease, and back pain, just to name a few. In Ms. L's case, she had a history of back pain before her fall, and a multitude of psychological factors that have 1) increased her pain and pain-related distress and 2) shaped maladaptive behaviors that have promoted the persistence of pain. It is likely that Ms. L is not aware of her contribution to her pain and suffering. Like most people with chronic pain, Ms. L has never been given accurate information to understand how she could help herself suffer less, function better, and live a higher-quality life.

Potent psychological predictors for pain and outcomes may be independent of a psychiatric diagnosis. Such factors include pain catastrophizing, pain-related anxiety, and kinesiophobia (fear of movement). By measuring these factors, you can help steer your patients to appropriate treatment.

Pain catastrophizing.   Pain catastrophizing is a pattern of negative cognitive and emotional responses to pain and includes rumination on pain, magnification of pain, and feelings of helplessness about pain. Often there is a focus or rumination on a worst case scenario: "What happens if my pain gets worse?" or "What if something is seriously wrong with me?" Pain catastrophizing is most commonly measured with the Pain Catastrophizing Scale (PCS; Sullivan et al. 1995). Pain catastrophizing is associated with greater pain, cortical changes that reinforce pain, and poor response to medical treatments. Patients with chronic pain can be administered the 13-item self-report PCS in the office.

Information on how to score the PCS is available online (see "Resources" near the end of this chapter). Patients scoring above 15 are demonstrating room for improvement and treatment needs. If a pain psychologist is not available for local individual treatment, several of the recommended patient self-help books address pain catastrophizing, and the Darnall books focus on treatment approaches for catastrophizing (see "Resources"). Although pain catastrophizing is a scientific term, it is losing clinical utility due its stigma and patients feeling blamed for their pain. Gentler terms may be used to describe the phenomenon of pain catastrophizing with patients, such as "negative pain mindset" or "negative pain appraisal." Use of patient-friendly terminology may increase patient receptivity and engagement in treatment. While Ms. L needs a full workup for catastrophizing, her vignette suggests that nighttime pain catastrophizing is contributing to sleep interference, greater pain, and, in all likelihood, greater daytime fatigue and poor sleep habits.

Kinesiophobia. *Kinesiophobia,* or fear of movement, impedes functional restoration and recovery from pain. Skilled chronic pain physical therapists can work with patients to dually address the behavioral and psychological aspects of kinesiophobia in session. Treatment goals include helping patients to 1) slowly begin moving; 2) gain strength; 3) challenge their fear of movement and pain; 4) extinguish avoidance behaviors; 5) understand that movement is vital to recovery of function; 6) increase confidence that they can become more active and therefore begin to overcome pain-related interference and disability; and 7) become actively engaged in their pain self-management plan.

Addressing pain-specific psychological factors is crucial for helping patients develop pain self-efficacy—that is, the confidence that they can engage in activities *in spite of* their pain. Persistent kinesiophobia—such as Ms. L's—warrants referral to a specialty pain clinic for interdisciplinary evaluation and treatment.

Pain and Opioids

Up to 75% of adults age 65 years and older report living with persistent pain. The majority describe their pain as moderate, and about one-quarter report having severe pain. Older adults are more likely to have additional health problems that can cause or complicate chronic pain. Older adults are also more likely to have mobility and balance issues, both of which may impact their ability to engage in daily therapeutic exercise.

Opioids are one of the most commonly used treatments for chronic pain. Indeed, opioids are so commonly used that sales of prescription opioids quadrupled between 1999 and 2014 despite little evidence to show they are effective for chronic pain (Sun et al. 2016). In 2014, 5.4% of the entire U.S. population (17.8 million people) was prescribed long-term opioids (Mojtabai 2018).

One population-based study showed that across age groups, the prevalence of opioid prescriptions among women has been increasing at a rate similar to or greater than that among men, with as many as 8%–9% of women age 65 and older receiving long-term opioid therapy (Campbell et al. 2010). Despite the increasing rate of opioid prescription in women, the specific risks and consequences of opioids in women have not been reviewed comprehensively. In more recent years, the bulk of research on prescription opioids has focused on outcomes related to pain reduction and the associated risks of medication misuse or abuse, with less attention paid to the medical and psychological risks conferred by opioid therapy or to the specific risks in women (Darnall and Stacey 2012; Darnall et al. 2012).

While averages suggest little benefit of long-term opioid use, it is important to note that many patients do benefit from opioid therapy, and indeed rely on it to function every day. Opioids have a role in chronic pain care for some older adults. In fact, recent restrictions in opioid prescribing have led to another problem: patients being unable to access the opioid medications they need. Patients taking long-term opioids should not have opioids abruptly stopped because doing so can lead to patient distress, withdrawal symptoms, mood deterioration, and suicidal ideation and attempt in patients with major depression (Darnall et al. 2019; U.S. Food and Drug Administration et al. 2019). New research suggests that opioid dose changes—whether increasing or decreasing the dose—should be approached with caution because these changes confer risk for unintentional opioid overdose (Glanz et al. 2019). As such, it is important to be mindful of the risks and consequences of long-term opioid use, dose changes, and tapering (Table 6–2). As with all medications, the benefits should outweigh the risks. Risks and consequences of long-term opioid use include various side effects and polypharmacy (Figure 6–1). The goal is to treat pain comprehensively so that opioid use may be obviated or, when beneficial, minimized.

The Trap

Like most people, Ms. L is caught in the trap of the biomedical treatment model. She believes pain is purely a sensory experience that

TABLE 6–2. Opioid risks to consider

Injury and fracture risks exist for older adults taking opioids (Buckeridge et al. 2010; Miller et al. 2011; Saunders et al. 2010).

New-onset depression is noted after initiation of opioids (Salas et al. 2017; Scherrer et al. 2017).

Medical complexity and polypharmacy can result after opioid prescription due to multiple side effects (see Figure 6–1).

Disrupted sleep architecture (Dimsdale et al. 2007) and apnea (Guilleminault et al. 2010) are formidable opioid risks, with downstream effects contributing to daytime fatigue and depressed mood.

In older adults, benzodiazepine and opioid coprescription carries extreme risks for injury (Buckeridge et al. 2010), overdose, and unintentional death (Sun et al. 2017).

Prolonged opioid use after surgery is associated with psychological factors, such as pain catastrophizing (Khan et al. 2011, 2012; Pavlin et al. 2005) and depression (Sun et al. 2016).

Opioid misuse and opioid use disorder are negatively associated with age in older adults (Papaleontiou et al. 2010).

Opioid use is associated with poorer mental health functioning in older adults (Papaleontiou et al. 2010).

Abrupt opioid cessation is to be avoided (U.S. Food and Drug Administration et al. 2019). Particular caution should be used when involuntarily tapering long-term opioids in individuals with major depression because suicidal ideation and suicide are risks.

For patients taking long-term opioids, opioid dose increases or decreases in excess of 25 morphine equivalent daily doses are associated with unintentional opioid overdose. New research suggests that opioid dose changes—whether increasing or decreasing the dose—should be approached with caution because these changes confer risk for unintentional opioid overdose (Glanz et al. 2019).

should be fixed with a pill. She also believes that she should be pain-free and that if she has pain it is just a sign that she is not getting enough medication. None of this is true.

The Solution

The International Association for the Study of Pain defines *pain* as a negative sensory and emotional experience. Psychology is integral to the definition of pain, although pain is rarely treated as such. Patients

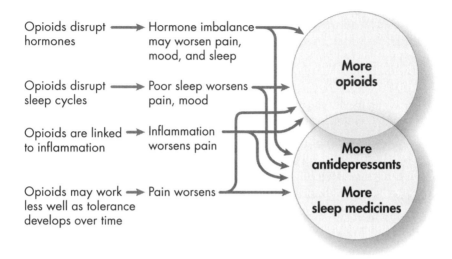

FIGURE 6–1. Opioid-related polypharmacy: how opioids can lead to more pain and more medications.

Source. Reprinted from Darnall B: Less Pain, Fewer Pills: Avoid the Dangers of Prescription Opioids and Gain Control Over Chronic Pain. Boulder, CO, Bull Publishing, 2014. Copyright © 2014 Beth Darnall. Used with permission.

receive suboptimal care and have suboptimal pain treatment outcomes when psychological factors are not addressed; Ms. L is a prime example. Untreated psychological factors undermine the effectiveness of pain treatments, including opioids or surgery (Abbott et al. 2011; Roh et al. 2014; Wertli et al. 2013). The first step is to recognize the profound influence that psychological factors have on the experience of physical sensation and the ongoing experience of pain (Figure 6–2).

Next, addressing psychological aspects of pain requires a comprehensive assessment, pain education, an integrative treatment approach, and focus on opioid-sparing strategies. Ultimately, treatment should emphasize self-management approaches that empower patients to engage in their own pain and symptom management. At each follow-up visit, the clinician should maintain consistent messaging and emphasize positive patient actions that serve to increase function and reduce pain and suffering.

Figure 6–3 illustrates how psychological and behavioral factors interact with physical and biological factors to maintain and amplify pain (i.e., the pain cycle). The psychobehavioral factors that are relevant to Ms. L include avoidance and disability, deconditioning, pain cognitive processes (dread and rumination), and depression and anxiety. Each

Pain Is Complex

Context

Meaning

Cognition

Emotion

Affect

Mood

Attention

Social factors

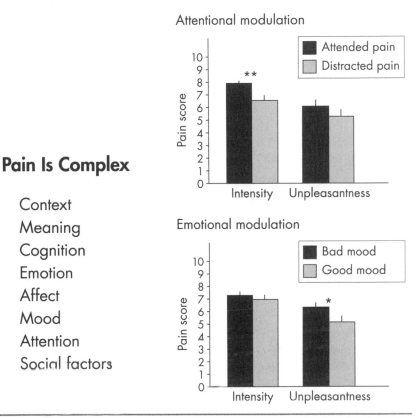

FIGURE 6–2. Complexity of pain and psychological modulation.

Source. Adapted with permission from Springer Nature: Bushnell MC, Ceko M, Low LA: Cognitive and emotional control of pain and its disruption in chronic pain. *Nature Reviews Neuroscience* 14(7):502–511, 2013. Copyright © 2013.

factor is an important therapeutic target that if effectively treated could reduce Ms. L's pain and suffering.

Treating Pain Better

Approaches to Minimizing Pain Interference, Loss of Physical Function, and Disability

Pain is a "harm alarm" that alerts individuals to danger or threats to survival. It works very well in acute situations because it motivates people to escape the pain and therefore the danger. Over time, pain loses its protective value as a harm alarm. Once chronic, pain becomes a dis-

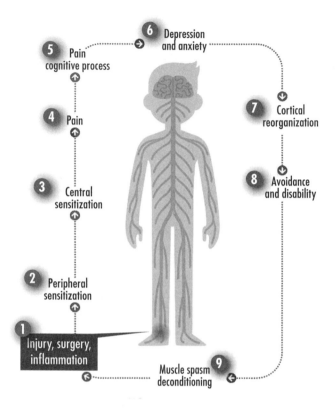

FIGURE 6–3. The cycle of pain.

Multiple peripheral, central, and behavioral factors modulate pain and contribute to its persistence.

Source. Image © 2016 Ming-Chih Koo, Ph.D. Used with permission.

tressing "false alarm" because there is no threat that the person can escape. Learning to calm this distressing false alarm is a critical aspect of psychological pain management.

All pain is processed in the nervous system, the brain, and the spinal cord. For this reason, psychological skills and techniques are particularly effective for reducing pain and distress. Importantly, when pain management skills are used regularly, patients gain self-efficacy in their ability to modulate their own pain and distress. Pain management skills can provide patients with a critical level of control over their experience; this serves to counteract feelings of helplessness that contribute to despair and depression. Patients can begin focusing on what they *can* do to help themselves.

Often individuals will say that the worst part of chronic pain is how the pain has interfered with their lives and robbed them of being able to engage with the things they love in life. Indeed, ongoing pain can cause people to become less active in an attempt to gain relief (so-called fear avoidance behavior). Fear avoidance behavior can lead people to do fewer activities that are enjoyable and meaningful to them. Participation in recreational and social activities may dwindle, and the patient can easily become socially withdrawn and isolated. As the patient's world becomes smaller and smaller, the pain and despair grow and may become the primary foci of his or her life. It is important to address fear avoidance behavior because it leads to greater disability. Doing less and less leads to depressive symptoms, deconditioning, and—paradoxically—greater pain over time. A major aspect of effective treatment for chronic pain involves encouraging clients to move beyond their fear of pain and to move forward again—*at an appropriate pace*—toward the goals that are meaningful to them and important for their health.

Table 6–3 provides tips for assessing psychological factors in older adults with pain. Table 6–4 provides tips on when to refer to a pain psychology specialist. Table 6–5 provides tips and scripts for enhancing patient receptivity to pain psychology treatment.

Evidence-Based Psychological Approaches

All psychological treatments for pain share a goal of improving self-regulation as a pathway to reduce pain and its negative impacts. All psychological treatment approaches offer somewhat different skills to improve self-regulation of thoughts, emotions, or physiological responses to pain and stress. Examples of self-regulatory skills include diaphragmatic breathing, progressive muscle relaxation, cognitive restructuring, mindfulness, meditation, hypnosis, distraction, and self-soothing strategies. All evidence-based psychological approaches also include education about pain and the role of psychological factors in the experience and treatment of pain. The following text provides detail on evidence-based behavioral treatments for pain.

Biofeedback. Biofeedback is a tool that uses a computer and biometrics to demonstrate to patients the physiological effects that the relaxation response has on heart rate, respiratory rate, muscle tension, and skin temperature. It is useful for establishing a rationale for the role of relaxation in pain management and for cultivating patients' self-efficacy in the skill set (for information on biofeedback, see "Resources" near the end of this chapter).

TABLE 6–3.   Assessment and referral tips for older adults with pain

Screen for depression. Depression is associated with greater pain intensity, likelihood of being prescribed opioids, and poor outcomes for pain.

Screen for alcohol use (Brennan et al. 2005). Although patients may believe alcohol is analgesic, high use of alcohol increases pain and can be a primary contributor to pain-inducing pathology, such as peripheral neuropathy.

Refer for addiction or substance use disorder if alcohol use is frequent or abuse is present, or if alcohol consumption is concomitant with opioid use. Red flag behaviors include doctor shopping or visiting emergency departments for opioid medication.

Assess for medication risks and patient safety.

Strongly caution against benzodiazepine and opioid coprescription due to risks noted above.

Assess for cognitive functioning to ensure patients have no memory impairment that would place them at increased risk for accidentally double-dosing opioids or other sedating medication.

Assess sleep. Refer for a sleep medicine evaluation or to cognitive-behavioral therapy for insomnia.

Assess for function and movement. Refer to a skilled chronic pain physical therapist for evaluation and development of a tailored movement program.

Refer to a comprehensive pain clinic for specialty, interdisciplinary pain evaluation. These clinics are usually located in academic centers and often offer evaluation and treatment with a pain physician, pain physical therapist, pain psychologist, and possibly additional professionals (nurse practitioners, occupational therapists).

Refer for psychological treatment for pain. Beware of older patients with either moderate pain and severe psychological symptoms or severe pain and moderate psychological symptoms. Research shows these combinations of pain and psychological symptoms predict poor outcomes (Larsson et al. 2017). As such, consider a specialty referral to address the individual patient's treatment needs.

Cognitive-behavioral therapy for pain.   CBT for pain (pain-CBT) is considered the gold-standard psychological treatment for pain because it has been studied the longest and has the best evidence to support it (Cherkin et al. 2016). Pain-CBT incorporates pain education, including

TABLE 6–4. When to refer to a pain psychologist

The patient is stuck in a passive role; they want their pain fixed or cured.

The patient is focused on medications and procedures.

Active self-management is lacking.

The patient displays overdependence on family members.

Imbalanced activity levels (e.g., doing too little, or intermittently doing too much and causing pain flares) are present. Poor activity pacing contributes to feelings of helplessness and depressed mood; it is treatable with education and behavioral intervention.

The patient has a lack of active goals or is sedentary.

The patient believes that pain equals harm.

The patient believes that pain must be eliminated before life activity can resume.

The patient laments his or her loss of function but is unsure how to go forward.

Fear of pain is reducing the patient's movement and activity.

The patient has no pain and stress management skills and therefore no ability to self-regulate.

Feelings of helplessness and despair about pain are present.

Psychological distress or anger is present.

The patient is socially isolated.

Anxiety or depression is present.

the connection between mood and pain and the connections among thoughts, emotions, and pain. The focus is on stressing activity pacing within the context of pain; addressing maladaptive pain beliefs and pain catastrophizing; reducing pain behaviors; setting appropriate activity goals and gradually increasing activity; and increasing general wellness and self-care behaviors. In short, the pain-CBT protocol centers around the self-management of chronic pain, including related distress. Pain-CBT is delivered by a psychologist or skilled mental health professional to individuals or groups and is typically covered by most insurance, including Medicare.

Mindfulness-based stress reduction. Recent research on mindfulness-based stress reduction (MBSR) for chronic low back pain showed equivalence with pain-CBT. Mindfulness teaches nonreactivity and nonjudgment of pain and other stimuli, with an awareness and accep-

TABLE 6–5.   Tips and scripts for enhancing patient receptivity to pain psychology treatment

Assure the patient that his or her pain is real, is valid, and has a medical basis.

Explain to the patient that despite pain having a medical basis, psychological and behavioral factors can make it better or worse.

Point out that pain psychology focuses on learning skills and techniques that will give better control over the experience of pain and a way to self-soothe and reduce suffering.

Emphasize that evidence-based psychological strategies, when used regularly over time, lead to prolonged dampening of pain processing in the nervous system. Research suggests that psychological treatment for pain enhances medical treatment outcomes.

Remind patients that they are the most important person on their pain care team. What they do on a daily basis can alter the trajectory of their pain and their health.

tance of the present moment. MBSR is a 9-week course delivered to groups of individuals. It is rarely covered by insurance, and course fees typically run about $350 (see "Resources").

Ms. L could have benefited from any of these evidence-based pain treatment approaches. Given her constellation of psychological and behavioral factors, pain-CBT would be the best place to start. If she evidenced resistance or difficulty with the relaxation skills, biofeedback could be engaged for a higher level of care and support.

KEY POINTS

- Psychological factors profoundly influence pain perception and pain treatment outcomes.
- While pain typically has a medical basis, attending to psychological factors and needs can reduce suffering and improve medical treatment response.
- Engaging patients as active participants in their pain care is vitally important. Behavioral pain medicine and self-management education help patients learn what they can do to help themselves.
- A key aspect of patient care is helping patients shift their focus to steps they can take to achieve their functional goals.
- Specific communications strategies can enhance patient engagement in behavioral pain medicine or pain psychology treatment.

- Numerous evidence-based behavioral pain treatments exist. Offer patients print, internet, and local resources based on availability in the community.
- Opioids may be one aspect of a comprehensive pain care plan. Specific risks for older adults should be appreciated and patients monitored closely.

Resources

Resources for Clinicians

Resource Guides

American Chronic Pain Association: ACPA Resource Guide to Chronic Pain Management: An Integrated Guide to Medical, Interventional, Behavioral, Pharmacologic and Rehabilitation Therapy. Rocklin, CA, American Chronic Pain Association, 2018. Available at: www.theacpa.org/wp-content/uploads/2018/05/ACPA_Resource_Guide_2018-Final_Feb.pdf.

Assessment Resource

Sullivan MJL: Pain Catastrophizing Scale and User Manual. Montreal, Quebec, Canada, McGill University, 2009. Available at: http://sullivan-painresearch.mcgill.ca/pdf/pcs/PCSManual_English.pdf.

Biofeedback

Biofeedback Certification International Alliance (BCIA): https://bcia.org. To locate a certified biofeedback therapist, go to "Find a Practitioner" tab. Conduct a radius search based on the patient's zip code.

Mindfulness-Based Stress Reduction

Palouse Mindfulness: http://palousemindfulness.com. Offers a free online MBSR course.

Books

American Pain Society: Principles of Analgesic Use, 7th Edition. Glenview, IL, American Pain Society, 2016

Darnall B: Psychological Treatment for Patients With Chronic Pain. Washington, DC, American Psychological Association, 2018

Thorn BE: Cognitive Behavioral Therapy for Chronic Pain: A Step by Step Guide, 2nd Edition. New York, Guilford, 2017

Websites (Containing Handouts and Videos)

The American Chronic Pain Association: www.theacpa.org
Pain Toolkit: www.paintoolkit.org. Excellent resource for clinicians
  who wish to integrate resources for chronic pain self-management
  into their practice.

Articles

Molton IR, Terrill AR: Overview of persistent pain in older adults. Am
  Psychol 69(2):197–207, 2014
Sturgeon JA: Psychological therapies for the management of chronic
  pain. Psychol Res Behav Manag 7:115–124, 2014

Resources for Patients

Websites (Containing Handouts and Videos)

American Chronic Pain Association: www.theacpa.org
Arthritis Foundation: www.arthritis.org
Chronic Pain Self-Management Program: www.cdc.gov/arthritis/
  interventions/self_manage.htm. Offered free in some closed payor
  systems and in the senior centers of some municipalities.
Pain Toolkit: www.paintoolkit.org. Print resources and more than 50
  different videos.

Video

Painaustralia: "Understanding Pain: What You Can Do About It in Less
  Than Five Minutes" YouTube video, running time 5:00, July 16, 2012.
  Available at: www.youtube.com/watch?v=RWMKucuejIs.

Patient Books

*All are workbook format. Those marked with ** address pain catastro-
  phizing.*
Caudill MA: Managing Pain Before It Manages You, 4th Edition. New
  York, Guilford, 2016
**Darnall B: The Opioid-Free Pain Relief Kit: 10 Simple Steps to Ease
  Your Pain. Boulder, CO, Bull Publishing, 2016. Includes "Enhanced
  Pain Management Relaxation" MP3 audiofile/CD.
LeFort S, Webster L, Lorig K, et al: Living a Healthy Life With Chronic
  Pain. Boulder, CO, Bull Publishing, 2015. Includes "Moving Easy"
  program CD.
**Lewandowski MJ: The Chronic Pain Care Workbook: A Self-Treat-
  ment Approach to Pain Relief Using the Behavioral Assessment of
  Pain Questionnaire. Oakland, CA, New Harbinger, 2006

**Turk DC, Winter F: The Pain Survival Guide: How to Reclaim Your Life. Washington, DC, American Psychological Association, 2005

Book for Patients Taking Opioids and a Resource for Family Members

Darnall B: Less Pain, Fewer Pills: Avoid the Dangers of Prescription Opioids and Gain Control Over Chronic Pain. Boulder, CO, Bull Publishing, 2014. Includes Enhanced Pain Management Relaxation MP3 audiofile/CD.

References

Abbott AD, Tyni-Lenné R, Hedlund R: Leg pain and psychological variables predict outcome 2–3 years after lumbar fusion surgery. Eur Spine J 20(10):1626–1634, 2011 21311916

Amtmann D, Kim J, Chung H, et al: Comparing CESD-10, PHQ-9, and PROMIS depression instruments in individuals with multiple sclerosis. Rehabil Psychol 59(2):220–229, 2014 24661030

Brennan PL, Schutte KK, Moos RH: Pain and use of alcohol to manage pain: prevalence and 3-year outcomes among older problem and non-problem drinkers. Addiction 100(6):777–786, 2005 15918808

Buckeridge D, Huang A, Hanley J, et al: Risk of injury associated with opioid use in older adults. J Am Geriatr Soc 58(9):1664–1670, 2010 20863326

Bushnell MC, Ceko M, Low LA: Cognitive and emotional control of pain and its disruption in chronic pain. Nat Rev Neurosci 14(7):502–511, 2013 23719569

Campbell CI, Weisner C, Leresche L, et al: Age and gender trends in long-term opioid analgesic use for noncancer pain. Am J Public Health 100(12):2541–2547, 2010 20724688

Cherkin DC, Sherman KJ, Balderson BH, et al: Effect of mindfulness-based stress reduction vs. cognitive behavioral therapy or usual care on back pain and functional limitations in adults with chronic low back pain: a randomized clinical trial. JAMA 315(12):1240–1249, 2016 27002445

Darnall BD, Stacey BR: Sex differences in long-term opioid use: cautionary notes for prescribing in women. Arch Intern Med 172(5):431–432, 2012 22412108

Darnall BD, Stacey BR, Chou R: Medical and psychological risks and consequences of long-term opioid therapy in women. Pain Med 13(9):1181–1211, 2012 22905834

Darnall BD, Juurlink D, Kerns RD, et al: International Stakeholder Community of Pain Experts, Leaders, Clinicians, and Patient Advocates Call for an Urgent Action on Forced Opioid Tapering. Pain Med 20(3):429–433, 2019

Davis MJ, Livingston M, Scharf SM: Reversal of central sleep apnea following discontinuation of opioids. J Clin Sleep Med 8(5):579–580, 2012 23066372

Dimsdale JE, Norman D, DeJardin D, et al: The effect of opioids on sleep architecture. J Clin Sleep Med 3(1):33–36, 2007 17557450

Glanz JM, Binswanger IA, Shetterley SM, et al: Association Between Opioid
Dose Variability and Opioid Overdose Among Adults Prescribed Long-term
Opioid Therapy. JAMA Netw Open 2(4):e192613, 2019 31002325

Guilleminault C, Cao M, Yue HJ, et al: Obstructive sleep apnea and chronic opioid use. Lung 188(6):459–468, 2010 20658143

Helmes E, Nielson WR: An examination of the internal structure of the Center
for Epidemiological Studies–Depression Scale in two medical samples.
Pers Individ Dif 25(4):735–743, 1998

Institute of Medicine Committee on Advancing Pain Research, Care, and Education: Relieving Pain in America: A Blueprint for Transforming Prevention, Care, Education, and Research. Washington, DC, National Academies
Press, 2011

Khan RS, Ahmed K, Blakeway E, et al: Catastrophizing: a predictive factor for
postoperative pain. Am J Surg 201(1):122–131, 2011 20832052

Khan RS, Skapinakis P, Ahmed K, et al: The association between preoperative
pain catastrophizing and postoperative pain intensity in cardiac surgery
patients. Pain Med 13(6):820–827, 2012 22568812

Larsson B, Gerdle B, Bernfort L, et al: Distinctive subgroups derived by cluster
analysis based on pain and psychological symptoms in Swedish older
adults with chronic pain—a population study (PainS65+). BMC Geriatr
17(1):200, 2017 28865445

Miller M, Stürmer T, Azrael D, et al: Opioid analgesics and the risk of fractures
in older adults with arthritis. J Am Geriatr Soc 59(3):430–438, 2011
21391934

Mojtabai R: National trends in long-term use of prescription opioids. Pharmacoepidemiol Drug Saf 27(5):526–534, 2018 28879660

Papaleontiou M, Henderson CR Jr, Turner BJ, et al: Outcomes associated with
opioid use in the treatment of chronic noncancer pain in older adults: a systematic review and meta-analysis. J Am Geriatr Soc 58(7):1353–1369, 2010
20533971

Pavlin DJ, Sullivan MJ, Freund PR, et al: Catastrophizing: a risk factor for post-
surgical pain. Clin J Pain 21(1):83–90, 2005 15599135

Roh YH, Lee BK, Noh JH, et al: Effect of anxiety and catastrophic pain ideation
on early recovery after surgery for distal radius fractures. J Hand Surg Am
39(11):2258–2264, 2014 25283489

Salas J, Scherrer JF, Schneider FD, et al: New-onset depression following stable, slow, and rapid rate of prescription opioid dose escalation. Pain
158(2):306–312, 2017 28092649

Saunders KW, Dunn KM, Merrill JO, et al: Relationship of opioid use and dosage levels to fractures in older chronic pain patients. J Gen Intern Med
25(4):310–315, 2010 20049546

Scherrer JF, Salas J, Schneider FD, et al: Characteristics of new depression diagnoses in patients with and without prior chronic opioid use. J Affect Disord 210:125–129, 2017 28033519

Sharp TJ, Harvey AG: Chronic pain and posttraumatic stress disorder: mutual
maintenance? Clin Psychol Rev 21(6):857–877, 2001 11497210

Sterling S, Chi F, Weisner C, et al: Association of behavioral health factors and social determinants of health with high and persistently high healthcare costs. Prev Med Rep 11:154–159, 2018 30003015

Sullivan MJ, Bishop SR, Pivik J: The pain catastrophizing scale: development and validation. Psychol Assess 7:524–532, 1995

Sun EC, Darnall BD, Baker LC, et al: Incidence of and risk factors for chronic opioid use among opioid-naive patients in the postoperative period. JAMA Intern Med 176(9):1286–1293, 2016 27400458

Sun EC, Dixit A, Humphreys K, et al: Association between concurrent use of prescription opioids and benzodiazepines and overdose: retrospective analysis. BMJ 356:j760, 2017 28292769

Thakkar MM, Sharma R, Sahota P: Alcohol disrupts sleep homeostasis. Alcohol 49(4):299–310, 2015 25499829

U.S. Food and Drug Administration: Drug Safety Communications: FDA identifies harm reported from sudden discontinuation of opioid pain medicines and requires label changes to guide prescribers on gradual, individualized tapering. April 9, 2019. Available at: https://www.fda.gov/media/122935/download. Accessed May 4, 2019.

Weathers FW, Litz BT, Huska JA, et al: PTSD Checklist–Civilian Version, 1994. Available at: https://www.mirecc.va.gov/docs/visn6/3_ptsd_checklist_and_scoring.pdf. Accessed December 10, 2018.

Wertli MM, Burgstaller JM, Weiser S, et al: The influence of catastrophizing on treatment outcome in patients with non-specific low back pain: a systematic review. Spine (Phila Pa 1976) 39(3):263–273, 2013

Primary Sleep Disorders

"My Wife Says I Snore Loudly and Sometimes Stop Breathing While I'm Asleep"

Cathy I. Cheng, M.D., FACP
Clete A. Kushida, M.D., Ph.D.

CHAPTER 7

As individuals age, some changes to sleep occur as part of the normal aging process. In older adults, for example, their sleep architecture changes; more time is spent in lighter stages of sleep (non–rapid eye movement, or NREM, sleep, stages N1 and N2) than in deeper stages of sleep (NREM sleep stage N3 or rapid eye movement [REM] sleep). Older adults also often experience an increased sleep latency (time it takes to fall asleep) and increased sleep fragmentation (frequent waking up during the night).

However, there are multiple primary sleep disorders, which by definition are not caused by another medical or psychiatric condition, that are not a part of normal aging. Many of the primary sleep disorders affecting younger adults may not only continue into old age but also increase in prevalence. In this chapter, we discuss the following categories of primary sleep disorders: sleep-related breathing disorders (SRBDs; breathing-related sleep disorders in DSM-5 [American Psychiatric Association 2013]), sleep-related movement disorders (SRMDs), parasomnias, circadian rhythm sleep-wake disorders (CRSWDs), and hypersomnolence disorders. (Insomnia is addressed in Chapter 8, "Evaluation and Management of Insomnia.") Throughout this chapter, please note that *International Classification of Sleep Disorders,* 3rd Edition (ICSD-3), terminology is used instead of DSM-5 terminology (although there may be some shared terminology) for relevance of subject matter discussion and terms used throughout the literature.

Within each category of primary sleep disorders, there exist different types of sleep conditions, of which detailed discussion for each is outside the scope of this book. Therefore, for each of the five categories of primary sleep disorders, the accompanying chief complaint and clinical vignette will represent the most commonly encountered type of sleep disorder that the clinician may encounter, namely, obstructive sleep apnea (OSA) (for SRBD); restless legs syndrome (RLS) (for SRMD); REM sleep behavior disorder (RBD) (for parasomnia); advanced sleep phase syndrome (for CRSWD); and narcolepsy (for hypersomnolence).

Sleep-Related Breathing Disorders

Clinical Presentation

Chief Complaint

"My wife says I snore loudly and and sometimes stop breathing while I'm asleep."

Vignette

A 70-year-old man presents to the clinic and tells the examiner that he does not think he has a sleep problem. However, his wife insisted he see a doctor because she was tired of being woken up by his loud snoring and was scared seeing the patient not breathe for several seconds intermittently throughout the night. The patient later adds that he occasionally wakes up gasping or choking at night, gets up four times a night to urinate, has morning headaches, and wakes up feeling unrefreshed despite sleeping 8–9 hours daily. His wife has noticed that the patient has a decreased ability to concentrate, increased forgetfulness, and increased irritability. Pertinent past medical history includes resistant hypertension, type 2 diabetes mellitus, atrial fibrillation, congestive heart failure, obesity, and stroke. Physical examination is notable for blood pressure (BP) 155/95, oxygen saturation (SaO_2) 93%, body mass index (BMI) 37, Mallampati class 4 airway (soft palate is not visible at all), neck circumference of 43 cm, irregularly irregular heart rhythm, central adiposity, and pitting edema up to both ankles. Laboratory tests are notable for serum bicarbonate (HCO_3^-) of 30 and random glucose level of 250 mg/dL. Complete blood count (CBC) and thyroid-stimulating hormone (TSH), vitamin B_{12}, and folate levels are all normal.

The patient is recommended to have a polysomnogram (sleep study), which reveals an apnea-hypopnea index (AHI) of 35 (see "Differential Diagnosis" later in this section for definition), which indicates in the majority of cases obstructive apnea. The patient is thus diagnosed with OSA. He is started on continuous positive airway pressure (CPAP) therapy. After 3 months of nightly CPAP, his morning headaches resolve and he feels much more refreshed upon waking up. His wife is also happy because the patient no longer snores with the CPAP on, focuses better, and is less irritable.

Discussion

Diagnosis and Workup

SRBDs constitute a spectrum of sleep disorders that involve difficulty breathing during sleep. In addition to OSA, other SRBDs include snoring (noise caused by flow of air from breathing that vibrates the tissues in the back of the throat), central sleep apnea (when the brain does not send proper signals to respiratory muscles, and there is cessation of airflow and no respiratory effort), and sleep-related hypoventilation. Reviews of these various types of SRBD may be found elsewhere (Sateia 2014). The most common SRBD is OSA. As such, OSA is the focus of this section.

Differential Diagnosis

When a patient presents with snoring, other diagnoses to consider in addition to OSA include primary snoring, upper airway resistance syndrome, obesity hypoventilation syndrome, and overlap syndrome. Briefly, primary snoring is defined by an AHI of less than 5 and no daytime sleepiness. The AHI refers to the number of apneas and hypopneas per hour of sleep. The higher the AHI, the more severe the OSA. An *apnea* is defined as a 90% or greater decrease in airflow for 10 seconds or longer. A *hypopnea* is defined as a 30% or greater decrease in airflow for 10 seconds or longer that is associated with either 1) a 3% or more oxygen desaturation from pre-event baseline or an arousal (American Academy of Sleep Medicine 2014) or 2) a 4% or more oxygen desaturation (Centers for Medicare & Medicaid Services 2016). *Respiratory ef-*

fort–related arousals (RERAs) are respiratory events characterized by increasing respiratory effort leading to an arousal that do not meet criteria for an apnea or hypopnea. *Upper airway resistance syndrome* is characterized by sleepiness in patients in whom AHI is less than 5 when the hypopnea definition requires a 4% or greater desaturation but a respiratory disturbance index (RDI; mainly RERAs) of 5 or more. *Obesity hypoventilation syndrome* should be considered if BMI is more than 30 kg/m^2; daytime partial pressure of carbon dioxide (PCO_2) is greater than 45; hypoventilation is not explained by lower airway, parenchymal lung disease, thoracic cage disorder, or neuromuscular disorder; and HCO_3^- is greater than 27 mEq/L in an obese patient with OSA. *Overlap syndrome* is defined as OSA and chronic obstructive pulmonary disease (COPD) and often involves severe arterial oxygen desaturation at night.

Diagnosis of Obstructive Sleep Apnea

OSA occurs when complete or partial upper airway obstruction occurs repeatedly during sleep to cause oxygen desaturation and arousal that often result in snoring and daytime sleepiness. In older adults, loss of tissue elasticity from aging may worsen airway collapse. The prevalence of OSA among older adults age 60 and older in various studies is 1.7 to more than 4.0 times as high as it is in younger adults (Young et al. 2002a). When the clinician is evaluating patients for OSA, it is important to ask the patient—and the patient's bed partner—about any history of snoring, witnessed apneas, gasping or choking at night, unrefreshing sleep, sleepiness, nocturia, morning headaches, decreased concentration, memory loss, decreased libido, or increased irritability because these findings are commonly found in patients with OSA. To measure sleepiness, many clinics have patients complete the Epworth Sleepiness Scale (Johns 1993; see http://epworthsleepinessscale.com/about-the-ess), which is a series of eight questions that address how likely the patient is to doze off in various scenarios. A score of greater than 10 on this scale indicates excessive daytime sleepiness.

Medical comorbidities that increase the risk for OSA include obesity, congestive heart failure, atrial fibrillation, resistant hypertension, type 2 diabetes, nocturnal arrhythmias, stroke, and pulmonary hypertension. Untreated OSA can increase the risk of these same conditions.

In older adults with sleep-disordered breathing, nocturia, cognitive dysfunction (sleepiness, decreased vigilance, worsened executive function, and dementia), and cardiac disease (hypertension, atrial fibrillation, and stroke) are especially prominent. In one study, the report of nocturnal urination more than three times during the night was reported significantly more often by patients with severe OSA compared with patients who had primary snoring, mild OSA, or moderate OSA; such nocturia had a positive predictive value of 0.71 (Kaynak et al. 2004). Regarding OSA and cognitive dysfunction, one of many studies demonstrated that the presence of sleep-disordered breathing was associated with an earlier age at cognitive decline (Osorio et al. 2015). In terms of OSA and cardiovascular disease, severe sleep apnea is an independent risk factor for incident hypertension in older adults with a mean age of 68.2 years (Guillot et al. 2013). Moreover, sleep-disordered breathing is associated with a two- to fourfold increased risk of cardiac arrhythmias, most commonly atrial fibrillation (Mehra et al. 2006). CPAP use has been shown to improve nocturia (Guilleminault et al. 2004), cognition (Dalmases et al. 2015; Osorio et al. 2015), and cardiovascular health (Barbé et al. 2012).

Physical examination findings suggestive of OSA include a BMI greater than 30 kg/m^2, nasal obstruction, narrow oropharynx, high Mallampati score (classes 3 or 4; visualization of only the base of the uvula or no visualization of the soft palate, respectively), retrognathia, high-arched palate, increased neck circumference (>16 inches in women; >17 inches in men), and/or evidence of cor pulmonale.

One screening tool to help clinicians detect OSA is the updated STOP-BANG Questionnaire (available at: www.stopbang.ca/osa/screening.php). Each letter in the updated STOP-BANG acronym stands for a symptom or sign of OSA (**S**noring, **T**ired, **O**bserved, **P**ressure, **B**ody mass index, **A**ge older than 50, **N**eck size large, **G**ender) that has an associated yes/no question. Answering "yes" to three or more of these eight items indicates a high risk for OSA. Answering "yes" to fewer than three of these items indicates a low risk for OSA.

Note that in older adults, male gender is no longer an important risk factor for OSA after age 50; the 2:1 male:female predominance of OSA in younger patients becomes a 1:1 ratio for older adults (Tishler et al. 2003). This change in ratio is thought to be related to the increase in OSA in women as they undergo menopause. Also, witnessed apneas and snoring are reported less frequently in older patients compared with younger patients (Young et al. 2002b). In addition, obesity is a less important risk factor for OSA in older adults compared with younger adults.

Per the American Academy of Sleep Medicine (AASM; 2014) *International Classification of Sleep Disorders,* 3rd Edition (ICSD-3), there are two ways to diagnose OSA depending on what clinical and/or polysomnographic features are present. One way of diagnosing OSA is if the patient has at least one clinical symptom (e.g., sleepiness, unrefreshing sleep, fatigue, insomnia, gasping, choking, awakening with breath holding, snoring, witnessed apneas) or associated medical disorder (e.g., hypertension, cognitive dysfunction, a mood disorder, congestive heart failure, coronary artery disease, stroke, atrial fibrillation, type 2 diabetes) and an RDI (including apneas, hypopneas, and RERAs) of five or more per hour of sleep on either a polysomnogram or home sleep test. The other way to diagnose OSA is if the RDI is 15 or more per hour of sleep on either a polysomnogram or a home sleep test. Note that the latter way of diagnosing OSA does not necessitate the presence of any OSA symptoms.

In contrast to the ICSD-3 (American Academy of Sleep Medicine 2014) definition of OSA, the Centers for Medicare & Medicaid Services (2008) define OSA as either an AHI of 15 or more or both an AHI greater than 5 and the presence of sleepiness, hypertension, stroke, ischemic heart disease, or mood disorder.

Per the AASM 2017 clinical practice guideline (Kapur et al. 2017), polysomnography is the standard diagnostic test used to diagnose OSA in adults. A home sleep apnea test can be used for the diagnosis of uncomplicated adult patients whose presenting signs and symptoms are consistent with an increased risk of moderate to severe OSA. If patients have significant cardiorespiratory disease, respiratory muscle weakness due to a neuromuscular condition, awake hypoventilation or suspected sleep-related hypoventilation, chronic opioid use, history of stroke, or severe insomnia, polysomnography is recommended over home sleep apnea testing.

Once OSA is diagnosed, the severity of OSA can be classified as mild, moderate, or severe based on the value of the AHI. *Mild OSA* is defined as an AHI of 5 to less than 15; *moderate OSA* is defined as an AHI of 15–30; and *severe OSA* is defined as an AHI of more than 30. *Postural OSA* is defined as a supine AHI value more than two times the nonsupine AHI value.

Treatment of Obstructive Sleep Apnea

Treating OSA is crucial because untreated OSA can lead to death, cardiovascular disease, stroke, atrial fibrillation, diabetes, impaired cognition, nocturia, and increased motor vehicle crashes. Indeed, after controlling for age, BMI, preexisting cardiovascular disease, smoking, diabetes, sleepiness, gender, dyslipidemia, and respiratory failure, one study revealed a twofold increase in risk of death in patients with severe OSA (AHI ≥30) and mean age of 71 years when compared with the control group. CPAP use decreased the risk of all-cause mortality and cardiovascular death, as well as death from stroke and heart failure (Martínez-García et al. 2012). Another study of patients with OSA and coronary heart disease or cardiovascular risk factors found that CPAP improved health-related quality of life (vitality, sleepiness, mental health, and social functioning) and depressive symptoms (Lewis et al. 2017).

Currently, the Centers for Medicare & Medicaid Services (2008) covers treatment for patients with an AHI of 5 or more and symptoms (e.g., sleepiness) or comorbid medical conditions (e.g., hypertension), as well as for patients with an AHI of 15 or higher, regardless of symptoms. There are several types of treatment for OSA: conservative measures, positive airway pressure therapy (e.g., CPAP), oral appliances, surgery, upper airway stimulation therapy, pharmacological treatment, and positional therapy. For everyone with OSA, conservative measures such as receiving treatment for nasal congestion, obtaining adequate sleep time, losing weight (in obese patients), abstaining from alcohol, and smoking cessation should be undertaken. In older patients, the most effective treatment for OSA is CPAP. Unlike younger patients, older patients may require lower CPAP pressures. Older age does not affect adherence to CPAP therapy (Weaver and Chasens 2007). For patients who require higher pressures than offered by CPAP or who have hypoventilation, bilevel positive airway pressure may be used.

Oral appliances, which are best managed by a dentist specializing in sleep medicine, are not as effective as CPAP but can be used to treat mild to moderate OSA and snoring. They include mandibular advancement devices, which anteriorly position the mandible and genioglossus, as well as tongue-retaining devices. Common side effects of oral appliances include dry mouth, increased salivation, tooth soreness, jaw pain, and bite changes. Upper airway surgery (e.g., bimaxillary advancement, hyoid myotomy, genioglossus advancement, and uvulopalatopharyngoplasty) for the treatment of OSA can be very successful; however, it is less effective and associated with high morbidity in elderly patients (Jones et al. 2005). For patients with moderate to severe OSA who are unable to tolerate CPAP, upper airway stimulation therapy has been demonstrated to result in objective and subjective improvements in OSA (Strollo et al. 2014). Regarding pharmacological treatment of OSA, although there is no medication effective enough to be recommended as a first-line treatment, nasal steroids have modest efficacy in treating sleep-disordered breathing. Positional therapy can treat mild OSA in some older adults. Because the supine position exacerbates OSA by worsening airway collapse and reducing lung volume, some patients experience OSA only when sleeping supine. For such patients, sleeping on their side can help treat their OSA.

Sleep-Related Breathing Disorders: Key Points

- The most common type of sleep-related breathing disorder is obstructive sleep apnea (OSA), in which there is cessation of oronasal airflow despite continued respiratory effort.
- The prevalence of OSA is increased in middle-age and older adults compared with younger adults.
- OSA can manifest differently in older adults compared with younger adults; in older adults, nocturia, cognitive dysfunction, and cardiac disease are especially prominent, but witnessed apneas and snoring are less frequently reported.
- In older adults, obesity and male gender are less important risk factors for OSA than in younger adults.
- OSA can be diagnosed by polysomnography or home sleep testing with or without clinical symptoms.
- Treatment of OSA is crucial because untreated OSA can result in death, cardiovascular disease, stroke, impaired cognition, and increased motor vehicle crashes.
- The most common and effective treatment for OSA in the elderly is continuous positive airway pressure.

Sleep-Related Movement Disorders

Clinical Presentation

Chief Complaint

"I have uncomfortable, creepy-crawly sensations in my legs every night around 9:30 P.M. when I'm laying down in bed. I feel this urge to move my legs, and getting up to walk helps the sensations, but because of these feelings I have a hard time falling asleep."

Vignette

A 65-year-old Asian woman presents to the clinic for daily painful sensations in her legs that feel like unpleasant crawling and deep aches. Moving her extremities partially relieves these symptoms, but at rest, the symptoms worsen. These painful sensations occur in the evening and make it difficult for her to fall asleep at night, so the patient tried taking nightly diphenhydramine, which only worsened her leg symptoms. Her relevant comorbidities include iron-deficiency anemia and anxiety. Physical examination is remarkable for no abnormal leg or arm movements and normal muscle tone and bulk of her legs. Laboratory tests are notable for ferritin 15 ng/mL.

The patient is diagnosed with RLS. She is told to discontinue diphenhydramine, take warm baths, perform regular stretches, and start ferrous sulfate 325 mg three times a day with ascorbic acid 200 mg daily (to aid absorption of the iron). Months later, recheck of ferritin is 80 µg/L, and her uncomfortable leg sensations have decreased from daily to three times a week. She begins taking gabapentin enacarbil (Horizant) 600 mg daily at 5 P.M., with eventual resolution of her symptoms.

Discussion

Diagnosis and Workup

Sleep-related movement disorders refers to a group of disorders characterized by simple and stereotyped movements that occur during sleep onset or sleep and result in distress, sleep disturbance, and impaired function. These conditions include RLS, periodic limb movement disorder (PLMD), sleep-related leg cramps, sleep-related bruxism, sleep-related rhythmic movement disorder, and propriospinal myoclonus. In this section, we focus on RLS; review of the other types of SRMD may be found elsewhere (Trotti 2017).

RLS, also known as *Willis-Ekbom disease* (named after the two different physicians, Sir Thomas Willis and Dr. Karl-Axel Ekbom, who separately described the entity in 1685 and 1945, respectively), is characterized by an overwhelming urge to move the legs (or arms) at rest that is usually accompanied by unpleasant sensations. Common descriptions of abnormal sensations in RLS include creepy-crawly, ants crawling under the skin, worms crawling in the veins, Pepsi-Cola in the veins, and excited nerves. In 50% of patients, such sensations can also affect the arms. A family history of RLS is reported in up to 50% of patients. A response to dopaminergic treatment can support the diagnosis of RLS.

RLS has a prevalence of up to 7.2% in the elderly (Allen et al. 2005). The prevalence of RLS increases with age up to 60–70 years, except in Asians. The increasing prevalence may be associated with the increasing presence of RLS risk factors such as iron deficiency and chronic kidney disease. RLS prevalence is higher in women than in men (2:1), and much of this difference is thought to be related to the increased incidence of RLS in pregnancy. With age, the severity of RLS also increases; older patients have symptoms more often and for longer compared with younger patients with RLS.

In contrast to early-onset RLS, in which RLS occurs before age 50 years with insidious onset, less severity, and higher familial association, late-onset RLS occurs in adults older than 50, has a more abrupt onset, has more severe manifestations, and has lower ferritin levels. RLS can also be classified as primary RLS or secondary RLS. In *primary RLS,* the cause of RLS is idiopathic and often familial. *Secondary RLS* refers to RLS caused by another medical condition such as iron deficiency, pregnancy, diabetic neuropathy, multiple sclerosis, renal failure, or Parkinson's disease. Medications such as selective serotonin reuptake inhibitors (SSRIs), first-generation antihistamines (e.g., diphenhydramine), neuroleptics (e.g., olanzapine), and lithium may worsen RLS.

Differential Diagnosis

When patients report the urge to move their legs while at rest, it is important to consider the following mimics of RLS: leg cramps, positional discomfort, local leg injury, arthralgia or arthritis, leg edema, venous stasis, peripheral neuropathy, radiculopathy, habitual foot tapping, drug-induced akathisia, myelopathy, myopathy, and vascular claudication (Figorilli et al. 2015). A careful history and physical examination can help rule out these RLS mimics. For example, arthritic pain, vascular claudication, and neuropathy may be worse at night and at rest, but they are not improved by movement; habitual foot tapping occurs unconsciously, whereas RLS patients are aware of their leg movements; and symptoms that are present only in certain body positions (e.g., crossed legs) are more likely to represent positional discomfort rather than RLS.

Diagnosis of Restless Legs Syndrome

The diagnosis of RLS is made by history and does not require a polysomnogram. Polysomnography is only needed if another sleep disorder (or associated condition such as PLMD) is suspected. Physical examination, including neurological examination of the limbs, should be normal. The acronym URGE can be used to describe four essential diagnostic criteria for RLS: **U**rge to move, **R**est-induced, **G**ets better with activity, and **E**vening and night worse. Per the ICSD-3 diagnostic criteria for RLS, all of the following criteria must be present to diagnose RLS: 1) there is an urge to move the legs that may be caused by or associated with uncomfortable sensations in the leg that begin or worsen during periods of inactivity, be at least partially relieved by movement, and occur at least mostly in the evening or night; 2) these symptoms are not secondary to another medical or behavioral condition; and 3) these symptoms disturb or impair the patient's sleep or mental, physical, social, occupational, educational, or other important areas of functioning (American Academy of Sleep Medicine 2014).

Treatment of Restless Legs Syndrome

Treatment of RLS can be divided into nonpharmacological and pharmacological treatments. Nonpharmacological treatments include exercise, stretching, heating the extremities (e.g., taking a warm bath), avoiding alcohol and caffeine, smoking cessation, avoiding first-generation antihistamines, and iron supplementation if ferritin is less than 50 ng/mL. It is important to replenish low iron stores, not only because it can help reduce RLS symptoms but also because low iron stores increase the risk for a phenomenon called *augmentation*. Augmentation refers to a change in the efficacy of RLS treatment, specifically with dopaminergic medications (e.g., carbidopa-levodopa, pramipexole, ropinirole, rotigotine). Augmentation can manifest as a persisting paradoxical response to treatment (e.g., increasing treatment dosage increases RLS severity, and decreasing treatment dosage decreases RLS severity) and an earlier onset of symptoms that can also be associated with either a shorter latency to symptoms at rest, extension of symptoms to other body parts, greater intensity of symptoms, or shorter duration of relief from treatment. If augmentation occurs, the clinician should avoid high doses of dopaminergic medication, switch to a dopamine agonist if the patient developed augmentation on carbidopa-levodopa, split the dose and give half of the dopaminergic medication dosage earlier, switch to a different dopamine agonist medication, or reduce the dopamine agonist dosage and add gabapentin or an opioid. In cases of severe augmentation, the clinician should stop or wean the dopaminergic medication and add a high-potency opioid. It is also important to educate patients to perform sedentary tasks in the morning instead of in the evening. If a patient has depression and is taking an SSRI, which can worsen RLS symptoms, the clinician can consider switching the SSRI to bupropion, which does not worsen and can sometimes improve RLS symptoms.

Pharmacological treatments of RLS include the following medication classes: dopamine agonists (e.g., pramipexole, ropinirole, rotigotine), dopamine precursors (e.g., carbidopa-levodopa), α_2-delta ligands (e.g., gabapentin enacarbil, gabapentin, pregabalin), benzodiazepines (e.g., clonazepam), and opioids (e.g., tramadol, hydrocodone, oxycodone, methadone). The treatment of RLS varies depending on whether the RLS is intermittent, chronic, or refractory (Silber et al. 2004). *Intermittent RLS* occurring less than twice a week can be treated with the nonpharmacological measures described earlier, benzodiazepines, carbidopa-levodopa (which is short-acting and active within 30 minutes), or low-potency opioids. For *chronic RLS* that requires daily therapy to control symptoms causing moderate-severe distress at least twice a week, the clinician can use a dopamine agonist or α_2-delta ligand in addition to nonpharmacological measures. If one dopamine agonist is not tolerated, another dopamine agonist can be tried. If RLS occurs during the daytime, the clinician can consider using the rotigotine patch. For patients with comorbid pain, anxiety, or insomnia, side effects with dopamine agonists, or impulse-control disorder on dopamine agonists, the clinician should use an α_2-delta ligand. Regarding *refractory RLS*, which describes RLS that is unresponsive to monotherapy with a dopamine agonist or α_2-delta ligand, the clinician can 1) try an opioid alone or in combination with another medication; 2) try the combination of a dopamine agonist and an α_2-delta ligand; or 3) switch to another medication in the same class (e.g., from pramipexole to ropinirole). A benzodiazepine can also be added at bedtime to control nightly RLS symptoms.

Sleep-Related Movement Disorders: Key Points

- The prevalence of restless legs syndrome (RLS) increases in the elderly and may be related to the increased presence of RLS risk factors among the elderly, such as iron deficiency and chronic kidney disease.
- RLS is diagnosed based on clinical history. A polysomnogram is not needed unless other sleep disorders, such as periodic limb movement disorder, are suspected.
- The acronym URGE (**U**rge to move, **R**est-induced, **G**ets better with activity, **E**vening and night worse) can be used to help diagnose RLS.
- Treatment options for RLS include nonpharmacological and pharmacological measures, which can involve dopamine agonists, dopamine precursors, α_2-delta ligands, benzodiazepines, and/or opioids.
- Augmentation can occur when using dopaminergic medications. Low serum ferritin is also a risk factor for augmentation.

Parasomnias

Clinical Presentation

Chief Complaint

"My wife says that I act out my violent dreams and that I've woken her up several nights with my screaming and kicking."

Vignette

A 75-year-old man presents to the clinician's office at the request of his wife, who mentions that she has had to sleep in a separate bed from the patient because she is afraid of being hit by him again whenever he acts out his violent dreams. The patient remembers his dreams, which the wife says occur in the latter third of the night and seem violent and tense because the patient is often punching or kicking something and occasionally screams. The patient's brother used to sleepwalk and talk in his sleep.

The clinician orders a polysomnogram that includes electromyography for the arms and legs. This reveals abnormal muscle augmentation during REM sleep—in other words, a lack of normal REM sleep atonia—and no evidence of OSA. Video during the polysomnogram captures the patient, with his eyes closed, sitting up and punching in front of him and screaming late into the night during one of his last REM periods. The patient is diagnosed with having REM sleep behavior disorder, started on clonazepam 0.5 mg at bedtime, advised to sleep in a hospital-style bed with padded and raised side rails, and instructed to remove sharp or heavy objects from the sleeping area. With such interventions, the patient's wife reports that the patient's abnormal sleep behaviors greatly improve.

Discussion

Diagnosis and Workup

Parasomnias are abnormal and undesirable motor, verbal, or experiential phenomena that occur during sleep or the sleep-wake transition. Parasomnias can be divided into two groups: parasomnias occurring during NREM sleep and parasomnias occurring during REM sleep. *NREM parasomnias* include confusional arousals, sleepwalking, sleep terrors, and sleep-related eating disorder, and typically patients awaken confused and do not recall the preceding event. In contrast, *REM parasomnias* include RBD, recurrent isolated sleep paralysis, and nightmare disorder, and patients oftentimes can remember their last dream. In this subsection, we focus on RBD. Review of the other types of parasomnias may be found elsewhere (Malhotra and Avidan 2012).

RBD is characterized by 1) a loss of normal muscle atonia during REM sleep and 2) dream enactment behavior that is often violent or emotionally charged. Behaviors may include talking, singing, shouting, strangulating, jumping from bed, hitting a wall, and kicking. Because the behaviors are often associated with violent dream content, both the patient and bed partner can be harmed. The prevalence of RBD is higher in adults age 50 years and older and is estimated to be up to 0.5% (Ohayon and Schenck 2010). There is a strong male predilection, with one review citing a ninefold increased prevalence of RBD in men compared with women (Malhotra and Avidan 2012).

RBD can be classified into acute and chronic forms. *Acute RBD* can occur after the withdrawal of REM suppressants such as alcohol and after the abrupt discontinuation of sedative-hypnotic medications. In addition, certain medications can cause acute RBD; these drugs include SSRIs, tricyclic antidepressants, monoamine oxidase inhibitors, serotonin-norepinephrine reuptake inhibitors, beta-blockers (e.g., bisoprolol, atenolol), anticholinesterase inhibitors, and selegiline. Excessive caffeine and chocolate (Vorona and Ware 2002) may also acutely exacerbate RBD. Regarding chronic RBD, 60% of such cases are idiopathic. The other 40% of chronic RBD cases are often associated with conditions such as multiple sclerosis, subarachnoid hemorrhage, ischemic stroke, brainstem neoplasms, and neurodegenerative disorders such as Parkinson's disease, dementias (e.g., Lewy body dementia), and multiple system atrophy. Indeed, 65% of men age 50 or older with RBD will eventually develop, at a mean of 13 years, a parkinsonian disorder (Ohayon and Schenck 2010). Patients with narcolepsy also have a higher incidence of RBD. In addition to acute and chronic forms of RBD, there is a condition called *pseudo-RBD*. Pseudo-RBD refers to patients who have OSA and dream-enactment behavior but lack evidence of REM sleep without atonia on polysomnography. Treatment of such patients with CPAP eliminates the dream-enactment behavior. Even patients who have both OSA and true RBD have fewer RBD episodes when treated with CPAP.

Differential Diagnosis

The differential diagnosis of RBD includes sleep terrors, sleepwalking, confusional arousals, nocturnal frontal lobe epilepsy, posttraumatic stress disorder (PTSD), and nightmare disorder. Sleep terrors, sleepwalking, and confusional arousals are NREM parasomnias that typically occur in the first third of the night, in contrast to RBD. Nocturnal frontal lobe epilepsy is a seizure disorder characterized by stereotypical movements that most often occur in NREM sleep and rarely in REM sleep; these movements differ from the typically nonstereotypical dream enactment behavior that occurs in REM sleep in patients with RBD. Whereas nocturnal frontal lobe epilepsy is characterized by onset in infancy or childhood with persistence into adulthood, RBD is characterized by an older age at onset. PTSD occurs after exposure to an extremely traumatic stressor and is characterized by recurrent distressing dreams of the traumatic event. Unlike RBD, there are no consistent REM sleep abnormalities seen on polysomnography in patients with PTSD. Nightmare disorder is characterized by recurrent nightmares that generally occur during REM sleep and cause clinically significant impairment or distress in the patient's functioning. Although patients with nightmare disorder may vocalize or move minimally during their dreams, usually they do not have dream enactment with complex motor behaviors paralleling dream content (Silber et al. 2017).

Diagnosis of REM Sleep Behavior Disorder

Per the ICSD-3, for RBD to be diagnosed, all of the following criteria must be present: 1) there must be repeated episodes of vocalization and/or complex motor behaviors during sleep; 2) there is polysomnographic evidence or presumption based on clinical history of dream enactment that these behaviors occur during REM sleep; 3) REM sleep without atonia is seen on polysomnography; and 4) such behaviors are not explained by another disorder, medication, or substance (American Academy of Sleep Medicine 2014). To identify electromyographic activity associated with RBD, the polysomnogram should show either sustained muscle activity in REM sleep on chin electromyogram or excessive transient muscle activity during REM on the chin or limb electromyogram. *Sustained muscle activity* in REM sleep is defined as an epoch of REM sleep with at least 50% of the epoch having a chin electromyographic amplitude greater than the minimum amplitude in NREM sleep. *Excessive transient muscle activity* in REM sleep is defined as a 30-second epoch having at least 15 seconds (50%) of epochs containing bursts of transient muscle activity that are 0.1–5 seconds long and at least four times the amplitude of the background electromyographic activity.

Treatment of REM Sleep Behavior Disorder

The treatment goals of RBD are to reduce the frequency and severity of dream enactment behavior and to prevent injury to the patient and bed partner. All patients with RBD should be advised to take environmental precautions of having the bed partner sleep in another bed or room, locking windows and doors, removing sharp or heavy objects near the sleeping area, and padding the bed and floor near the bed or lowering the mattress to floor level to minimize fall-related injury.

The two medications most commonly used to pharmacologically treat RBD are clonazepam and melatonin. The usual dose of clonazepam ranges from 0.25 mg to 2 mg and is given 30 minutes before bedtime. Clonazepam has been found to dramatically reduce the severity and frequency of dream-enactment behavior, but in some studies it did not eliminate REM sleep without atonia. Because of its long half-life of 30–40 hours, clonazepam can cause side effects such as sedation, confusion, worsened sleep-disordered breathing (e.g., worsened OSA), and increased fall risk. Melatonin, in doses from 3 mg to 15 mg, with a median effective dose of 6 mg, can be used alone or in conjunction with clonazepam to treat RBD. Side effects of melatonin include sedation, hallucinations, morning headaches, and nightmares.

Parasomnias: Key Points

- Parasomnias are abnormal and undesirable motor, verbal, or experiential phenomena that occur during sleep or the sleep-wake transition. Parasomnias can be classified as non–rapid eye movement parasomnias or rapid eye movement (REM) parasomnias.
- REM sleep behavior disorder (RBD) is a REM parasomnia characterized by dream-enactment behavior that is often violent and the presence of REM sleep without atonia on polysomnography.
- The prevalence of RBD increases in adults age 50 years or older and is much more common in men than in women.
- For all patients with RBD, nonpharmacological treatment should include safeguarding the sleeping environment for both the patient and the bed partner. Regarding pharmacological treatment of RBD, the two most common medications used to reduce the frequency and severity of the dream enactment behavior are clonazepam and melatonin.

Circadian Rhythm Sleep-Wake Disorders

Clinical Presentation

Chief Complaint

"I get sleepy early in the evening and awaken earlier in the morning. Then I try falling back asleep but I can't."

Vignette

A 68-year-old woman presents to the clinician's office because she is frustrated with how her sleep schedule has changed in recent years as she has gotten older. When she was younger, she used to get tired around 10 P.M. and wake up around 7 A.M., but over the past few years, her sleep-wake patterns have shifted earlier; she starts feeling tired after eating dinner, goes to sleep around 7 P.M. and wakes up around 3 A.M. When she wakes up around 3 A.M., she is unable to fall back asleep. She denies depression or snoring. Her physical examination and laboratory tests are unremarkable.

The clinician diagnoses the patient with advanced sleep-wake phase disorder (ASWPD). With bright light therapy at 5 P.M., the patient is able to stay awake enough for a few more hours before falling asleep at 9 P.M. and waking up at 5 A.M.

Discussion

Diagnosis and Workup

Circadian rhythms are intrinsic physiological cycles lasting approximately 24 hours that control sleep-wake cycles and other physiological processes. Circadian rhythm sleep-wake disorders (CRSWDs) occur either as the result of a disrupted endogenous circadian clock or as the result of misalignment of the circadian clock and 24-hour social and physical environments. The different types of CRSWD include ASWPD, delayed sleep-wake phase disorder (DSWPD), non-24-hour sleep-wake disorder, irregular rhythm sleep-wake disorder, shift work disorder, and jet lag disorder. In the elderly, the most common circadian rhythm sleep-wake disorder is ASWPD, which is the focus of this section.

Differential Diagnosis

In ASWPD, habitual and involuntary sleep and wake times are typically more than 2 hours earlier compared with societal averages. Briefly, DSWPD occurs when there is a significant delay in the phase of sleep with respect to the required or desired sleep time and wake-up time; patients with DSWPD often have difficulty falling asleep and difficulty waking up at a required or desired clock time. Non-24-hour sleep-wake disorder occurs when there is a disruption in the normal entrainment and synchronization of a patient to a 24-hour circadian rhythm. The true intrinsic biological circadian period length for most people is 24.2 hours, not 24 hours. Normally, exposure of light, which is a strong zeitgeber (i.e., environmental cue that resets the internal body clock) to the suprachiasmatic nucleus, allows the hypothalamus to synchronize the patient's internal time period and entrain the patient to a shorter 24-hour clock day length; in patients who are blind, however, the retinohypothalamic tract is broken, and the subsequent absence of light input to the suprachiasmatic nucleus allows for an intrinsically longer circadian period that is misaligned to the clock day. Irregular rhythm sleep-wake disorder occurs when patients have difficulty synchronizing their sleep time with societal norms for sleep times, and patients often sleep during irregular times during the day or night; patients with neurodegenerative disorders such as dementia often have irregular sleep-wake rhythm disorder. More detailed discussions of the various types of CRSWD are available (Pavlova 2017; Zee et al. 2013). Clinical practice guidelines for the various CRSWDs may be found elsewhere (Auger et al. 2015).

It is important to recognize and treat ASWPD because it has been demonstrated that the shift to morningness with increasing age is associated with a significant worsening in sleep quality (Barbosa et al. 2016). As discussed elsewhere (Tranah et al. 2017), aging is associated with changes in circadian rhythm activity, and older adults with weaker and time-shifted circadian rhythms are at greater risk of death, mild cognitive impairment, dementia, and cardiovascular disease. The prevalence of ASWPD is generally stated to be around 1% in the middle-age population, and this increases with age. Many think that this 1% prevalence may be an underestimate because patients with ASWPD (compared with patients with DSWPD for example) are often better able to adapt to societal and social obligations, so ASWPD may be underrecognized and underreported. ASWPD affects men and women equally.

Diagnosis of Advanced Sleep-Wake Phase Disorder

Patients with ASWPD typically go to sleep between 6 P.M. and 8 P.M. and wake up between 1 A.M. and 3 A.M. despite attempts to delay their sleep-wake times. Polysomnography is not required for the diagnosis of ASWPD. Per the ICSD-3, all of the following criteria must be present to diagnose ASWPD: 1) there is a recurrent difficulty in staying awake or remaining asleep until the required or desired sleep or wake times for at least 3 months; 2) sleep quality and duration improve when patients are allowed to sleep by their own preferred schedule, with the sleep and wake times being consistently in advance of the required or desired conventional sleep or wake times; 3) sleep logs/diaries or actigraphy (wrist-worn devices that measure activity to estimate sleep-wake patterns over time) for at least 7 days (preferably 14 days) that include both work/school and free days demonstrate consistently advanced sleep and wake times; and 4) such advancement in the sleep/wake times is not better explained by another disorder, medication, or substance (American Academy of Sleep Medicine 2014).

Additional diagnostic measures that may be considered are continuous ambulatory monitoring of body temperature and collection of salivary melatonin samples to determine dim light melatonin onset. Body temperature and dim light melatonin onset are physiological markers of circadian timing, and the measurement of such markers in patients with ASWPD can help confirm an advance in circadian phase. Patients with

ASWPD are known to have a dim light melatonin onset and core body temperature minimum that are advanced several hours compared with those in control subjects. Another diagnostic tool that can help determine if patients are morning larks (ASWPD) or night owls (DSWPD) is the Morningness-Eveningness Questionnaire (Horne and Ostberg 1976), also known as the MEQ. The MEQ is composed of 19 questions that elicit responses from patients about their daily sleep-wake habits and the times of day they prefer to perform certain activities.

Treatment of Advanced Sleep-Wake Phase Disorder

Per the 2015 AASM Clinical Practice Guideline for the treatment of circadian rhythm sleep-wake disorder (Auger et al. 2015), one option for treating adult ASWPD is evening light therapy. Generally, recommendations for light therapy are to administer bright light (approximately 4,000 lux) in the evening from 7 P.M. to 9 P.M. The results of another study (Campbell et al. 1993) indicated that the "largest effects were seen after a 12-day treatment of 2 hours of bright white broad spectrum light (~4,000 lux) from 2 light boxes (proximity to source not specified), timed to occur daily between 20:00 and 23:00, and ending before habitual bedtime" (Auger et al. 2015, p. 1210). Light boxes are available over the counter in the United States. There is no evidence to support the use of sleep-promoting medications, melatonin, melatonin agonists, alertness-promoting medications, or combination therapy for patients with ASWPD (Auger et al. 2015). Patients with ASWPD should also avoid exposure to bright light in the morning hours after awakening to avoid further phase advancement of their sleep-wake cycle.

Circadian Rhythm Sleep-Wake Disorders: Key Points

- Advanced sleep-wake phase disorder (ASWPD) is a circadian rhythm sleep-wake disorders characterized by habitual and involuntary sleep and wake times that are typically more than 2 hours earlier compared to societal averages.
- The prevalence of ASWPD increases in the elderly.
- Treatment of ASWPD is the administration of bright light (approximately 4,000 lux) in the evening, typically from 7 P.M. to 9 P.M., and to avoid exposure to bright light in the morning hours after awakening. Melatonin, other medications, and combination therapy have not been supported by evidence to be effective in treating patients with ASWPD.

Hypersomnolence Disorders

Clinical Presentation

Chief Complaint

"A few times a year for the past several years, whenever I hear a particularly funny joke, my knees buckle, I feel really weak in my legs, and then I fall. I remain aware of my surroundings during these episodes."

Vignette

A 65-year-old man presents to the clinician's office with a several-year history of leg weakness and falls that are always precipitated by strong emotions such as laughter. On further history, despite obtaining 7 hours of sleep a night, he also endorses years of excessive daytime sleepiness, which he fights off by drinking 10 cups of coffee daily. The patient also has noticed that when he is about to fall asleep, he occasionally has hallucinations and temporary paralysis. The patient is otherwise healthy, with a normal physical examination and unremarkable laboratory tests. An overnight polysomnogram followed by a multiple sleep latency test (MSLT) are notable for one sleep-onset REM period (SOREMP) in the polysomnogram and another SOREMP on the MSLT. The mean sleep latency from the MSLT is 6 minutes.

The clinician diagnoses the patient with narcolepsy type 1. In addition to scheduling naps, the clinician starts the patient on sodium oxybate (Xyrem) 2.25 grams at bedtime and another 2.25 grams 2–3 hours later. The patient thereafter experiences significant improvement in his symptoms.

Discussion

Diagnosis and Workup

Excessive daytime sleepiness (EDS) is defined as the inability to maintain alertness during waking episodes of the day, with sleep occurring unintentionally or at inappropriate times almost daily for at least 3 months and interfering with the patient's functioning. *Hypersomnia* is a disorder characterized by EDS.

Differential Diagnosis

When a patient presents with EDS, disorders to consider in the differential diagnosis include narcolepsy type 1, narcolepsy type 2, idiopathic hypersomnia, Kleine-Levin syndrome, hypersomnia due to a medical disorder, hypersomnia due to a medication or substance, hypersomnia associated with a psychiatric disorder, and insufficient sleep syndrome. These various types of hypersomnolence of central origin are reviewed elsewhere (Drakatos and Leschziner 2014). In this section we focus on narcolepsy.

Diagnosis of Narcolepsy

Narcolepsy is characterized by EDS and a short REM latency and intrusion of features of REM sleep into wakefulness. The four most common symptoms of narcolepsy are 1) **excessive sleepiness,** which is defined by irrepressible lapses into sleep; 2) **cataplexy,** which is defined as more than one episode of brief (less than 2 minutes), usually bilaterally symmetrical, sudden loss of muscle tone with retained consciousness that is precipitated by strong emotions; 3) **hypnagogic or hypnopompic hallucinations,** which are often bizarre dreamlike images; and 4) **sleep paralysis,** which can be either partial or complete and usually occurs on awakening. Not all narcoleptics have all four of these symptoms, and cataplexy is the only symptom that is specific for narcolepsy. In patients with narcolepsy age 65 or older, cataplexy is significantly less severe compared with that in patients younger than age 65 (Furuta et al. 2001).

In North America and Europe, the prevalence of narcolepsy is 1 in 2,000 (Chakravorty and Rye 2003). Narcolepsy symptoms appear in a bimodal distribution, with most narcoleptic patients experiencing symptoms around the teenage years and a second, smaller peak occurring in older patients around ages 40s to 50s (Quick et al. 2006) or after age 60 (Berry and Wagner 2014). Because narcolepsy is a lifelong disorder, narcolepsy can be seen in older individuals who have had symptoms for many years. As the authors of a review on narcolepsy in older adults concluded, "Elderly narcoleptic patients, despite age-related decrements in sleep quality, are generally less sleepy and less likely to evidence REM sleep dyscontrol" (Chakravorty and Rye 2003, p. 362).

Narcolepsy can be classified as type 1 or type 2, partly depending on whether cataplexy is present or whether there is a deficiency of hypocretin. Hypocretin is produced by cells in the posterolateral hypothalamus and is thought to stabilize wakefulness and sleep transitions and prevent intrusion of REM sleep into wakefulness. It is perhaps not surprising, then, that certain medical disorders can cause narcolepsy. Such disorders include tumors, sarcoidosis, and arteriovenous malformations affecting the hypothalamus; multiple sclerosis plaques impairing the hypothalamus; Parkinson's disease; and multiple system atrophy, to name a few. Per the ICSD-3, there are two ways to diagnose type-1 narcolepsy (American Academy of Sleep Medicine 2014). One way is if the patient has daily lapses into sleep for at least 3 months, cataplexy, an MSLT showing a mean sleep latency of ≤8 minutes, and two SOREMPs on the MSLT (or one SOREMP on an MSLT and one SOREMP that occurs within 15 minutes of sleep onset during the preceding night of polysomnography). The other way to diagnose type-1 narcolepsy is if cerebrospinal fluid hypocretin-1 concentration is ≤110 pg/mL or less than one-third of the mean values obtained in normal subjects with the same standardized assay.

For a diagnosis of narcolepsy type 2 to be made, the following must be present: daily lapses into sleep for at least 3 months, an MSLT showing a mean sleep latency of ≤8 minutes, and two SOREMPs on the MSLT (or one SOREMP on an MSLT and one SOREMP that occurs within 15 minutes of sleep onset during the preceding night of polysomnography). However, in contrast to type-1 narcolepsy, in type-2 narcolepsy, there must also be the absence of cataplexy; cerebrospinal fluid hypocretin-1 concentration has not been measured or is greater than 110 pg/mL (or greater than one-third of the mean values obtained in normal subjects with the same standardized assay); and hypersomnolence or MSLT findings are not better explained by other causes, such as insufficient sleep or OSA.

Treatment of Narcolepsy and Hypersomnias

Treatment of narcolepsy involves treating excessive sleepiness, cataplexy, sleep-related hallucinations, and sleep paralysis. Nonpharmacological measures include 7–8 hours of sleep nightly and scheduled daytime naps to improve symptoms. Pharmacological treatment of narcolepsy includes sodium oxybate (Xyrem), which is the only medication approved by the U.S. Food and Drug Administration (FDA) to treat both excessive sleepiness and cataplexy. Sodium oxybate is also known as γ-hydroxybutyrate or the "date-rape drug." As such, sodium oxybate is dispensed only from one central pharmacy and, because of its short half-life, must be given in divided doses; the first dose is at bedtime and the second dose is taken 2–3 hours later. Because sodium oxybate is rich in sodium, sodium oxybate is contraindicated in patients with heart failure. Alerting agents such as modafinil and armodafinil, as well as stimulants such as methylphenidate and dextroamphetamine, are FDA approved to treat excessive sleepiness. Aside from sodium oxybate, various types of antidepressants, such as fluoxetine and venlafaxine, may be used to treat cataplexy. Tricyclic antidepressants can also treat cataplexy; however, associated anticholinergic side effects such as dry mouth, blurred vision, urinary retention, constipation, and orthostatic hypotension may limit their use in the elderly population (Wolkove et al. 2007). Treatment of sleep-related hallucinations and sleep paralysis is the same as that for cataplexy.

Hypersomnolence Disorders: Key Points

- Narcolepsy is a disorder of hypersomnolence characterized by excessive sleepiness, cataplexy, hypnagogic or hypnopompic hallucinations, and sleep-related paralysis.
- Cataplexy is the only symptom specific for narcolepsy. One study suggests that cataplexy is less severe in patients age 65 or older compared with patients younger than 65.
- Narcolepsy symptoms appear in a bimodal distribution, with most narcoleptic patients experiencing symptoms during their teenage years, but others experiencing symptoms in older age (age 40s or older than 60 depending on the reference).
- In contrast to type-2 narcolepsy, type-1 narcolepsy is a disorder that includes cataplexy and hypocretin deficiency
- Sodium oxybate (Xyrem) is the only medication that is approved by the U.S. Food and Drug Administration to treat excessive sleepiness and cataplexy. Alerting agents and stimulants can also be used to treat excessive daytime sleepiness. Antidepressants, including fluoxetine and venlafaxine, are effective in treating cataplexy, sleep-related hallucinations, and sleep paralysis.

KEY POINTS

- Sleep disorders in the elderly are often increased in prevalence compared to that in younger adults.
- Although older adults experience some changes to their sleep that are part of normal aging, many sleep disorders exist that do not constitute normal aging and can significantly affect the quality of life of older adults.
- Sleep disorders prevalent in the elderly include obstructive sleep apnea and other sleep-related breathing disorders, restless legs syndrome and other sleep-related movement disorders, rapid eye movement sleep behavior disorder and other parasomnias, advanced sleep-wake phase disorder and other circadian rhythm sleep-wake disorders, and narcolepsy and other hypersomnolence disorders.

Sleep-onset and sleep-maintenance insomnia are also prevalent in older adults and are discussed further in Chapter 8, "Evaluation and Management of Insomnia."

- These various sleep disorders not only have clear-cut diagnostic criteria but also have effective treatments.
- If untreated, sleep disorders can increase the risk of falls and depression, among other ailments, in the elderly. Understanding the diverse spectrum of sleep disorders that can affect older adults is therefore crucial to optimizing the physical and emotional health of the elderly population. By improving the sleep quality of older adults, clinlicians can also improve their quality of life.

Resources

Organizations With Educational Resources for Clinicians and Patients

American Academy of Sleep Medicine: https://aasm.org (sleep education at www.sleepeducation.org)
American Sleep Association: www.sleepassociation.org
National Health Sleep Awareness Project: www.sleepeducation.org/healthysleep
National Sleep Foundation: https://sleepfoundation.org
Sleep Research Society: www.sleepresearchsociety.org

Patient Advocacy Organizations

American Sleep Apnea Association: www.sleepapnea.org
Circadian Sleep Disorders Network: www.circadiansleepdisorders.org
Narcolepsy Network: http://narcolepsynetwork.org
Restless Legs Syndrome Foundation: www.rls.org
Wake Up Narcolepsy: www.wakeupnarcolepsy.org

References

Allen RP, Walters AS, Montplaisir J, et al: Restless legs syndrome prevalence and impact: REST general population study. Arch Intern Med 165(11):1286–1292, 2005 15956009
American Academy of Sleep Medicine: International Classification of Sleep Disorders, 3rd Edition. Darien, IL, American Academy of Sleep Medicine, 2014
American Psychiatric Association: Diagnostic and Statistical Manual of Mental Disorders, 5th Edition. Arlington, VA, American Psychiatric Association, 2013

Auger RR, Burgess HJ, Emens JS, et al: Clinical practice guideline for the treatment of intrinsic circadian rhythm sleep-wake disorders: advanced sleep-wake phase disorder (ASWPD), delayed sleep-wake phase disorder (DSWPD), non-24-hour sleep-wake rhythm disorder (N24SWD), and irregular sleep-wake rhythm disorder (ISWRD). An update for 2015: an American Academy of Sleep Medicine Clinical Practice Guideline. J Clin Sleep Med 11(1):1199–1236, 2015 26414986

Barbé F, Durán-Cantolla J, Sánchez-de-la-Torre M, et al: Effect of continuous positive airway pressure on the incidence of hypertension and cardiovascular events in nonsleepy patients with obstructive sleep apnea: a randomized controlled trial. JAMA 307(20):2161–2168, 2012 22618923

Barbosa AA, Miguel MAL, Tufik S, et al: Sleep disorder or simple sleep ontogeny? Tendency for morningness is associated with worse sleep quality in the elderly. Braz J Med Biol Res 49(10):e5311, 2016 27737315

Berry RB, Wagner MH: Hypersomnolence of Central Origin—I, in Sleep Medicine Pearls, 3rd Edition. Philadelphia, PA, Saunders, 2014, pp 477–483

Campbell SS, Dawson D, Anderson MW: Alleviation of sleep maintenance insomnia with timed exposure to bright light. J Am Geriatr Soc 41(8):829–836, 1993 8340561

Centers for Medicare & Medicaid Services: Continuous Positive Airway Pressure (CPAP) Therapy for Obstructive Sleep Apnea (OSA)—JA6048. Medicare Learning Network, Provider Inquiry Assistance. Baltimore, MD, Centers for Medicare and Medicaid Services, October 15, 2008. Available at: https://www.cms.gov/Medicare/Medicare-Contracting/ContractorLearningResources/downloads/JA6048.pdf. Accessed October 26, 2018.

Centers for Medicare & Medicaid Services: CPAP for Obstructive Sleep Apnea. Baltimore, MD, Centers for Medicare and Medicaid Services, 2016. Available at: https://www.cms.gov/Medicare/Coverage/Coverage-with-Evidence-Development/CPAP.html. Accessed July 2, 2018.

Chakravorty SS, Rye DB: Narcolepsy in the older adult: epidemiology, diagnosis and management. Drugs Aging 20(5):361–376, 2003 12696996

Dalmases M, Solé-Padullés C, Torres M, et al: Effect of CPAP on cognition, brain function, and structure among elderly patients with OSA: a randomized pilot study. Chest 148(5):1214–1223, 2015 26065720

Drakatos P, Leschziner GD: Update on hypersomnias of central origin. Curr Opin Pulm Med 20(6):572–580, 2014 25165990

Figorilli M, Puligheddu M, Ferri R: Restless legs syndrome/Willis-Ekbom disease and periodic limb movements in sleep in the elderly with and without dementia. Sleep Med Clin 10(3):331–342, xiv–xv, 2015 26329443

Furuta H, Thorpy MJ, Temple HM: Comparison in symptoms between aged and younger patients with narcolepsy. Psychiatry Clin Neurosci 55(3):241–242, 2001 11422857

Guilleminault C, Lin CM, Gonçalves MA, et al: A prospective study of nocturia and the quality of life of elderly patients with obstructive sleep apnea or sleep onset insomnia. J Psychosom Res 56(5):511–515, 2004 15172207

Guillot M, Sforza E, Achour-Crawford E, et al: Association between severe obstructive sleep apnea and incident arterial hypertension in the older people population. Sleep Med 14(9):838–842, 2013 23831239

Horne JA, Ostberg O: A self-assessment questionnaire to determine morning-ness-eveningness in human circadian rhythms. Int J Chronobiol 4(2):97–110, 1976 1027738

Johns MW: Daytime sleepiness, snoring, and obstructive sleep apnea. The Epworth Sleepiness Scale. Chest 103(1):30–36, 1993 8417909

Jones TM, Earis JE, Calverley PM, et al: Snoring surgery: a retrospective review. Laryngoscope 115(11):2010–2015, 2005 16319615

Kapur VK, Auckley DH, Chowdhuri S, et al: Clinical practice guideline for diagnostic testing for adult obstructive sleep apnea: an American Academy of Sleep Medicine clinical practice guideline. J Clin Sleep Med 13(3):479–504, 2017 28162150

Kaynak H, Kaynak D, Oztura I: Does frequency of nocturnal urination reflect the severity of sleep-disordered breathing? J Sleep Res 13(2):173–176, 2004 15175098

Lewis EF, Wang R, Punjabi N, et al: Impact of continuous positive airway pressure and oxygen on health status in patients with coronary heart disease, cardiovascular risk factors, and obstructive sleep apnea: A Heart Biomarker Evaluation in Apnea Treatment (HEARTBEAT) analysis. Am Heart J 189:59–67, 2017 28625382

Malhotra RK, Avidan AY: Parasomnias and their mimics. Neurol Clin 30(4):1067–1094, 2012 23099130

Martínez-García MA, Campos-Rodríguez F, Catalán-Serra P, et al: Cardiovascular mortality in obstructive sleep apnea in the elderly: role of long-term continuous positive airway pressure treatment: a prospective observational study. Am J Respir Crit Care Med 186(9):909–916, 2012 22983957

Mehra R, Benjamin EJ, Shahar E, et al: Association of nocturnal arrhythmias with sleep-disordered breathing: The Sleep Heart Health Study. Am J Respir Crit Care Med 173(8):910–916, 2006 16424443

Ohayon MM, Schenck CH: Violent behavior during sleep: prevalence, comorbidity and consequences. Sleep Med 11(9):941–946, 2010 20817553

Osorio RS, Gumb T, Pirraglia E, et al: Sleep-disordered breathing advances cognitive decline in the elderly. Neurology 84(19):1964–1971, 2015 25878183

Pavlova M: Circadian rhythm sleep-wake disorders. Continuum (Minneap Minn) 23(4, Sleep Neurology):1051–1063, 2017 28777176

Quick AD, Black DN, Attarian HP: New-onset narcolepsy with cataplexy in a geriatric patient. Sleep Med 7(6):533, 2006 16931149

Sateia MJ: International classification of sleep disorders-third edition: highlights and modifications. Chest 146(5):1387–1394, 2014 25367475

Silber MH, Ehrenberg BL, Allen RP, et al: An algorithm for the management of restless legs syndrome. Mayo Clin Proc 79(7):916–922, 2004 15244390

Silber MH, St. Louis EK, Boeve BF: Rapid eye movement sleep parasomnia, in Principles and Practice of Sleep Medicine, 6th Edition. Edited by Kryger M, Roth T, Dement WC. Philadelphia, PA, Elsevier, 2017, pp 993–1001

Strollo PJJr, Soose RJ, Maurer JT, et al: Upper-airway stimulation for obstructive sleep apnea. N Engl J Med 370(2):139–149, 2014 24401051

Tishler PV, Larkin EK, Schluchter MD, et al: Incidence of sleep-disordered breathing in an urban adult population: the relative importance of risk factors in the development of sleep-disordered breathing. JAMA 289(17):2230–2237, 2003 12734134

Tranah GJ, Stone KL, Ancoli-Israel S: Circadian rhythms in older adults, in Principles and Practice of Sleep Medicine, 6th Edition. Edited by Kryger M, Roth T, Dement WC. Philadelphia, PA, Elsevier, 2017, pp 1510–1515

Trotti LM: Restless legs syndrome and sleep-related movement disorders. Continuum (Minneap Minn) 23(4, Sleep Neurology):1005–1016, 2017 28777173

Vorona RD, Ware JC: Exacerbation of REM sleep behavior disorder by chocolate ingestion: a case report. Sleep Med 3(4):365–367, 2002 14592201

Weaver TE, Chasens ER: Continuous positive airway pressure treatment for sleep apnea in older adults. Sleep Med Rev 11(2):99–111, 2007 17275370

Wolkove N, Elkholy O, Baltzan M, et al: Sleep and aging: 2. Management of sleep disorders in older people. CMAJ 176(10):1449–1454, 2007 17485699

Young T, Peppard PE, Gottlieb DJ: Epidemiology of obstructive sleep apnea: a population health perspective. Am J Respir Crit Care Med 165(9):1217–1239, 2002a 11991871

Young T, Shahar E, Nieto FJ, et al: Predictors of sleep-disordered breathing in community-dwelling adults: The Sleep Heart Health Study. Arch Intern Med 162(8):893–900, 2002b 11966340

Zee PC, Attarian H, Videnovic A: Circadian rhythm abnormalities. Continuum (Minneap Minn) 19(1 Sleep Disorders):132–147, 2013 23385698

Evaluation and Management of Insomnia

"My Sleeping Pill Isn't Working Anymore"

Erin L. Cassidy-Eagle, Ph.D., CBSM, DBSM
Laura B. Dunn, M.D.
Oxana Palesh, Ph.D., M.P.H.

Clinical Presentation

Chief Complaint

"My sleeping pill isn't working anymore."

Vignette

Mr. V is a 76-year-old divorced man. He was referred by his primary care physician, who reports that the patient is experiencing insomnia and desires behavioral treatment because his zolpidem "is no longer working."

Mr. V retired approximately 1 year ago from his 30-year career as an engineer for a large technology company. He was married for 25 years, has two grown sons, and was divorced about 10 years ago. He is currently living alone in his home. He previously enjoyed playing tennis and serving on the boards of other local organizations, though for both physical and cognitive reasons (e.g.,"I don't feel as sharp as I used to"), he has stopped doing both.

Two months into his retirement, about 10 months ago, he went to the emergency department with complaints of dizziness and shortness of breath. After heart monitoring uncovered an irregular heartbeat, he underwent surgery to have a pacemaker placed. He recovered well, and he reports that he is in otherwise good health.

He reports that his sleep really began to deteriorate about 6 months ago. His primary care physician initiated zolpidem (5 mg), which appeared to help him to sleep for about 2 months. However, despite an increase of the zolpidem dosage to 10 mg after 2 months, he now states that he gets in bed at 11 P.M., spends several prolonged periods at night awake, and has to force himself to get out of bed at 10 A.M. He reports that he doesn't intentionally nap during the day. However, he does acknowledge that he frequently falls asleep while watching television in the evening.

Interdisciplinary Team Commentary

Psychiatrist: I would like to know whether Mr. V's symptoms may meet criteria for another psychiatric disorder, particularly depression or anxiety, because both of these (or the combination) could certainly affect his sleep. I would also like to know whether he may have symptoms of another primary sleep disorder such as obstructive sleep apnea (OSA). However, even if I diagnose him with a depressive or anxiety disorder, we still will need to address his sleep habits, rather than assume that they will "fix themselves" if his depression or anxiety is treated. Mr. V's comment that the zolpidem "isn't working anymore" makes me worry that he wants a "magic pill" for his sleep, so I would want to try to address this in the first visit. I would want to know more about what goes through his head when he is awake in the middle of the night, as well as what he actually does during this time. (Does he stay in bed or move to another room? Does he take some other type of medication or drink?) From a medication perspective, I would want to gradually wean him off the zolpidem, with his agreement (over a few weeks or months), while working collaboratively with the rest of the team—particularly the psychologist or other behavioral provider with expertise in sleep—on addressing his sleep-related thoughts and behaviors. What I would *not* want to do is replace his zolpidem with another sedative-hypnotic, because then the cycle will just be perpetuated. Moreover, giving him another hypnotic would work to counteract the efforts of the psychologist and send the wrong message.

Clinical psychologist: I would want to do a thorough evaluation of Mr. V's sleep and wakefulness patterns. It is particularly helpful if the patient can fill out a "sleep log" for the 1–2 weeks prior to the intake appointment. Key elements of the schedule include when he typically goes to bed, wakes up, and actually gets up out of bed. This is particularly important for Mr. V, because he is clearly spending much more time in bed than he could reasonably be expected to sleep, so it is not surprising that he is awake for extended periods. I would want to know about the quality of his sleep, such as how much time he spends awake after falling asleep and the estimate of total time spent sleeping. I would ask about behavioral and environmental factors, such as whether he engages in other activities in bed (e.g., watching television) and the qualities of the sleep environment, such as temperature, light, and noise. I would ask about daytime functioning, in particular whether he is physically active, withdrawing socially, or spending time napping, intentionally or unintentionally. Screening for other primary sleep disorders (e.g., sleep apnea, restless legs syndrome [RLS], parasomnias, or circadian rhythm disorders) as well as comorbid mood, anxiety, or substance use disorders would also be part of my intake. I would work closely with my psychiatrist or primary care colleague to make sure we had some behavioral sleep recommendations on board before Mr. V attempted to decrease or change his sleep medication. An important part of the intake is finding out whether the patient is sufficiently motivated and committed to trying behavioral interventions, because there are some patients who are seeking a "magic pill," as my psychiatrist colleague mentioned. Helpful tools for assessing sleep are also used prospectively to monitor progress and adjust recommendations over time (see the subsection "Helpful Sleep Assessment Tools" later in this chapter).

Discussion

Diagnosis

Sleep disturbances, and insomnia specifically, are often a leading complaint of older adults, who may also be experiencing comorbid mood and anxiety symptoms. They are both cause and consequence of a multitude of medical, social, and age-related factors. The American Psychiatric Association's (2013) *Diagnostic and Statistical Manual of Mental Disorders,* 5th Edition (DSM-5), defines *insomnia* as dissatisfaction with the quality or quantity of sleep manifested as difficulty with sleep initiation, maintenance, or waking earlier than planned. These difficulties occur despite the opportunity for adequate sleep, occur 3 or more nights per week over the course of at least 3 months, and cause the individual distress or other symptoms of impairment, such as excessive daytime sleepiness and daytime fatigue. The *International Classifica-*

tion of Sleep Disorders, 3rd Edition (ICSD-3; American Academy of Sleep Medicine 2014), which has considerable overlap with the DSM-5 criteria, includes difficulty initiating or maintaining sleep, daytime consequences, and symptoms not attributable to an inadequate opportunity for sleep. Patients taking hypnotic medications to aid their sleep may report symptoms that meet these criteria when not taking their medication and, as such, also meet criteria for chronic insomnia, particularly if these patients are presenting clinically with complaints and request for treatment.

Causes and Consequences

Insomnia is a treatable condition and the most frequently encountered sleep disorder in primary care settings. One in five patients has a lifetime risk of experiencing a diagnosable level of insomnia at some point, with half of those experiencing a chronic course. Increasing age, female gender, comorbid medical and mental disorders, and lower socioeconomic status all serve as risk factors for developing insomnia, so it is not surprising that almost 40% of those age 65 years and older report experiencing some form of sleep disruption (Foley et al. 2004). Increasing rates of comorbid psychiatric and medical illnesses, side effects from the medications used to treat these problems, increased nocturia, and other primary sleep disorders, such as sleep apnea and RLS, serve to further complicate the clinical picture of the older patient with insomnia. Persistent insomnia also puts the individual at risk of developing neuropsychiatric disorders (Spiegelhalder et al. 2013), depression, suicidal ideation and behavior (Pigeon et al. 2012), alcohol dependence, metabolic syndrome, hypertension, and cardiac disease. Importantly, chronic insomnia also increases the rate of all-cause mortality (Parthasarathy et al. 2015), even after control for variables including age, gender, marital status, hypnotic use, body mass index, habitual snoring, smoking, sleep opportunity (>7 hours), diabetes mellitus, serum C-reactive protein levels, and baseline heart disease.

Table 8–1 lists key factors that may precipitate onset of insomnia in older adults, and Table 8–2 lists the key elements in the assessment and comprehensive evaluation of insomnia.

Insomnia is also associated with negative consequences, including depressive symptoms, daytime impairment, decreased quality of life, and increased health care utilization (Foley et al. 2004; Hatoum et al. 1998). McKinnon et al. (2014) found that depression symptoms, impaired cognition, antidepressant use, and alcohol consumption, in addition to age and education, were all significant predictors of poor sleep

TABLE 8–1. Key factors that may precipitate onset of insomnia

Life changes (e.g., retirement, move to senior housing)

Serious health events (e.g., pacemaker)

Withdrawal from or lack of engagement in social and or physical activities (e.g., stopped tennis, stopped part-time work)

Loss of a loved one

Possible in-visit follow-up questions:

What activities are you currently engaging in both inside and outside of your home?

What is a typical day like?

Are you experiencing daytime symptoms, such as sleepiness (i.e., struggling to stay awake while at the movies or riding on a bus to community activities)?

Are you willing to fill out a sleep log so that we may better understand your sleep patterns?

quality. Sleep problems can occur in the context of declining health status and acute and chronic stressors caused by life transitions and loss. In addition, environmental factors such as light, noise, and the lack of a set schedule in senior residential settings can also disrupt the individual's sleep schedule and result in new concerns. Older patients frequently attempt to combat these shifts by engaging in what are believed to be sleep compensatory behaviors, such as spending more time in bed, as well as having more intense feelings of worry with regard to their health and what amount of sleep they "should" be getting. Decreased activity levels, napping (both planned and unplanned), and comorbid medical conditions are three of the most common variables that fuel daytime sleepiness and disrupt the sleep schedule across the entire 24 hours of each day (Martin et al. 2006).

Key Factors That May Perpetuate Insomnia

Factors that serve to perpetuate insomnia can include a wide range of efforts, both behavioral and cognitive, that may have some short-term efficacy but over time accumulate into a set of efforts that further fuel patients' frustration as they stop helping. For example, while gathering the patient history and details of their symptoms, the clinician may dis-

TABLE 8–2.   Key elements in the assessment and comprehensive evaluation of insomnia

History and nature of sleep complaints

Typical sleep-wake schedule (i.e., bedtime/rise time, latency, time spent awake, total sleep time)

Onset, duration, frequency, severity, course, and perpetuating factors

Sleep environment

Daytime/wake consequences (i.e., fatigue, depression) and behaviors (i.e., napping, canceling activities, using bed for other activities besides sleep and sex)

Screen for other primary sleep disorders (e.g., sleep apnea, restless legs syndrome) and refer to sleep center, if suspected.

Medical (e.g., neurological, pulmonary, cardiovascular) and psychiatric (e.g. mood disorders, anxiety disorders) comorbid conditions

History of sleep assessments ("sleep study") and what type

Pain

Medications (both prescribed and over-the-counter)

Alcohol and drugs

The patient's current approach to "treating" symptoms (e.g., Is the patient consuming more alcohol or over-the-counter sleep aids, or using other prescription medication [e.g., those targeting another symptom such as anxiety] to aid sleep?)

cover that the patient has developed conditioned arousal around sleep preparation and processes (i.e., connecting being awake with being in bed), a range of cognitive distortions around sleep expectations and norms, and sleep behaviors that negatively impact the ability to sleep. Although particular behaviors, such as staying in bed while awake for extended periods or extending the sleep window in hopes of obtaining more sleep, feel initially useful, they serve to perpetuate the patient's difficulties in obtaining adequate and consolidated sleep over time.

Helpful Sleep Assessment Tools

Subjective Self-Report Measures

The cornerstone of any sleep assessment and treatment is the prospective sleep diary. A snapshot of a sleep diary, adapted from the consensus sleep diary (Carney et al. 2012) used with our population of older adults, is shown in Figure 8–1.

Subject ID: _____

Sleep log	Sample	Day 1	Day 2	Day 3	Day 4	Day 5	Day 6	Day 7
1. What time did you get into bed?	10:15 pm							
2. What time did you try to go to sleep?	11:30 pm							
3. How long did it take you to fall asleep (minutes)?	55 min.							
4. How many times did you wake up, not counting your final awakening?	3 times							
5. In total, how long did these awakenings last?	1 hour 10 min.							
6. What time was your final awakening?	6:35 am							
7. What time did you get out of bed for the day?	7 am							
8. How much alcohol did you drink last night?	2 drinks							
9. Did you take over-the-counter or prescription medication to help you sleep?	No							
10. How many times did you nap?	2 times							
11. How would you rate the quality of your sleep?	☐ Very poor ☐ Poor ☐ Fair ☐ Good ☐ Very good	☐ Very poor ☐ Poor ☐ Fair ☐ Good ☐ Very good	☐ Very poor ☐ Poor ☐ Fair ☐ Good ☐ Very good	☐ Very poor ☐ Poor ☐ Fair ☐ Good ☐ Very good	☐ Very poor ☐ Poor ☐ Fair ☐ Good ☐ Very good	☐ Very poor ☐ Poor ☐ Fair ☐ Good ☐ Very good	☐ Very poor ☐ Poor ☐ Fair ☐ Good ☐ Very good	☐ Very poor ☐ Poor ☐ Fair ☐ Good ☐ Very good

For office use only | SOL | WAKE | WASO | TST | TIB | SE |

FIGURE 8–1. Sample sleep log.

SE = sleep efficiency; SOL = sleep onset latency; TIB = time in bed; TST = total sleep time; WAKE = last awakening/time of rise; WASO = wake after sleep onset.

In addition, screening the patient for other possible primary sleep disorders, many of which increase in prevalence along with increasing age, is an essential part of an assessment. There are some useful tools the clinician can use to screen for the presence of other primary sleep disorders: the Global Sleep Assessment Questionnaire (GSAQ; Roth et al. 2002) for multiple sleep disorders and STOP-BANG for OSA (Chung et al. 2008) are two frequently relied on measures.

The need to identify comorbid psychiatric disorders, such as depression and anxiety, is also a standard part of the intake. Quick and easy-to-score measures include the Patient Health Questionnaire (PHQ)–9 and PHQ-2 (Kroenke et al. 2001) and the Geriatric Depression Scale (Yesavage et al. 1982–1983) for depression and the Generalized Anxiety Disorder (GAD)–7 for anxiety (Spitzer et al. 2006).

The clinician could also consider using a common screening measure to get a baseline snapshot of the presence of insomnia. The Insomnia Severity Index (ISI; Morin et al. 2011) is a quick seven-item survey that helps to determine whether the patient's symptoms meet diagnostic levels of impairment. It can be administered over time to assess the patient's overall response to treatment and the degree of subjective change experienced. This is a key consideration because the diagnosis of insomnia is based on subjective patient reports, and hence, so is the success of the chosen intervention.

Finally, the Epworth Sleepiness Scale (Johns 1991) is used primarily in sleep clinics and research to assess daytime sleepiness, a commonly reported correlate of disrupted sleep in the elderly.

Wrist Actigraphy

Actigraphy is increasing in popularity in both clinical and research endeavors and provides an objective assessment of sleep parameters, such as time in bed, number and length of nighttime awakenings, and sleep efficiency (proportion of actual sleep time relative to intended sleep time/time in bed). An actigraph device is worn on the wrist for the purpose of recording activity counts that can be used to approximate sleep parameters; these devices provide a useful alternative to laboratory sleep studies for older adults (Morgenthaler et al. 2007) because they are cheaper than the sleep study, can be used over longer periods of time, and are generally more acceptable to patients. Actigraphy is particularly useful when combined with the use of a sleep diary, which is daily recording of approximate sleep schedules by the individual or their caregivers (Carney et al. 2012). However, the use of actigraphy remains largely in the research domain because there is a large effort involved in the data extraction, data cleaning, and scoring.

Polysomnography

Polysomnography, also called an *overnight sleep study*, is a test used to diagnose primary sleep disorders. The equipment records the patients' brain waves, oxygen level in the blood, heart rate, and breathing, as well as eye and leg movements, over the course of one night in the sleep center. If the patient is suspected of having another primary sleep disorder (e.g., OSA), then a referral to a sleep center for an overnight study (i.e., polysomnography) is necessary. Polysomnography can be also conducted at home depending on the rule-out diagnosis.

Insomnia Interventions

There are two main treatment options for insomnia: 1) multicomponent cognitive-behavioral interventions and 2) pharmacotherapy. Cognitive-behavioral therapy for insomnia (CBT-I) has considerable support as the recommended first-line treatment (Qaseem et al. 2016), although actual studies of interventions used in primary care settings reveal that implementation of such strategies by non–sleep specialists remains limited.

A consensus conference focused on insomnia, organized by the National Institutes of Health in 2005, found that both CBT-I and benzodiazepine agonists were effective short-term treatments of insomnia. More recently, in 2016, the American College of Physicians produced their own clinical practice guideline, in which they recommended multicomponent CBT-I as the first-line treatment for insomnia for all patients (Qaseem et al. 2016). They emphasized that pharmacotherapy, which has insufficient efficacy for insomnia, should only be considered as an option when patients are unable to participate in CBT-I; as adjunctive treatment for those with residual symptoms who are receiving, or have received, CBT-I; or, in rare cases, as an initial adjunct to those currently starting CBT-I. See Figure 8–2 for a basic treatment algorithm for patients with insomnia.

Cognitive and Behavioral Treatments

Multicomponent CBT-I addresses the behavioral and cognitive factors that serve to fuel insomnia. After starting with sleep education around the mechanisms underlying sleep, CBT-I includes some combination of relaxation training, sleep restriction therapy, stimulus control therapy, cognitive therapy, and sleep hygiene. CBT-I focuses on developing healthy sleep behaviors, addressing thought processes that interfere with sleep, and giving patients a set of skills that can be utilized whenever they face a prolonged period of sleep issues.

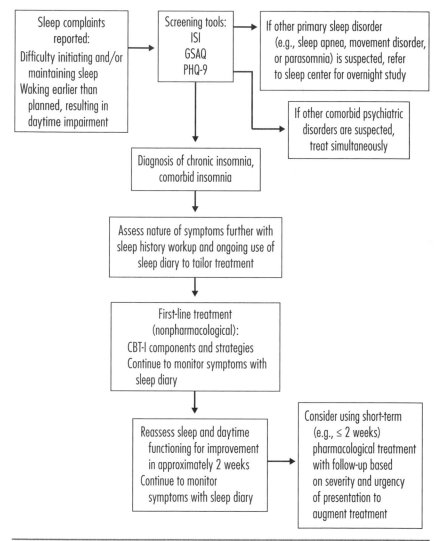

FIGURE 8–2.   Treatment algorithm for insomnia.

CBT-I=cognitive-behavioral therapy for insomnia; GSAQ=Global Sleep Assessment Questionnaire; ISI=Insomnia Severity Index; PHQ=Patient Health Questionnaire.

   Meta-analyses illustrate the effectiveness of CBT-I in the treatment of a range of parameters involved in insomnia in both adult (Geiger-Brown et al. 2015; Trauer et al. 2015) and older adult populations. Specifically, CBT-I has been shown to improve sleep latency (e.g., shorten the time it takes to fall asleep), sleep maintenance (e.g., decrease the amount of time spent awake in the middle of the night), sleep efficiency (e.g., increase the time spent asleep/time spent in bed), and, to a lesser degree, total sleep time. In fact, a study comparing 6–10 weeks of CBT-I with pharmacotherapy revealed that CBT-I had equal to superior effects, with improvements holding steady for many participants at a 3-year follow-up (Mitchell et al. 2012).

One of the core behavioral components of CBT-I is sleep restriction (Spielman et al. 1987), which involves looking at the amount of time the patient actually spends asleep and working to sync that up with the amount of time the patient spends in bed. This approach is one that the provider needs to monitor, because it often results in some sleep deprivation, which can initially worsen daytime symptoms (e.g., sleepiness, decreased reaction time) and is not recommended in some populations (e.g., those with certain psychiatric conditions such as bipolar disorder).

In older adults, a more gradual approach, known as sleep compression, can be especially useful in those with comorbid medical conditions and those who present safety issues (e.g., mobility limitations that place the patient at risk of falling). The other key behavioral component that has been found effective with older adults, stimulus control (Engle-Friedman et al. 1992), involves efforts to strengthen the association of the bed with sleeping. As older adults spend more time in bed awake and engaging in other activities, due to pain or fatigue, they begin to associate being in bed with being awake. Recommendations include 1) going to bed only when sleepy; 2) getting out of bed when unable to sleep; 3) using the bed/bedroom only for sleep and sex (i.e., no reading, watching television); 4) arising at the same time every morning; and 5) avoiding naps. Cognitive techniques, similar to methods with other psychiatric disorders, aim to correct faulty underlying beliefs and attitudes about sleep and teach patients methods to control their active minds to the extent that such cognitive activity interferes with sleep. Relaxation therapy and meditation work to decrease physiological and mental arousal. Finally, sleep hygiene ensures that the patient is not engaging in sleep-interfering behaviors. Although this element is not effective in isolation from the other components and techniques, it is considered necessary to improving sleep and can include recommendations around exercise, caffeine, and the sleep environment.

For the primary care setting, or when time with the patient is limited, brief behavioral treatment for insomnia (BBT-I) is the recommended choice because of its simplicity and established effectiveness (Buysse et al. 2011). This version emphasizes sleep education and four main behavioral recommendations, including to 1) reduce time in bed; 2) get up at the same time every day, regardless of sleep duration; 3) not go to bed unless sleepy; and 4) not stay in bed unless asleep. Napping is also discouraged in BBT-I. See Table 8–3 for specific behavioral treatment recommendations to use with patients who have insomnia, based on presenting complaint.

In addition to a greater reliance on pharmacotherapy (discussed below), non–sleep specialists/providers often include recommendations around optimal or healthy sleep hygiene practices (e.g., decreasing caffeine, optimizing the sleep environment) that have been found to be "necessary but not sufficient" in treating insomnia if recommended in isolation from the other components of CBT-I (Irish et al. 2015). These findings create an exciting target for change in primary care settings.

Pharmacological Treatments

As stated earlier, both behavioral and pharmacological agents are indicated for management of insomnia that is of new onset or acute. Pharmacological agents are effective particularly for insomnia that is precipitated by a transient trigger and that is unlikely to become chronic. However, there are several concerns associated with use of sleep medication, and they center on issues of safety, habit formation, and dependency (Bertisch et al. 2014). In addition, sleep medications do not address the underlying cause of insomnia and only work for addressing the symptoms. Once the medications are stopped, patients might experience a return of insomnia symptoms or rebound insomnia. Despite the low quality of evidence in support of pharmacotherapy, particularly beyond a few months, national surveys have reported monthly use of hypnotic medications that range from 2% to 7%, with older adults reporting the highest usage (Chong et al. 2013). Therefore, providers need to be informed regarding the evidence around specific medications.

For a detailed review of pharmacological agents used to treat insomnia, including graded quality of evidence, see the American Academy of Sleep Medicine's recently published clinical practice guideline (Sateia et al. 2017). In brief, the convened task force of experts in sleep medicine found only "weak" evidence for recommending a number of pharmacological agents for sleep-onset and sleep-maintenance insomnia, indicating less certainty than a "strong" recommendation about the appropriateness of the treatment, although not a statement regarding ineffectiveness. These recommendations are listed below; however, it should be noted that they were made for adults, not for older adults. Therefore, additional caution in prescribing any of these agents to older adults is extremely important. The guidelines stress the importance of assessing risk of harm on an individual basis. Therefore, although the guidelines found weak evidence for two benzodiazepines (triazolam and

TABLE 8–3. Nonpharmacological/behavioral patient care guide for insomnia

Patient complaint	What to ask	Possible strategies to recommend
Possible cause: Unhelpful sleep behaviors		
"I have trouble falling asleep." "I wake up in the middle of the night and remain awake." "I wake up too early." "I'm tired and have difficulty concentrating during the day."	Utilize a sleep diary: How much time do you spend in bed vs. actually sleeping? When is your usual bedtime and rise time?	Consider sleep restriction/compression. Aim to shrink time spent in bed to align more closely to the time spent sleeping in order to strengthen homeostatic sleep drive and consolidate sleep.
Possible cause: Circadian misalignment		
"I fall asleep too early and wake up in the middle of the night almost every day."	Utilize a sleep diary: Is the sleep time consistently shifted earlier or later? Is the amount of sleep you're getting interfering with your work or quality of life (i.e., who is it a problem for)?	Regulate sleep schedule. Time bright-light exposure: in the evening if falling asleep too early, in the morning if tending to sleep too late. Get up at the same time 7 days a week, regardless of sleep amount. Establish a nighttime wind-down period before bedtime. Remove electronics from bedroom.

TABLE 8–3. Nonpharmacological/behavioral patient care guide for insomnia (*continued*)

Patient complaint	What to ask	Possible strategies to recommend
Possible cause: Conditioned arousal		
"I can't shut my mind off when I get in bed or when I wake up in the middle of the night."	What are you thinking about (i.e., stressors or reviewing your day)?	Strengthen the association of bed with sleep and reduce arousal (stimulus control). Only go to bed when sleepy. If awake in the middle of the night, get out of bed and do something (preferably something relaxing and boring). Go back to bed when sleepy enough to fall back asleep. Only use the bed for sleep and sex.
Possible cause: Negative thinking, stress, worry, faulty beliefs about the consequences of poor sleep		
"I feel overwhelmed and tense throughout the day and can't relax at bedtime; I'm worried that I will negatively impact my health; I don't think I can make it through the day if I don't get sleep."	What stressful life events, loss, or transitions are you facing? (Look for comments/decision making based on perceived consequences of poor sleep that are catastrophic vs. realistic.)	Use cognitive therapy. Try constructive worry technique—write down worrisome issues and identify solutions and next steps. Challenge underlying beliefs and worries about impact of sleep loss through psychoeducation. Use relaxation training. Incorporate breathing exercises and/or progressive muscle relaxation. Try meditating daily. Don't "clock-watch."

temazepam), geriatric psychiatrists and internists tend to be very concerned about these agents in older adults, given the increased risk of adverse events, particularly falls and hip fractures (Donnelly et al. 2017).

The American Academy of Sleep Medicine, in its clinical practice guideline for pharmacological treatment of chronic insomnia in adults (Sateia et al. 2017), recommended the following, but only after noting that the evidence for such recommendations was judged to be "weak":

- For insomnia involving sleep onset difficulty: eszopiclone, zaleplon, zolpidem, triazolam, temazepam, ramelteon
- For insomnia involving difficulty with sleep maintenance (which is prevalent in older adults as sleep becomes more fragmented with aging): suvorexant, eszopiclone, zolpidem, temazepam, doxepin

In contrast, they recommended that clinicians *not* use the following agents, again with only "weak" quality of evidence, for either sleep-onset or sleep-maintenance insomnia: trazodone, tiagabine, and popular over-the-counter medications/supplements such as diphenhydramine, melatonin, tryptophan, and valerian root.

Vignette *(continued)*

When the team started treatment for Mr. V, they first targeted the amount of time he was spending in bed. They set up an initial sleep schedule of 12 A.M. to 8 A.M., with plans to shrink that time if he was still finding himself awake a lot in the middle of the night. He was to get up at the same time every day, regardless of how he slept that night. The team focused on simultaneously increasing his homeostatic sleep drive (increasing his hunger for sleep) and regulating his circadian rhythm by sticking to a set schedule. They also encouraged him to drink his morning coffee in his sun room in order to increase his bright light exposure in the morning to help with his alertness.

Pharmacologically, the psychiatrist worked with him over time to decrease the zolpidem. It also was found at the time of the intake that Mr. V had symptoms that met criteria for a mild depression, so an antidepressant was started and Mr. V was encouraged to increase his engagement with pleasant activities during the day (e.g., behavioral activation strategies), particularly those that would connect him with family and friends. It was also hoped that this increase in physical activity would also help him to strengthen his homeostatic sleep drive and avoid napping during the day more successfully. Although he struggled some with the recommendation to get up at the same time every day and find ways to stay awake until midnight, his sleep did improve and become more consolidated. As providers, the treatment team members were pleased to see this improvement and continued to follow up with him over the next 6 months in monthly clinic visits.

KEY POINTS

- Insomnia is defined as difficulty with sleep initiation, maintenance, or waking earlier than planned.
- Insomnia is a treatable condition and the most frequently encountered sleep disorder in primary care settings.
- There are two main treatment options for insomnia: multicomponent cognitive-behavioral interventions and pharmacotherapy.
- Cognitive-behavioral therapy for insomnia (CBT-I) has considerable support as the recommended first-line treatment.
- CBT-I focuses on developing healthy sleep behaviors, addressing thought processes that interfere with sleep, and giving patients a set of skills that can be used whenever they face a prolonged period of sleep issues.

Resources

CBT-I Free Mobile App

Cognitive Behavioral Therapy for Insomnia (CBT-I) Coach, a mobile application originally designed as a companion for in-person therapy for promoting better sleep for veterans, available now to the general public at no cost.

CBT-I Fee-Based Online Courses

Sleepio: www.sleepio.com
SHUTi (Sleep Healthy Using the Internet): www.myshuti.com

Free (or Available for a Free Trial) Relaxation and Meditation Apps

Numerous apps are available; here are some examples:
  Insight Timer
  Calm
  Breathe2Relax
  Headspace

Practice Guidelines

American Academy of Sleep Medicine: https://aasm.org/clinical-resources/practice-standards/practice-guidelines

Books for Patients

Carney C, Manber R: Quiet Your Mind and Get to Sleep: Solutions to Insomnia for Those With Depression, Anxiety, or Chronic Pain (New Harbinger Self-Help Workbook). Oakland, CA, New Harbinger Publications, 2009

Jacobs GD: Say Good Night to Insomnia: The Six-Week, Drug-Free Program Developed at Harvard Medical School. New York, St. Martin's Griffin/Henry Holt, 2009

Helpful Tools and Websites (Free): Sleep Scheduling

Jet Lag Rooster: www.jetlagrooster.com

Entrain: http://entrain.math.lsa.umich.edu

Links to sleep diaries, constructive worry worksheets, progressive muscle relaxation example, thought trackers, etc.: http://drcolleencarney.com/resources

References

American Academy of Sleep Medicine: International Classification of Sleep Disorders, 3rd Edition. Darien, IL, American Academy of Sleep Medicine, 2014

American Psychiatric Association: Diagnostic and Statistical Manual of Mental Disorders, 5th Edition. Arlington, VA, American Psychiatric Association, 2013

Bertisch SM, Herzig SJ, Winkelman JW, et al: National use of prescription medications for insomnia: NHANES 1999–2010. Sleep 37(2):343–349, 2014 24497662

Buysse DJ, Germain A, Moul DE, et al: Efficacy of brief behavioral treatment for chronic insomnia in older adults. Arch Intern Med 171(10):887–895, 2011 21263078

Carney CE, Buysse DJ, Ancoli-Israel S, et al: The consensus sleep diary: standardizing prospective sleep self-monitoring. Sleep 35(2):287–302, 2012 22294820

Chong Y, Fryer CD, Gu Q: Prescription sleep aid use among adults: United States, 2005–2010. NCHS Data Brief (127):1–8, 2013 24152538

Chung F, Yegneswaran B, Liao P, et al: STOP questionnaire: a tool to screen patients for obstructive sleep apnea. Anesthesiology 108(5):812–821, 2008 18431116

Donnelly K, Bracchi R, Hewitt J, et al: Benzodiazepines, Z-drugs and the risk of hip fracture: a systematic review and meta-analysis. PLoS One 12(4):e0174730, 2017 28448593

Engle-Friedman M, Bootzin RR, Hazlewood L, et al: An evaluation of behavioral treatments for insomnia in the older adult. J Clin Psychol 48(1):77–90, 1992 1556221

Foley D, Ancoli-Israel S, Britz P, et al: Sleep disturbances and chronic disease in older adults: results of the 2003 National Sleep Foundation Sleep in America Survey. J Psychosom Res 56(5):497–502, 2004 15172205

Geiger-Brown JM, Rogers VE, Liu W, et al: Cognitive behavioral therapy in persons with comorbid insomnia: A meta-analysis. Sleep Med Rev 23:54–67, 2015 25645130

Hatoum HT, Kong SX, Kania CM, et al: Insomnia, health-related quality of life and healthcare resource consumption. A study of managed-care organisation enrollees. Pharmacoeconomics 14(6):629–637, 1998 10346415

Irish LA, Kline CE, Gunn HE, et al: The role of sleep hygiene in promoting public health: a review of empirical evidence. Sleep Med Rev 22:23–36, 2015 25454674

Johns MW: A new method for measuring daytime sleepiness: the Epworth sleepiness scale. Sleep 14(6):540–545, 1991 1798888

Kroenke K, Spitzer RL, Williams JB: The PHQ-9: validity of a brief depression severity measure. J Gen Intern Med 16(9):606–613, 2001 11556941

Martin JL, Webber AP, Alam T, et al: Daytime sleeping, sleep disturbance, and circadian rhythms in the nursing home. Am J Geriatr Psychiatry 14(2):121–129, 2006 16473976

McKinnon A, Terpening Z, Hickie IB, et al: Prevalence and predictors of poor sleep quality in mild cognitive impairment. J Geriatr Psychiatry Neurol 27(3):204–211, 2014 24687189

Mitchell MD, Gehrman P, Perlis M, et al: Comparative effectiveness of cognitive behavioral therapy for insomnia: a systematic review. BMC Fam Pract 13:40, 2012 22631616

Morgenthaler T, Alessi C, Friedman L, et al: Practice parameters for the use of actigraphy in the assessment of sleep and sleep disorders: an update for 2007. Sleep 30(4):519–529, 2007 17520797

Morin CM, Belleville G, Bélanger L, et al: The Insomnia Severity Index: psychometric indicators to detect insomnia cases and evaluate treatment response. Sleep 34(5):601–608, 2011 21532953

National Institutes of Health: National Institutes of Health State of the Science Conference statement on Manifestations and Management of Chronic Insomnia in Adults, June 13–15, 2005. Sleep 28(9):1049–1057, 2005 16268373

Parthasarathy S, Vasquez MM, Halonen M, et al: Persistent insomnia is associated with mortality risk. Am J Med 128(3):268–275, 2015 25447616

Pigeon WR, Pinquart M, Conner K: Meta-analysis of sleep disturbance and suicidal thoughts and behaviors. J Clin Psychiatry 73(9):e1160–e1167, 2012 23059158

Qaseem A, Kansagara D, Forciea MA, et al: Management of Chronic Insomnia Disorder in Adults: A Clinical Practice Guideline From the American College of Physicians. Ann Intern Med 165(2):125–133, 2016 27136449

Roth T, Zammit G, Kushida C, et al: A new questionnaire to detect sleep disorders. Sleep Med 3(2):99–108, 2002 14592227

Sateia MJ, Buysse DJ, Krystal AD, et al: Clinical practice guideline for the pharmacologic treatment of chronic insomnia in adults: an American Academy of Sleep Medicine clinical practice guideline. J Clin Sleep Med 13(2):307–349, 2017 27998379

Spiegelhalder K, Regen W, Nanovska S, et al: Comorbid sleep disorders in neuropsychiatric disorders across the life cycle. Curr Psychiatry Rep 15(6):364, 2013 23636987

Spielman AJ, Saskin P, Thorpy MJ: Treatment of chronic insomnia by restriction of time in bed. Sleep 10(1):45–56, 1987 3563247

Spitzer RL, Kroenke K, Williams JB, Löwe B: A brief measure for assessing generalized anxiety disorder: the GAD-7. Arch Intern Med 166(10):1092–1097, 2006 16717171

Trauer JM, Qian MY, Doyle JS, et al: Cognitive behavioral therapy for chronic insomnia: a systematic review and meta-analysis. Ann Intern Med 163(3):191–204, 2015 26054060

Yesavage JA, Brink TL, Rose TL, et al: Development and validation of a geriatric depression screening scale: a preliminary report. J Psychiatr Res 17(1):37–49, 1982–1983 7183759

Bipolar Disorder

"What's Wrong With Mom— Is It Dementia?"

Barbara R. Sommer, M.D.

CHAPTER 9

Clinical Presentation

Chief Complaint

"What's wrong with Mom—is it dementia?"

Vignette 1

A primary care physician referred Ms. D, a 75-year-old woman with no previous psychiatric care. Over the previous 18 months, psychiatric symptoms had slowly emerged, beginning with anxiety, which slowly escalated over time, such that over the preceding few months she had become frankly irascible. She had also begun to experience the following: very low energy, markedly decreased motivation, and insomnia. Around that time, she also had stopped talking and lost her appetite, losing more than 20 pounds. By the time Ms. D presented to her primary care physician, her daughter needed to hire a caregiver to help with laundry, housework, and driving—activities Ms. D had always performed without assistance. She had always been quick-tempered, labile, and at times verbally abusive, periodically not needing sleep and misusing alcohol, but she had had many friends and activities. Lately, however, she had lost friendships because of her insults and quick temper.

The primary care physician performed routine laboratory tests and physical exam, both of which were normal; Mini-Mental State

Exam (MMSE; Folstein et al. 1975) was 28, and neurological examination was nonfocal. Because of the new changes in mental status, part of her evaluation included a noncontrast brain magnetic resonance imaging (MRI) scan, which showed symmetrical ventricles and periventricular white matter ischemic changes without pronounced atrophy in the frontal or temporal area. She was prescribed risperidone 2 mg and zolpidem, which she began to use in combination with diphenhydramine for extra sleep.

Discussion

Diagnosis and Workup

This case highlights the difficulties in assessing older patients with symptoms consistent with several possible psychiatric diagnoses. The clinician must prioritize which symptoms to treat first, in order of acuity. Often, the treatment of one symptom may temporarily exacerbate another. While rating instruments are able to quantify symptoms, it is the mental status examination that enables the clinician to arrive at working diagnoses that in the end will inform the long-term treatment. In this case, the treatment team prioritized symptom reduction even before arriving at a formal diagnosis, and the problem list included the following:

- *History of alcohol misuse.* Her use of alcohol was sporadic, such that over the course of her adult life she may have often had withdrawal syndromes. Without knowing the frequency and quantity of alcohol consumed, it was not possible to distinguish between withdrawal, delirium, and "self-treated" affective symptoms.
- *Effects of anticholinergic medications on cognitive impairment.* The team felt that she had subsyndromal delirium (Cole et al. 2013), rather than frank dementia.
- *Effects of antipsychotic medication.* The flatness that the psychiatrist was to notice upon referral could have been induced by or exacerbated by dopamine D_2 receptor-blocking antipsychotics such as risperidone, or could have been a symptom of depression or dementia.

Differential Diagnosis

The psychiatry treatment team entertained the following additional diagnoses at this point in Ms. D's presentation:

- Alcohol use disorder
- Delirium

- Bipolar disorder (While the treatment team members were not certain at first, as they got to know the patient, they made it a working diagnosis.)
- Major neurocognitive disorder (It was not possible to make a diagnosis of major neurocognitive impairment on the first visit, but the concern was great enough that the team continued to evaluate her over time with periodic neuropsychological testing.)

Vignette 1 *(continued)*

During the course of the evaluations by psychiatry, Ms. D's primary care physician had also referred her to the neurology group because of her apparent cognitive deficits. Her flatness and amotivation were prominent, and neurology gave her a presumptive diagnosis of frontotemporal dementia (FTD), with the thought that future MRIs would show the changes usually seen in the frontal and temporal lobes. Although the psychiatry team agreed that FTD could have explained some of her symptoms, they also were impressed by her histories of affective lability, decreased need for sleep, and alcohol misuse. Furthermore, they felt the exacerbation of symptoms may have resulted from diphenhydramine, zolpidem, and risperidone, which they discontinued. With diagnoses of bipolar disorder, "subsyndromal delirium," and alcohol use disorder, the psychiatry team prescribed low-dose lithium and quetiapine, targeting affective symptoms, sleep, and appetite, and referred Ms. D for treatment of her alcohol problem.

Alcohol Use Disorder

The treatment team first began by addressing Ms. D's alcohol use, with the thinking that it contributed significantly to her behavior, which by the time they saw her was so unacceptable that she was disruptive in the waiting room. Thus, even before treating for bipolar disorder, the team referred her to a specialty addictions clinic, where she was prescribed gabapentin, topiramate, and group therapy; while she achieved mastery of her addiction, cognitive impairment remained. Nonetheless, the alcohol use had been considered so important that the team thought they could attend at a future date to possible effects on cognition of the medications used to treat the alcohol problem.

Substance misuse may become prominent over time in older adults, and older women may be particularly susceptible to abusing (Gurnack and Hoffman 1992; Wetterling et al. 2003). Living alone may confer a greater risk of alcohol and sedative overuse. At times, the team wondered about the concept of "inadvertent alcohol abuse" (their term) in patients without a previous history who slowly acquire psychological dependence and tolerance over time. These patients may underestimate their consumption when providing their medical history, and upon admission to the hospital for surgical procedures, for example, they may undergo acute alcohol withdrawal postoperatively (Moss and Burnham 2006).

Delirium

Frequent alcohol withdrawal and bipolar disorder both may have played a role in Ms. D's insomnia, leading to zolpidem and diphenhydramine use. In turn, these medications may have induced "subsyndromal delirium," possibly confounding her diagnosis and worsening her overall prognosis (Cole et al. 2003, 2013). The patient had not listed diphenhydramine on her medication list. This highlights why it is so important to ask the patient and family to bring in all medications, including over-the-counter preparations, for the most comprehensive list possible.

Bipolar Disorder

The treatment team obtained the past psychiatric history first from the patient alone and then from family members, who stated that as they were growing up, she often had been irascible, short-tempered, and "downright scary," but that in the past year her behavior had escalated. The patient did not recognize these difficulties herself and thought that others were "bossy" and that she needed to protect herself from their intimidating personalities, demonstrated when they tried to help her with activities of daily living (ADLs). It was important to ascertain if her present symptoms were similar to those of her past, because even if patients have a past history of psychiatric disorders, new symptoms may arise, suggesting new pathology. In this case, the team learned that after each of her pregnancies, she had experienced either profound lethargy or an increase in energy, at times doing household chores in the middle of the night. Over the course of her life, she had had discrete periods in which she seemed to need almost no sleep at all. This information helped the team to diagnose bipolar disorder.

To diagnose an affective disorder whose symptoms wax and wane over the course of a lifetime, it is important to get a detailed past history, which the patient may be able to document prior to the first appointment. In this case, Ms. D's children were able to chronicle her symptoms after the death of her husband. In general, for patients with long-standing psychiatric histories, it is important for the patient or family to document the symptoms and duration of each episode, what medications and dosages were prescribed, and whether these could establish a treatment effect.

Studies of older women with bipolar disorder have found that the index episode is often depressed rather than manic and that the average duration of affective illness is 20 years (Depp and Jeste 2004). Comorbid anxiety, panic, or dysphoria may make the diagnosis of bipolar disorder difficult to make, because mood elevation symptoms may be overshadowed (Goldstein et al. 2006). Although the euphoria of mania makes a diagnosis easier to make, the prominent depressive symptoms of dysphoric mania and mixed episodes may resemble agitated depression (for a full review of the differential diagnosis among mixed episodes, dysphoric mania, and major depression with irritability, see Ketter 2010).

Major Neurocognitive Disorder

After Ms. D became abstinent, the medications therapeutic for acute alcoholism but thought to contribute to cognitive changes were tapered and discontinued. The team tapered gabapentin and discontinued topiramate, hoping that the adjustments to these medications (which have potentially severe adverse side effects in the older adult) would enable more definitive ascertainment of her diagnosis. She remained labile in terms of mood, however. Although risperidone 2 mg usually is well tolerated by younger adults, older patients, particularly those with ischemic brain changes and decreased metabolism, may need and tolerate lower doses (Uchida et al. 2009). In this case, low-dose risperidone was unable to help her control her behaviors. Although her daughter thought she "was starting to clear" cognitively, Ms. D's aggressive behaviors resulted in a number of caregivers quitting, and the team continued to worry that she had both an underlying major neurocognitive disorder and bipolar disorder, with symptoms having been compounded by medications.

Vignette 1 *(continued)*

Over the ensuing 8 years, neither Ms. D's MRI findings nor her neuropsychological testing results changed. She had resolution of mood lability and did not want to be followed in the psychiatry clinic. However, she requested that the neurology service, whose clinicians saw her in routine follow-up, discontinue lithium and quetiapine because of a 30-pound weight gain. Within a few months, though, the patient became severely agitated and verbally and physically threatening, and had poor sleep. Referred back to geriatric psychiatry, Ms. D was once again prescribed lithium and quetiapine, with nutritional counseling for weight management, and a diagnosis of bipolar disorder was definitively made, with symptoms having been exacerbated by chronic alcoholism and the "deliriogenic" effects of medications. She is now well, having reestablished her friendships, and no longer in need of a caregiver.

History and Assessment

Rating Scales

Optimally, while in the waiting room the patient and family would fill out questionnaires on mood, such as the Patient Health Questionnaire–9 (PHQ-9; Kroenke and Spitzer 2002) or Geriatric Depression Scale (Yesavage et al. 1982–1983), and objective instruments may be administered during the interview. The Montgomery-Åsberg Depression Rating Scale (MADRS; Montgomery and Åsberg 1979) is a clinician-administered scale that quantifies the symptom list that diagnoses depression. The Activities of Daily Living (ADLs) and Instrumental ADLs (IADLs) scales (Katz 1983; Kempen and Suurmeijer 1990) assess routine self-care abilities. Studies of the Young Rating Scale (Young et al. 1978) and Hypomania Checklist–32 (HCL-32; Angst et al. 2005) for mania are limited in older adults but nonetheless may be useful for documenting symptoms in this age group. During the first interview, cognition should be assessed using either the Montreal Cognitive Assessment (MoCA; Nasreddine et al. 2005) or an alternate instrument such as the St. Louis University Mental Status (SLUMS; Tariq et al. 2006) examination to minimize practice effects (Goldberg et al. 2015). When the differential diagnosis includes a neurodegenerative disorder, longitudinal follow-up with imaging and cognitive testing is important. If English is not the patient's first language or if the patient has not completed high school, the Mini-Cog (Borson et al. 2000) has been found valid and reliable. Cognitive examinations should be performed without the family present. Less structured examinations also may assess cognition in the course of the interview. For example, if a patient states that he or she watches the news channel every day, asking about the day's news may help to rule out confabulation or problems with memory and concentration.

Mental Status Examination

As the patient enters the office, there is opportunity to evaluate balance, gait, posture, presence of pendular arm movements, and balance. In Ms. D, masked face, bradykinesia, and mild tremor were noticeable, suggesting that risperidone was either causing or exacerbating her emotionless appearance.

When patients are being escorted to the office, talking to them with social pleasantries (e.g., where were you driving from, how long did it take to get here) will relax them and give a sense of conversational abilities and affect before anxiety arises during a more formal interview. The team finds that although time-consuming, performing the interview while writing notes has yielded more clinical information than sitting at a computer, which may be off-putting to an older patient and may impede evaluation of the patient's eye contact and presence of abnormal movements.

The exact words in the chief complaint are important, revealing subjective priorities and insight into the disorder. For example, if the patient states, "I don't know, my daughter brought me," such a response speaks to insight or impairment, and at that point, it is advisable to ensure that the patient knows what kind of professional you are. If the chief complaint is "I can't sleep," obtaining a complete history of sleep habits may be a good place to begin the interview, ruling out not only sleep disorders but bipolar disorder as well. An Epworth Sleepiness Scale (Johns 1991) may also be helpful in ruling out sleep disorders such as obstructive sleep apnea.

During the initial interview, it is important to ask some questions of the patient without the presence of family members—for example, if the patient has suicidal feelings, whether the patient feels he or she is a burden to the family, and whether there has been physical or emotional abuse. If the patient otherwise cannot provide an accurate history, the clinician may want to bring family in early in the interview. Assessments for mood should be performed at each visit if affective lability is present, and studies suggest that cognitive testing should be repeated at least twice per year (Suh et al. 2004).

The team finds that a comprehensive social history is equivalent to the medical review of systems (see Table 9–1 for questions to consider). In the case of bipolar disorder, it may be useful to ask about the longest-held job, the number of times a patient has moved, and how many marriages he or she has had. When the clinician asks about financial well-being, it would be important to learn whether a patient has few resources despite a profitable job history, suggesting having spent to excess. It is important to address all safety issues with the patient and family. Specifically, if the patient drives, when was the last time a family member was a passenger with him or her? Have there been any recent near-miss accidents or tickets? Do other drivers honk at the patient? Does the patient leave the burners of the stove on? Does he or she forget to take medications? How does the patient remember to take medications properly? Does he or she ever feel that his or her life is no longer worth living? If the spouse has recently died, does the patient ever feel like joining the spouse in heaven? The patient's spiritual life needs examination. Some patients with bipolar disorder have grandiose feelings, thinking that they have a special relationship with God. If such feelings are present, these patients may want to die in an effort to get to heaven to join God.

Pitfalls in a Confusing History

Coordination of care is often difficult when another department does not have access to psychiatric records that require a double layer of security. Thus, it may be wise to verbally discuss the patient with the other service. For the professional treating a psychiatric disorder, electronic health records (EHRs) are important in the treatment of a complicated patient with multiple diagnoses, allowing the clinician to examine laboratory, radiological, and neuropsychological testing prior to the interview, the results of which would be important to other providers. However, this case exemplifies the effects on patient care if two fields in medicine cannot coordinate care to treat all aspects of the patient's symptoms.

It is important to personally examine and document all medications rather than to assume that those mentioned in the EHR are the only ones taken. In this way, double prescriptions, over-the-counter medications, and adherence to the regimen can all be assessed.

Medical Workup

Late-onset bipolar disorder is not usually associated with a family history of psychiatric disorder, consistent with the hypothesis that organic, genetic, and psychosocial factors play different roles in the disorder depending on the age at onset (Table 9–2). Vascular disease and psychosocial factors are key elements in both affective and cognitive disorders in older adults (Aziz and Steffens 2013; Krishnan 2002). Studies on the natural course of early-onset bipolar disorder suggest that over a lifetime, manic and depressive episodes generally remain stable, but that women have more depressions later in life than do men. Even when the disorder is treated, it has been suggested that residual symptoms remain between episodes in many cases (Angst and Sellaro 2000).

The thorough psychiatric examination should include a complete blood count and comprehensive metabolic panel (many psychiatric medications result in hyponatremia; albumin of less than 3.0 may reflect poor nutritional intake; and kidney and liver function and calcium and magnesium may influence affective state, consistent with medical etiologies). Thyroid function studies and vitamins D, B_{12}, and folate should all be assessed, and urine toxicology screening should be obtained. If a patient has risk factors for sexually transmitted diseases (possible in older adults, especially those with bipolar disorder and/or

TABLE 9–1. A concise social history

This should take around 10 minutes—the clinician should ask specific questions and warn the patient that he or she may interrupt the patient at times:

1. Where were you born? (The clinician may ask about family history for psychiatric or neurological illness here.)

2. What did your parents do for work? (This gives insight into the life the patient led as a child.)

3. How many siblings did you have? What are their ages, and are they doing well? Do you keep in touch? (If a sibling has a well-treated psychiatric disorder, try to find out what medication regimen he or she takes, which may be a guide to prescribing for the patient.)

4. If you could describe in just one word how your childhood was, what would that one word be? (If there is a history of physical abuse, the clinician can interrupt here, stating that the issue is too important to pursue at this time. Would you like to see a therapist to discuss it further?)

5. How much education do you have? (The clinician may want to get the history of substance use here.) What kind of student were you?

6. When was the first time you saw a mental health professional? What was the diagnosis? What treatments did you receive? Were there any subsequent assessments and treatments? (Either here or in the past psychiatric history it is important to elicit this information. Most psychiatric syndromes occur episodically throughout life, with long intervals of psychological wellness. Those whose initial onset is followed by a chronic, downhill course may have diagnoses other than affective illnesses.)

7. What did you do after your education? When did you marry? How many spouses have you had? Do you have children and grandchildren? (Have the patient give as much of this history as possible because it will speak to cognitive impairment. If their eyes do not light up in speaking about grandchildren, then something is wrong [e.g., depression, cognitive problems, something with the relationship].)

8. Military history? Highest rank? Honorably discharged? Did you see combat? If so, do you have nightmares?

9. When and why did you move to your present residence?

10. What is your work history? How long was your longest-held job? How did retirement go for you? How did you deal with the stress of retirement? Do you have financial worries?

11. The clinician can get the activities of daily living (ADLs) and independent ADLs history here, asking where the patient lives and with whom. The family will need to corroborate the patient's statements.

TABLE 9–1. A concise social history *(continued)*

12. Is there anything else about you that I should know to better treat you?

Note. When the family aids in the diagnosis, it is recommended to ask about their own well-being as caregivers and if they are getting enough support and respite. In the case of bipolar disorder, many families find it helpful to join the National Alliance on Mental Illness (see the section "Resources" at the end of this chapter). It has been found that if there is ample caregiver support at home, assisted living admissions can be staved off (Mittelman et al. 1996).

living in retirement communities, where condoms may not be used), appropriate testing should be acquired. If concomitant cognitive deficits are present, or if symptoms are new in later life, brain imaging should be acquired, looking for ischemic disease or atrophy. Electrocardiograms are important, because QTc prolongation may result from selective serotonin reuptake inhibitors, particularly if these medications are given concomitantly with antipsychotic drugs. See Table 9–3 for recommended follow-up laboratory tests.

Pharmacological and Other Biological Treatments

General principles for administering pharmacotherapy for bipolar disorder in older adults are presented in Table 9–3.

Antidepressants

Antidepressant therapy for patients with bipolar depression may have limited effectiveness, making the diagnosis essential for treatment (Sidor and MacQueen 2011). For example, the difference between "agitated depression" and "dysphoric mania" is important. Sedating antidepressants such as trazodone and mirtazapine may improve the symptoms of the former but not the latter (Ghaemi et al. 2003; Sidor and MacQueen 2011). Irritability and cognitive dysfunction also may indicate major neurocognitive disorder with behavioral changes or delirium. Treating agitation, irritability, and insomnia with sedating medications associated with fall risk needs to be weighed against the risk of falling as a result of insomnia and agitation (Lavsa et al. 2010). In particular, zolpidem and benzodiazepines, whether short- or long-acting, are associated with both cognitive impairment and falling (American Geriatrics Society 2015 Beers Criteria Update Expert Panel 2015; MacFarlane et al. 2014; Wang et al. 2001; Woolcott et al. 2009).

TABLE 9–2. **Possible causes of secondary mania in older adults**

Neurological diseases
  Cerebral tumor (particularly temporal, orbitofrontal, or thalamic)
  Cerebrovascular accident
  Delirium
  Dementia (major neurocognitive disorder)
  Multiple sclerosis
  Seizure disorder
  Traumatic brain injury
Endocrine diseases
  Addison's disease
  Cushing's syndrome
  Hyperthyroidism
  Hypothyrsoidism
Infectious diseases
  HIV/AIDS
  Tertiary syphilis
Nonpsychiatric medications
  Anticholinergics (e.g., diphenhydramine)
  Baclofen
  Bromides
  Captopril
  Dopamine agonists (e.g., levodopa)
  Hydralazine
  Metrizamide
  Phenytoin
  Procainamide
  Steroids
  Thyroxine
  Yohimbine
Psychiatric medications and somatic therapies
  Antidepressants
  Electroconvulsive therapy
  Phototherapy
  Stimulants

TABLE 9–2. **Possible causes of secondary mania in older adults** *(continued)*

Substances

  Alcohol

  Cocaine

  Illicit stimulants

Source. Reprinted from Brooks JO III, Sommer BR, Ketter TA: "Management of Bipolar Disorders in Older Adults," in *Handbook of Diagnosis and Treatment of Bipolar Disorders.* Edited by Ketter TA. Washington, DC, American Psychiatric Publishing, 2010, p. 456. Copyright © 2010 American Psychiatric Publishing. Used with permission.

In the subsections that follow, the limited number of treatments indicated for bipolar disorder in older adults is discussed. Table 9–4 provides dosing guidelines.

Lithium

Although lithium is considered the treatment of choice for patients with bipolar disorder, its narrow therapeutic index and medical side effects often make clinicians leery of prescribing it to older adults. Hypothyroidism and nephrogenic diabetes insipidus, known side effects, can easily be monitored and are not considered absolute contraindications to continued treatment. Other side effects include tremor, exacerbated by antipsychotic medications that are often simultaneously prescribed; weight gain; and ataxia, especially at higher dosages. Changes in glomerular filtration rate (GFR), however, constitute the most worrisome potential adverse side effect and may be one of the main reasons for discontinuation. Lithium carries a black box warning because of the small margin between therapeutic and toxic levels. A recent observational study following younger and older patients over a 6-year period found that GFR had declined after long-term use, even with mean lithium dosages lower than the usual in each age group (Bocchetta et al. 2017).

These findings need to be weighed against the poor quality of life that lithium responders may experience without it, because patients with bipolar disorder may be expected to have recurrent symptoms, with episodes usually continuing into older adulthood and with residual hypomanic or depressed symptoms occurring between major episodes (Angst and Sellaro 2000). Moreover, more recent evidence suggests that lithium may be neuroprotective, making it unique among mood stabilizers. One observational study reported greater white matter in-

TABLE 9–3. **Principles of pharmacotherapy of bipolar disorder in older adults**

1. Start with a careful diagnostic evaluation: complete medical and psychiatric history, physical examination, mental status examination (including cognition), and baseline laboratories as indicated. Head imaging may be indicated for first onset of symptoms in older age.

2. Perform ongoing careful psychiatric, medical, and cognitive clinical monitoring and laboratory monitoring.

3. Give highest priority to psychiatric medications with proven effectiveness and tolerability in mixed-aged populations with bipolar disorder.

4. Consider concurrent medical conditions and other medications when selecting psychiatric medication.

5. Start psychiatric medications one at a time at low dosages (e.g., 10%–50% of young adult full dosage) and gradually increase the dosage (e.g., in increments of 5%–10% of young adult full dosage every 4–7 days) as necessary and tolerated.

    • Initial target dosage is 10%–50% of young adult full dose in "frail" older adults (e.g., with substantive medical or neurological comorbidity); 50% of young adult dosage in "nonfrail" older adults (e.g., without significant medical or neurological comorbidity).

    • Higher subsequent dosages: 75% of young adult full dosage may be necessary and tolerated in some patients (e.g., "nonfrail" older adults with acute mania).

6. Remember that dosages during acute depression and maintenance may be as much as 50% lower than during acute mania.

7. Carefully explore dosage range of individual agents before prescribing combinations.

8. Ensure that medications are taken as prescribed, assigning a family member to supervise if warranted.

9. For follow-up laboratory tests, include the following (Sommer et al. 2003):

    Metabolic panel, observing for hyponatremia

    Complete blood count, observing for pancytopenia

    Electrocardiogram, observing for QT prolongation

Source. Adapted from Brooks JO III, Sommer BR, Ketter TA: "Management of Bipolar Disorders in Older Adults, in *Handbook of Diagnosis and Treatment of Bipolar Disorders.* Edited by Ketter TA. Washington, DC, American Psychiatric Publishing, 2010, p. 459. Copyright © 2010 American Psychiatric Publishing. Used with permission.

TABLE 9–4.   Dosing guidelines for older adults with bipolar disorder

Medication	Starting dosage (mg/day)	Dosage increment[a] (mg/day)	Initial target (mg/day and/or level)
Mood stabilizers			
Lithium	150[b]	150	Dosage varies with renal clearance (0.3–0.6 mEq/L)
Divalproex	250[b]	125–250	250–1,000 (30–60 µg/mL)
Carbamazepine	100[b]	100	400–800[c] (3–6 µg/mL)
Lamotrigine	12.5–25[b]	12.5–25	50–100
Second-generation antipsychotics			
Olanzapine	1.25–2.5	1.25–2.5	2.5–10
Risperidone	0.25–0.5[b]	0.25–0.5	0.5–2[c]
Quetiapine	25–50[b]	25–50	200–400[c]
Ziprasidone[d]	20	20	40–80
Aripiprazole	2–5	2–5	2–15[c]
Clozapine	6.25–25[b]	6.25–25	112.5–225[c]

Note.   Except for lamotrigine, dosages are for acute agitation/mania, and doses for bipolar depression and maintenance may be up to 50% lower. Dosages are guidelines only—concurrent medications (e.g., carbamazepine-related enzyme induction, or valproate-related enzyme inhibition), medical comorbidity, and genetic variation in metabolism will affect dosing in individual patients.

[a]Increase every 4–7 days, except for lamotrigine (12.5–25 mg/day for 2 weeks, 25–50 mg/day for 2 weeks, then increasing weekly by 12.5–25 mg/day).

[b]In divided doses to avoid adverse side effects.

[c]"Frail" older adults may only tolerate even lower dosages (i.e., carbamazepine 100–300 mg/day, risperidone 0.5–1.5 mg/day, quetiapine 50–200 mg/day, aripiprazole 2–10 mg/day, clozapine 25–100 mg/day).

[d]Low dosages may cause akathisia, and higher dosages may be sedating.

Source.   Adapted from Brooks JO III, Sommer BR, Ketter TA: "Management of Bipolar Disorders in Older Adults, in *Handbook of Diagnosis and Treatment of Bipolar Disorders.* Edited by Ketter TA. Washington, DC, American Psychiatric Publishing, 2010, p. 460. © 2010 American Psychiatric Publishing. Used with permission.

tegrity among bipolar patients who had received lithium compared with nonbipolar control subjects (Gildengers et al. 2015). A growing literature also attests to the possibility that lithium may delay the clinical symptoms of dementia (reviewed in Forlenza et al. 2012).

One of the more comprehensive analyses of Canadian inpatient prescribing habits for older patients with bipolar disorder has found that lithium was prescribed only 1.4% of the time, when perhaps 30%–50% of patients could potentially have responded (Rej et al. 2017), and most of the patients were prescribed multiple medications, including antipsychotics, benzodiazepines, and antidepressants, without concomitant mood stabilizers, contrary to expert guidelines recommending primarily mood stabilizers (Yatham et al. 2013). This implies that in order to quickly stabilize acutely symptomatic patients, inpatient units may prescribe a regimen that must be carefully streamlined on discharge. Psychiatrists rather than internists may be best suited for this process, which often requires weekly outpatient visits.

Valproate

Valproate was approved for the treatment of seizure disorders in 1978, yet it is not considered the drug of choice in older adults because of risks of tremor, weight gain, and osteoporosis and its ability to affect drug-metabolizing enzymes (Perucca et al. 2006). Furthermore, other antiepileptic drugs have similar effectiveness with a more favorable side-effect profile. However, fewer medication options are available to treat bipolar disorder, and although lithium remains the treatment of choice in both young adults and older patients, valproate, which is also approved by the U.S. Food and Drug Administration (FDA) for bipolar disorder and often perceived to have a safer profile, has become the default first-choice medication (Bowden et al. 1994; Pope et al. 1991). However, a large retrospective study has found that the rate of medical hospitalizations in patients with bipolar disorder was the same whether lithium, valproate, or nonlithium/nonvalproate groups were used (Rej et al. 2015). In one of the few prospective studies assessing efficacy and tolerability in older patients with bipolar disorder (blood levels 0.80–0.99 mEq/L for lithium, 80–99 µg/mL for valproate), tolerability was similar in both groups, and lithium had superior efficacy after 9 weeks (Young et al. 2017).

Lamotrigine

The 2002 revision of the bipolar disorder practice guideline from the American Psychiatric Association recommended lamotrigine as a first-line treatment for acute depressive episodes in bipolar patients (American Psychiatric Association 2002), and around that time the FDA approved it for maintenance treatment. In contrast to valproate, lamotrigine affects depression more than the manic component (Ketter et al. 2005). It is well tolerated and, unlike valproate, does not appear to have drug interactions (Messenheimer et al. 1998). Perhaps the most worrisome potential adverse event is the risk of rash. The incidence, prevalence, and severity of any rash during treatment with lamotrigine is no greater in older adults than in younger individuals, and the management is identical. A simple morbilliform rash can occur within the first 8 weeks of treatment (Messenheimer et al. 1998), and although the incidence of potentially life-threatening serious rash (i.e., Stevens-Johnson syndrome and toxic epidermal necrolysis) is low, in new users the risk of such occurrence warrants specific dosing guidelines (Mockenhaupt et al. 2005). Guidelines for prescribing lamotrigine are presented in Table 9–5.

Second-Generation (Atypical) Antipsychotic Medications

Second-generation antipsychotic (SGA) medications are often used as treatments for acute mania and for bipolar depression (specifically, quetiapine and the combination of olanzapine and fluoxetine; see Meltzer 2004 for a definition of what makes an antipsychotic atypical). Olanzapine and aripiprazole as monotherapies and quetiapine as adjunctive therapy all have indications for maintenance treatment, and some authors have suggested that the other SGAs may ultimately prove to have utility in not only acute mania but also bipolar depression (Jarema 2007). Lurasidone, with few drug interactions, has also been demonstrated as effective both as monotherapy and as adjunctive therapy with mood stabilizers in the treatment of bipolar depressed patients, but there are few data on prescribing recommendations for the older patient (Loebel et al. 2014).

A crucial safety concern with SGAs in older adults with dementia is the increase in mortality. Seventeen controlled trials of olanzapine, risperidone, quetiapine, and aripiprazole in 5,106 older adult patients with neurocognitive disorders and behavioral changes found an approximately 1.7-fold increase in mortality when compared with placebo (typically increased from 2.6% to 4.5% after a 10-week exposure), primarily due to cardiovascular events (e.g., heart failure, stroke, sudden death) or infections (mostly pneumonia) (Kuehn 2005). The FDA imposed a black box warning for all SGAs, including clozapine and ziprasidone. In 2008, a similar warning was applied to first-generation antipsychotics,

TABLE 9-5. **Guidelines for prescribing lamotrigine in older adults**

1. Advise the patient and family to monitor for rash closely as the dosage is increased.

2. Introduce lamotrigine gradually, starting with 25 mg/day for 2 weeks, then 50 mg/day for 2 weeks, then 100 mg/day for 1 week, and then 200 mg/day. Additional weekly increases of 100 mg/day to 300 or 400 mg/day may be necessary and tolerated in some patients.
   In patients taking valproate, these dosages must be halved. In patients taking carbamazepine, these dosages may need to be doubled.

3. Monitor for adverse events, especially rash and central nervous system effects, when lamotrigine is given in combination with valproate.

4. In patients who have not taken lamotrigine for 5 days or more, restart lamotrogine slowly, as in point 2.

Source. Fenn et al. 2006.

which have similar effects (Herrmann et al. 2004). It is unclear if these same risks occur in older patients with bipolar disorder without dementia as well.

Patients should also be warned of the risk of hyperglycemia and diabetes mellitus—with clozapine and olanzapine being the most commonly associated, risperidone and quetiapine less so, and ziprasidone and aripiprazole being the least implicated (Physicians' Desk Reference 2008). (See Brooks et al. 2010 for descriptions of other antipsychotic drugs in older patients with bipolar disorder).

Electroconvulsive Therapy

While the evidence is clear on the positive effects of electroconvulsive therapy (ECT) for major depressive disorder, patients with bipolar disorder have not been as rigorously studied (Brooks et al. 2010). Yet despite the limited information on ECT use in bipolar disorder, retrospective analyses have shown dramatic improvement, especially of rapid cycling (Frasca et al. 2003). The most common and severe side effect of ECT is cognitive, with other adverse effects including headache, muscle or jaw pain, and nausea. Although verbal learning is affected, even with right unilateral ECT, a specific deficit in delayed learning may be the most significant deficit (Frasca et al. 2003). One study comparing cognitive outcome among patients without cognitive impairment and those with mild neurocognitive impairment and patients with frank dementia found that depressed patients in all three groups had improvement in depression symptoms after ECT and that this modality was safe, with generally transient cognitive decline from baseline (Hausner et al. 2011). Taken together, the limited efficacy data of ECT in older adults with bipolar disorder and its adverse effects on cognition may lead clinicians to hold this option in reserve for cases of treatment-resistant illnesses. On the other hand, ECT may carry a lower risk for complications than some forms of pharmacotherapy among older adults (Herrmann et al. 2004; Kamat et al. 2003). ECT remains the treatment of choice when the acuteness of affective illness compromises the patient's medical stability.

Benzodiazepines

As a class, benzodiazepines, ranging from shorter-acting agents such as alprazolam and lorazepam to longer-acting agents such as clonazepam and diazepam, should be avoided in treating elderly patients, particularly when prescribed with other centrally active medications (American Geriatrics Society 2015 Beers Criteria Update Expert Panel 2015). Even younger patients are advised to take benzodiazepines with caution, given adverse effects such as cognitive impairment, oversedation, and gait instability (Ketter and Wang 2010). The 2015 Beers Criteria provide a comprehensive review of medications and drug interactions to be avoided in older adults (American Geriatrics Society 2015 Beers Criteria Update Expert Panel 2015).

Psychotherapy and Social Interventions

It is difficult to overstate the importance of the social atmosphere of any patient, and there is evidence that cognitive-behavioral, supportive, problem-solving, and interpersonal therapies are all useful in the multidisciplinary treatment of patients with depression. However, there are few studies in bipolar disorder in general and fewer still in older adults (Swartz and Frank 2001). The following case highlights the need for an integrated approach in obtaining treatment remission in an older patient.

Vignette 2

Ms. K was a 75-year-old widowed woman with a lifelong history of rapid-cycling bipolar disorder, characterized by protracted periods of grandiosity, decreased need for sleep, racing thoughts, and overspending. Over the course of her life she began to have protracted periods of depression, and during a particularly debilitating depression, she became more dependent on her very busy son, who placed her in a residential facility for more care. Her daughter in California asked that the patient move to be closer to her, with medical management at a treatment center. After a long hospitalization, ECT, and a change of medications from carbamazepine to valproate and low-dose olanzapine, Ms. K did quite well. Over the course of the next 15 years she remained stable, and while her daughter believes this has been due to medications, the treatment team thinks that the real difference has been in the support and love her daughter provides and living in an apartment with a loving and attentive caregiver. Ms. K has had interpersonal, supportive therapy, and now at 90 years old she is more stable than ever in her life.

KEY POINTS

- Substance misuse may become prominent over time in older adults, and older women may be particularly susceptible to abusing. Patients may underestimate their consumption when providing their medical history, and on admission to the hospital for surgical procedures, for example, they may undergo acute alcohol withdrawal postoperatively. Acquiring a history from the patient and family may aid in quantifying the contribution of substances to the symptom complex.
- Even if patients have a past history of psychiatric disorders, new symptoms may arise, suggesting new pathology and requiring a new medical workup.
- A comprehensive analysis of Canadian inpatient prescribing habits for older patients with bipolar disorder has found that lithium was prescribed only 1.4% of the time, when perhaps 30%–50% of patients could potentially have responded (Rej et al. 2017), and most of the patients were prescribed multiple medications, including antipsychotics, benzodiazepines, and antidepressants, without concomitant mood stabilizers, contrary to expert guidelines recommending primarily mood stabilizers (Yatham et al. 2013). The implications are as follows:
  - Lithium in general may be underprescribed; and
  - In order to quickly stabilize acutely symptomatic patients, inpatient units may prescribe a regimen that must be carefully streamlined upon discharge. Psychiatrists rather than internists may best be suited for this process, which often requires weekly outpatient visits.
- Most psychiatric syndromes occur episodically throughout life, with long intervals of psychological wellness. Those whose initial onset is

followed by a chronic, downhill course may have diagnoses other than affective illnesses.

*   The 2015 Beers Criteria (American Geriatrics Society 2015 Beers Criteria Update Expert Panel 2015) provide a comprehensive review of medications and drug interactions to be avoided in older adults.

Resources

Resources for Clinicians

Bauer M, McBride L: Structured Group Psychotherapy for Bipolar Disorder: The Life Goals Program. New York, Springer, 1996

Kay SR, Fiszbein A, Opler LA: The positive and negative syndrome scale (PANSS) for schizophrenia. Schizophr Bull 13 (2):261–276, 1987

Lam DH, Jones SH, Hayward P, et al: Cognitive Therapy for Bipolar Disorder: A Therapist's Guide to Concepts, Methods, and Practice. Chichester, UK, Wiley, 1999

Overall JE, Gorham DR: The brief psychiatric rating scale. Psychological Reports 10:799–812, 1962

Ramirez Basco M, Rush A (eds): Cognitive-Behavioral Therapy for Bipolar Disorder, 2nd Edition. New York, Guilford, 2005

Rating scales and safety measurements in bipolar disorder and schizophrenia—a reference guide. Psychopharmacol Bull 47(3):77–109, 2017 (Provides the following scales to assess affective disorders: Montgomery-Åsberg Depression Rating Scale, Clinical Global Impression–Bipolar Version–Severity of Illness, Young Mania Rating Scale, Hamilton Rating Scale for Anxiety, Quick Inventory of Depressive Symptomatology–Self-Report)

Resources for Patients

Jamison JR: An Unquiet Mind. New York, Knopf, 1995

Phelps J: Why am I Still Depressed? Recognizing and Managing the Ups and Downs of Bipolar II and Soft Bipolar Disorder. New York, McGraw-Hill, 2006

Resources for Patients and Families

Depression and Bipolar Support Alliance, 55 E Jackson Blvd., Suite 490, Chicago, IL 60604; (800) 826-3632; www.dbsalliance.org

National Alliance on Mental Illness (NAMI), Colonial Place Three, 3803 N. Fairfax Dr., Suite 100, Arlington, VA 22203; (800) 950-6264; www.nami.org

References

American Geriatrics Society 2015 Beers Criteria Update Expert Panel: American Geriatrics Society 2015 updated Beers criteria for potentially inappropriate medication use in older adults. J Am Geriatr Soc 63(11):2227–2246, 2015 26446832

American Psychiatric Association: Practice guideline for the treatment of patients with bipolar disorder (revision). Am J Psychiatry 159 (4 suppl):1–50, 2002 11958165

Angst J, Sellaro R: Historical perspectives and natural history of bipolar disorder. Biol Psychiatry 48(6):445–457, 2000 11018218

Angst J, Adolfsson R, Benazzi F, et al: The HCL-32: towards a self-assessment tool for hypomanic symptoms in outpatients. J Affect Disord 88(2):217–233, 2005 16125784

Aziz R, Steffens DC: What are the causes of late-life depression? Psychiatr Clin North Am 36(4):497–516, 2013 24229653

Bocchetta A, Cabras F, Pinna M, et al: An observational study of 110 elderly lithium-treated patients followed up for 6 years with particular reference to renal function. Int J Bipolar Disord 5(1):19, 2017 28393327

Borson S, Scanlan J, Brush M, et al: The mini-cog: a cognitive 'vital signs' measure for dementia screening in multi-lingual elderly. Int J Geriatr Psychiatry 15(11):1021–1027, 2000 11113982

Bowden CL, Brugger AM, Swann AC, et al: Efficacy of divalproex vs lithium and placebo in the treatment of mania. JAMA 271(12):918–924, 1994 8120960

Brooks JO III, Sommer BR, Ketter TA: Management of bipolar disorders in older adults, in Handbook of Diagnosis and Treatment of Bipolar Disorders. Edited by Ketter TA. Washington, DC, American Psychiatric Publishing, 2010, pp 453–497

Cole M, McCusker J, Dendukuri N, et al: The prognostic significance of subsyndromal delirium in elderly medical inpatients. J Am Geriatr Soc 51(6):754–760, 2003 12757560

Cole MG, Ciampi A, Belzile E, et al: Subsyndromal delirium in older people: a systematic review of frequency, risk factors, course and outcomes. Int J Geriatr Psychiatry 28(8):771–780, 2013 23124811

Depp CA, Jeste DV: Bipolar disorder in older adults: a critical review. Bipolar Disord 6(5):343–367, 2004 15383127

Fenn HH, Sommer BR, Ketter TA, et al: Safety and tolerability of mood-stabilising anticonvulsants in the elderly. Expert Opin Drug Saf 5(3):401–416, 2006 16610969

Folstein MF, Folstein SE, McHugh PR: "Mini-mental state." A practical method for grading the cognitive state of patients for the clinician. J Psychiatr Res 12(3):189–198, 1975 1202204

Forlenza OV, de Paula VJ, Machado-Vieira R, et al: Does lithium prevent Alzheimer's disease? Drugs Aging 29(5):335–342, 2012 22500970

Frasca TA, Iodice A, McCall WV: The relationship between changes in learning and memory after right unilateral electroconvulsive therapy. J ECT 19(3):148–150, 2003 12972984

Ghaemi SN, Hsu DJ, Soldani F, et al: Antidepressants in bipolar disorder: the case for caution. Bipolar Disord 5(6):421–433, 2003 14636365

Gildengers AG, Butters MA, Aizenstein HJ, et al: Longer lithium exposure is associated with better white matter integrity in older adults with bipolar disorder. Bipolar Disord 17(3):248–256, 2015 25257942

Goldberg TE, Harvey PD, Wesnes KA, et al: Practice effects due to serial cognitive assessment: Implications for preclinical Alzheimer's disease randomized controlled trials. Alzheimers Dement (Amst) 1(1):103–111, 2015 27239497

Goldstein BI, Herrmann N, Shulman KI: Comorbidity in bipolar disorder among the elderly: results from an epidemiological community sample. Am J Psychiatry 163(2):319–321, 2006 16449489

Gurnack AM, Hoffman NG: Elderly alcohol misuse. Int J Addict 27(7):869–878, 1992 1618585

Hausner L, Damian M, Sartorius A, et al: Efficacy and cognitive side effects of electroconvulsive therapy (ECT) in depressed elderly inpatients with coexisting mild cognitive impairment or dementia. J Clin Psychiatry 72(1):91–97, 2011 21208587

Herrmann N, Mamdani M, Lanctôt KL: Atypical antipsychotics and risk of cerebrovascular accidents. Am J Psychiatry 161(6):1113–1115, 2004 15169702

Jarema M: Atypical antipsychotics in the treatment of mood disorders. Curr Opin Psychiatry 20(1):23–29, 2007 17143078

Johns MW: A new method for measuring daytime sleepiness: the Epworth sleepiness scale. Sleep 14(6):540–545, 1991 1798888

Kamat SM, Lefevre PJ, Grossberg GT: Electroconvulsive therapy in the elderly. Clin Geriatr Med 19(4):825–839, 2003 15024814

Katz S: Assessing self-maintenance: activities of daily living, mobility, and instrumental activities of daily living. J Am Geriatr Soc 31(12):721–727, 1983 6418786

Kempen GIJM, Suurmeijer TP: The development of a hierarchical polychotomous ADL-IADL scale for noninstitutionalized elders. Gerontologist 30(4):497–502, 1990 2394384

Ketter TA (ed): Handbook of Diagnosis and Treatment of Bipolar Disorders. Washington, DC, American Psychiatric Publishing, 2010

Ketter TA, Wang PW: Antidepressants, anxiolytics/hypnotics, and other medications, in Handbook of Diagnosis and Treatment of Bipolar Disorders. Edited by Ketter TA. Washington, DC, American Psychiatric Publishing, 2010, pp 611–660

Ketter TA, Sach GS, Bowden CL, et al (eds): Advances in the Treatment of Bipolar Disorder, Washington, DC, American Psychiatric Publishing, 2005

Krishnan KRR: Biological risk factors in late life depression. Biol Psychiatry 52(3):185–192, 2002 12182925

Kroenke K, Spitzer RL: The PHQ-9: A new depression diagnostic and severity measure. Psychiatr Ann 32(9):509–515, 2002

Kuehn BM: FDA warns antipsychotic drugs may be risky for elderly. JAMA 293(20):2462, 2005 15914734

Lavsa SM, Fabian TJ, Saul MI, et al: Influence of medications and diagnoses on fall risk in psychiatric inpatients. Am J Health Syst Pharm 67(15):1274–1280, 2010 20651318

Loebel A, Cucchiaro J, Silva R, et al: Lurasidone as adjunctive therapy with lithium or valproate for the treatment of bipolar I depression: a randomized, double-blind, placebo-controlled study. Am J Psychiatry 171(2):169–177, 2014 24170221

MacFarlane J, Morin CM, Montplaisir J: Hypnotics in insomnia: the experience of zolpidem. Clin Ther 36(11):1676–1701, 2014 25455931

Meltzer HY: What's atypical about atypical antipsychotic drugs? Curr Opin Pharmacol 4(1):53–57, 2004 15018839

Messenheimer J, Mullens EL, Giorgi L, et al: Safety review of adult clinical trial experience with lamotrigine. Drug Saf 18(4):281–296, 1998 9565739

Mittelman MS, Ferris SH, Shulman E, et al: A family intervention to delay nursing home placement of patients with Alzheimer disease. A randomized controlled trial. JAMA 276(21):1725–1731, 1996 8940320

Mockenhaupt M, Messenheimer J, Tennis P, et al: Risk of Stevens-Johnson syndrome and toxic epidermal necrolysis in new users of antiepileptics. Neurology 64(7):1134–1138, 2005 15824335

Montgomery SA, Åsberg M: A new depression scale designed to be sensitive to change. Br J Psychiatry 134:382–389, 1979 444788

Moss M, Burnham EL: Alcohol abuse in the critically ill patient. Lancet 368(9554):2231–2242, 2006 17189035

Nasreddine ZS, Phillips NA, Bédirian V, et al: The Montreal Cognitive Assessment, MoCA: a brief screening tool for mild cognitive impairment. J Am Geriatr Soc 53(4):695–699, 2005 15817019

Perucca E, Aldenkamp A, Tallis R, et al: Role of valproate across the ages. Treatment of epilepsy in the elderly. Acta Neurol Scand Suppl 184:28–37, 2006 16776494

Physicians' Desk Reference. Montvale, NJ, Thomson PDR, 2008

Pope HG Jr, McElroy SL, Keck PE Jr, et al: Valproate in the treatment of acute mania. A placebo-controlled study. Arch Gen Psychiatry 48(1):62–68, 1991 1984763

Rej S, Yu C, Shulman K, et al: Medical comorbidity, acute medical care use in late-life bipolar disorder: a comparison of lithium, valproate, and other pharmacotherapies. Gen Hosp Psychiatry 37(6):528–532, 2015 26254672

Rej S, Hermann N, Shulman K, et al: Current psychotropic medication prescribing patterns in late-life bipolar disorder. Int J Geriatr Psychiatry 32(12):1459–1465, 2017 27911003

Sidor MM, MacQueen GM: Antidepressants for the acute treatment of bipolar depression: a systematic review and meta-analysis. J Clin Psychiatry 72(2):156–167, 2011 21034686

Sommer BR, Fenn H, Pompei P, et al: Safety of antidepressants in the elderly. Expert Opin Drug Saf 2(4):367–383, 2003 12904093

Suh GH, Ju YS, Yeon BK, et al: A longitudinal study of Alzheimer's disease: rates of cognitive and functional decline. Int J Geriatr Psychiatry 19(9):817–824, 2004 15352138

Swartz HA, Frank E: Psychotherapy for bipolar depression: a phase-specific treatment strategy? Bipolar Disord 3(1):11–22, 2001 11256459

Tariq SH, Tumosa N, Chibnall JT, et al: Comparison of the Saint Louis University mental status examination and the mini-mental state examination for detecting dementia and mild neurocognitive disorder—a pilot study. Am J Geriatr Psychiatry 14(11):900–910, 2006 17068312

Uchida H, Mamo DC, Mulsant BH, et al: Increased antipsychotic sensitivity in elderly patients: evidence and mechanisms. J Clin Psychiatry 70(3):397–405, 2009 19192476

Wang PS, Bohn RL, Glynn RJ, et al: Zolpidem use and hip fractures in older people. J Am Geriatr Soc 49(12):1685–1690, 2001 11844004

Wetterling T, Veltrup C, John U, et al: Late onset alcoholism. Eur Psychiatry 18(3):112–118, 2003 12763296

Woolcott JC, Richardson KJ, Wiens MO, et al: Meta-analysis of the impact of 9 medication classes on falls in elderly persons. Arch Intern Med 169(21):1952–1960, 2009 19933955

Yatham LN, Kennedy SH, Parikh SV, et al: Canadian Network for Mood and Anxiety Treatments (CANMAT) and International Society for Bipolar Disorders (ISBD) collaborative update of CANMAT guidelines for the management of patients with bipolar disorder: update 2013. Bipolar Disord 15(1):1–44, 2013 23237061

Yesavage JA, Brink TL, Rose TL, et al: Development and validation of a geriatric depression screening scale: a preliminary report. J Psychiatr Res 17(1):37–49, 1982–1983 7183759

Young RC, Biggs JT, Ziegler VE, et al: A rating scale for mania: reliability, validity and sensitivity. Br J Psychiatry 133(5):429–435, 1978 728692

Young RC, Mulsant BH, Sajatovic M, et al: GERI-BD: A randomized double-blind controlled trial of lithium and divalproex in the treatment of mania in older patients with bipolar disorder. Am J Psychiatry 174(11):1086–1093, 2017 29088928

Posttraumatic Stress Disorder

"My Stomach Hurts"

Kelli M. Smith, M.D.
Aazaz U. Haq, M.D.

CHAPTER 10

Clinical Presentation

Chief Complaint

"My stomach hurts."

Vignette

Mr. M was a 93-year-old World War II combat veteran with no prior psychiatric history who presented to the emergency department with 2 weeks of upset stomach, bloating, and queasiness, ever since his nephew had been cooking for him. He had become convinced that his nephew was trying to poison him to inherit the family estate.

Mr. M was admitted to inpatient psychiatry because of concerns for psychosis. On the unit, Mr. M's concerns were felt to be nonpsychotic in nature, but his admission became prolonged because of concerns about his ability to live independently, given his advanced age and mild cognitive slowing. Throughout his stay, he consistently denied depressive, anxious, or psychotic symptoms and remained pleasant and social.

During one of his evaluations, Mr. M was asked about his experience in World War II. He began to slowly and cautiously recount the experience, including his experience as a prisoner of war locked in a cold, dark, underground cell without food for a month. For the first time in his life, he talked about his difficulties with transition back to civilian life, his anger about the way he had been treated by the government, his ongoing nightmares about his experiences, and the shame he felt for the violence he had committed.

Discussion

Assessment

Like Mr. M in the case vignette, some trauma survivors may experience chronic symptoms of posttraumatic stress disorder (PTSD) that begin shortly after the trauma and persist well into older adulthood. For these individuals, stress-related symptoms may become a "part of life" that is not recognized as problematic or treatable (Richmond and Beck 1986). For others, PTSD may become salient for the first time in advanced age, after they have been relatively symptom free for years, or even decades, after a trauma (Cook 2011; Van Dyke et al. 1985). In fact, symptom-free intervals of 15–30 years are not uncommon. Generally, PTSD symptoms are most severe immediately after a trauma, tend to remit, and then often reemerge later in life (Port et al. 2001). Other older adults may have experienced distress immediately after the trauma, which becomes masked throughout middle adult life until the eventual "reactivation" of symptoms in senescence (Macleod 1994). Psychosocial stressors and symptoms from any recent trauma may compound the impact of previous trauma (Higgins and Follette 2002; Macleod 1994). Among older U.S. veterans, approximately 1 in 10 experiences a clinically significant exacerbation of PTSD in late life (Mota et al. 2016).

The diagnosis of PTSD in older adults is challenging for several reasons. Older adults may be less likely to present for psychiatric care because of a stigma toward mental illness among members of their generation (Thorp et al. 2011). As a cohort, older adults experience a culture that has traditionally stigmatized both older age and mental illness. They may be less able to self-identify psychological distress or interpret problems using a psychological framework due to a lack of awareness of mental health terminology (Thorp et al. 2011). They commonly misattribute symptoms of PTSD to somatic complaints or aging (Owens et al. 2005). Psychological symptoms are overshadowed by vague complaints of pain, insomnia, gastrointestinal distress, or feeling "sick" (Macleod 1994; Norris 1992).

It follows then that most older adults with mental health complaints present to their primary care provider for help. The long-term nature of a

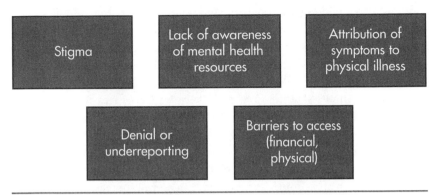

FIGURE 10–1. Barriers to mental health care among older adults.

primary care relationship makes it ideal for providing the safe and supportive environment in which the patient may be able to express vulnerabilities and concerns. If the patient has been seen longitudinally, the primary care provider has the advantage of being able to assess whether the individual's current physical or mental functioning deviates significantly from baseline. There is generally less stigma associated with going to a primary care provider than to a mental health specialist, and the patient may be more likely to discuss distress in this setting (Figure 10–1).

The primary care setting can be the most likely place to start the conversation around PTSD symptoms, clarify the diagnosis, initiate treatment, and, when necessary, make appropriate referrals. Anger, guilt, and anxiety are common features of PTSD, and providers should be mindful of the possibility of triggering these emotions when starting discussions about traumatic events. Trauma victims often experience intense emotions around their trauma, and probing into long-standing painful feelings of trauma before the patient is ready can lead to an overwhelming emotional response by the patient. One way to start a discussion in a sensitive and productive manner is to inquire about current symptoms of PTSD that the patient may be experiencing, while only touching briefly on the trauma itself. Delving into the details of the trauma should be avoided until appropriate comfort is established, and, in the case of complex or severe trauma, ideally in the context of an ongoing psychotherapeutic relationship.

Evaluation and Diagnosis

Several validated PTSD screening tools are available for identifying individuals at risk for PTSD, although none have been studied specifically among older adults. A widely used tool is the four-item Primary Care PTSD screen (PC-PTSD; Prins et al. 2003), which asks yes/no questions about the presence of symptoms over the past month (nightmares, avoidance, hypervigilance, detachment) that are related to any "frightening, horrible, or upsetting" experience over the lifespan. Other validated PTSD screening tools include the PTSD Brief Screen (Leskin and Westrup 1999) and the seven-item Short Screening Scale for PTSD (Breslau et al. 1999).

Screening for PTSD is meant to identify those individuals likely or unlikely to have the condition, but it is not a substitute for comprehensive assessment. Positive screening results should increase the clinician's index of suspicion and should be followed by a comprehensive clinical evaluation. Negative results are in no way "rule outs" and should not deter the clinician from further evaluation of risk factors and symptoms.

If a patient screens positive for PTSD, a comprehensive psychiatric follow-up should be performed. Any prior or current episodes of abuse, including sexual, physical, or emotional, should be identified. Prior hospitalizations, episodes of depression, psychotic symptoms, substance use, and cognitive status should also be assessed, as should medical comorbidities. Current stressors in domains of health (diagnoses, change in function, loss of independence), psychosocial status (relationships, death or illness of loved ones, interpersonal conflict), and identity (retirement, relocation, financial concerns) should be identified. These issues can commonly precipitate PTSD symptoms by triggering memories of past losses of functionality related to the traumatic experience. The gold standard in structured diagnostic interviews is the Clinician-Administered PTSD Scale (CAPS; Blake et al. 1995).

The clinical interview can be supplemented by symptom-based self-report scales, such as the PTSD Checklist, which has been validly used in older adults, especially with appropriate adjustment of cutoff scores to account for age-related differences (Cook et al. 2003; Thorp et al. 2011; Weathers et al. 1993). Collateral information from the patient's relatives or friends can be useful to corroborate the history, especially in patients with comorbid cognitive impairments or those who have difficulty discussing their symptoms.

The mnemonic TRAUMA can be used to outline the elements of a comprehensive clinical evaluation (Figure 10–2):

Trauma history.   Any experience that threatens an individual's physical or psychological integrity may constitute a traumatic event. Common examples of trauma include combat exposure, sexual assault, motor vehicle accident, physical violence, terrorism, and natural disasters. It is known that trauma exposure at a younger age is associated

Trauma history

Assess for trauma history. Any experience that threatens an individual's physical or psychological integrity may constitute a traumatic event, including but not limited to combat exposure, sexual assault, motor vehicle accident, physical violence, terrorism, and natural disasters.

Risk factors

Identify risk factors for suicidal and homicidal behavior. If there is imminent risk, call authorities who can place the patient on a psychiatric hold and facilitate transfer to an emergency department for psychiatric evaluation.

Active symptoms

Elicit current symptoms. Ask about the patient's mood, sleep quality, nightmares, flashbacks, self-blame and guilt, irritability, aggression, hypervigilance, paranoia, and avoidance behaviors.

Underlying conditions

Review past medical and psychiatric history. Ensure that the patient has had appropriate lab workup for possible medical etiologies of psychiatric symptoms (e.g., vitamin B_{12}, syphilis, HIV, cognitive impairment).

Mental status exam

Obtain mental status exam. Mental status examinations with evidence of cognitive deficits should be referred for comprehensive diagnostic evaluation. Patients with evidence of delirium should be referred for medical workup.

ADLs

Understand level of functioning. Ask about symptom-related distress, such as impairment in occupational functioning or avoidance of socialization.

FIGURE 10–2. "TRAUMA" mnemonic for evaluating posttraumatic stress disorder.

ADLs = activities of daily living.

with poorer outcomes, and younger age at entry into the military has been linked to greater risk of PTSD development (Kang et al. 2016).

Risk factors. All older patients with symptoms of PTSD should be assessed for safety regarding suicidal and homicidal ideation. Suicide risk is increased among older adults, and particularly in those with trauma history. Routine screening is paramount because research shows suicide is often committed shortly after contact with clinicians. Among older adults who died by suicide, 20% had seen their primary care physician the day of the suicide, 40% had been seen within 1 week of their suicide, and 70% had been seen within 1 month of committing suicide (National Institute of Mental Health 2007). In screening for suicidality, the clinician should start by asking the patient about any feelings of despair or hopelessness, thoughts of death or suicide, any plans the patient has considered, and whether the patient has had intent to carry the plan out. Hopelessness, recent stressors, and command auditory hallucinations are associated with increased risk of suicide (Hirschfeld and Russell 1997). The mnemonic "SADPERSONS" can be helpful in screening older adults for suicide risk (Table 10–1).

Active symptoms.   Particularly in the older population, the provider should be aware of atypical presentations of psychological distress, such as memory problems, noncompliance with medications, and frequent visits (Davidson et al. 1990; Frueh et al. 2008). Although more typical PTSD symptoms, such as nightmares and irritability, may be reported, their presentations are typically less dramatic in older adults. Somatic complaints, or vague complaints of "issues" or "stress" rather than "depression" or "anxiety," are common (Aldwin et al. 1996). In addition to the patient's chief complaint, the clinician should inquire about the patient's mood; sleep quality, including presence of nightmares; flashbacks; negative cognitions, such as self-blame and guilt; irritability or aggression; hypervigilance or exaggerated startle response; avoidance behaviors; and any trauma-related thoughts or feelings.

Underlying conditions.   The clinician should assess past medical and psychiatric history. Previous psychiatric diagnoses, history of suicide attempts, prior hospitalizations, and treatment can inform the clinician about the patient's risk. The clinician should also ask about current and past substance use, which can often serve as a coping tool for PTSD symptoms. Medical conditions, and specifically neurocognitive comorbidities, should be explored.

Mental status examination.   PTSD is rarely the only psychiatric diagnosis in an older adult and is generally comorbid with substance use and mood and anxiety disorders (Averill and Beck 2000; Durai et al. 2011; Pietrzak et al. 2012). The risk of dementia is twofold in patients with PTSD, so the mental status examination should include a thorough cognitive screening (Lohr et al. 2015).

TABLE 10–1. Suicide risk factors: remember "SADPERSONS"

Sex (male)

Age (>60)

Depression

Previous suicide attempts

EtOH (ethyl alcohol)/substance abuse

Rational thinking loss (psychosis)

Social support lacking

Organized plan to commit suicide

No spouse (divorced/widowed/single)

Sickness (physical illness)

Activities of daily living. Evaluations of geriatric patients should include assessment of the patient's global functioning, including their ability to tend to activities of daily living (e.g., ambulating, feeding, transfers, changing clothes, bathing, toileting) and instrumental activities of daily living (e.g., medication management, driving, grocery shopping, cleaning, cooking, laundry, using the telephone). Severe PTSD, particularly when accompanied by cognitive impairments, can have a negative impact on one or more of these functional abilities.

Diagnostic Criteria

While symptom patterns and severity will vary among individuals, to meet DSM-5 criteria for PTSD (Table 10–2; American Psychiatric Association 2013), these symptoms must be present for at least 1 month, cause significant distress or functional impairment, and not be attributed to medication, substance use, or other mental illness. Figure 10–3 provides an overview of the DSM-5 criteria for PTSD.

Vignette *(continued)*

Mr. M reported regularly hearing the screams and smelling the blood of his fellow soldiers as they endured bullet wounds and lay dying around him. He spoke about how, when he had come back from war, he felt estranged from his family, and how he had been too nervous to go to the movie theater due to the dimmed lighting. He had difficulty with close relationships, so he never married. From 1949 to 2017, he had lived a life

TABLE 10–2. Summary of DSM-5 criteria for posttraumatic stress disorder

History of exposure to a traumatic event. The patient describes exposure to actual or threatened death, serious injury, or sexual violence.

Intrusion symptoms. Despite the patient's best efforts, the traumatic event is persistently re-experienced in at least **one** of the following ways:

1. Recurrent, involuntary, and intrusive distressing memories.
2. Recurrent distressing dreams with content or affect related to the traumatic event.
3. Dissociative reactions in which the patient is mentally transported back to the scene (e.g., flashbacks).
4. Intense or prolonged distress after exposure to reminders of the trauma.
5. Marked physiological reactivity after exposure to trauma-related stimuli.

Avoidance. Some avoidance may be deliberate and conscious, but part is involuntary. The patient avoids at least **one** of the following:

1. Thoughts and feelings related to the trauma.
2. External reminders (e.g., people, places, conversations, objects).

Negative cognitions and mood. Despite the patient's best efforts, he or she experiences negative alterations in cognition and mood that started or worsened after the event in at least **two** of the following ways:

1. Inability to recall features of the traumatic event.
2. Persistent, exaggerated negative beliefs or expectations of oneself or the world.
3. Persistent, distorted blame toward self or others for causing the event or for the resulting consequences.
4. Persistent negative trauma-related emotions (e.g., fear, guilt, anger, shame).
5. Loss of interest in pleasurable activities (e.g., hobbies, relationships).
6. Feelings of alienation from others (e.g., detachment).
7. Persistent inability to experience positive emotions; constricted affect.

TABLE 10–2. Summary of DSM-5 criteria for posttraumatic stress disorder (continued)

Alterations in arousal. The patient experiences increased arousal or reactivity since the traumatic event in the form of at least **two** of the following:

1. Irritable behavior and angry outbursts, typically expressed as aggressive behavior.

2. Reckless or self-destructive behavior.

3. Hypervigilance.

4. Exaggerated startle response.

5. Problems with concentration.

6. Disturbed sleep.

Source. Adapted from American Psychiatric Association: *Diagnostic and Statistical Manual of Mental Disorders*, 5th Edition. Arlington, VA, American Psychiatric Association, 2013. Copyright © 2013 American Psychiatric Association. Used with permission.

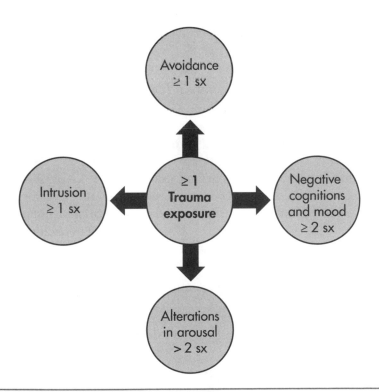

FIGURE 10–3. Overview of DSM-5 criteria for posttraumatic stress disorder.

that continued to be shaped by his war experience, rarely discussing it with anyone and never seeking treatment.

Subsyndromal PTSD

Not all traumatic experiences result in PTSD. PTSD is formally diagnosed if the patient's trauma-related symptoms cause a diminished ability to participate in typical activities (e.g., socialization, sleep, work/occupational function). However, posttraumatic stress symptoms may be present without significant functional impairment, or individuals may experience clinically significant impairment without experiencing all the symptoms mandated by the DSM-5 criteria for PTSD. These individuals should be diagnosed with other specified or unspecified trauma- and stressor-related disorder (Yaffe et al. 2010).

Differential Diagnosis of PTSD

The identification of PTSD among older adults can be complicated by the co-occurrence of other medical and psychiatric conditions as well as the overlap of symptoms between PTSD and other diseases. PTSD is commonly comorbid with depression and anxiety. It also confers an increased risk of development of dementia (Blake et al. 1995). Moreover, older adults with PTSD have higher rates of physical health conditions (Pietrzak et al. 2012).

Major or mild neurocognitive disorders.   Behavioral disturbances such as suspiciousness and irritability are not specific to PTSD and in older adults often herald a neurocognitive disorder. Changes in sleep patterns as well as vivid hallucinations are common. Assessments for PTSD should include formal cognitive testing as part of the mental status examination. The diagnostic interview should aim to clarify whether symptoms are related to past trauma or are without an identifiable prior experience.

Phobias.   Hypervigilance and physiological distress, as well as avoidance, are common features of phobias as well as PTSD. The distinction between phobias and PTSD-related avoidance can be made by deciphering the motivation for the individual's avoidance behavior. For example, if the avoidance is related to the traumatic experience, it is more suggestive of a PTSD-related behavior than a specific phobia. Individuals with PTSD tend to be in a state of constant hyperarousal, whereas those with phobias tend to become aroused in anticipation of exposure to a feared stimulus.

Psychotic disorders. Patients with psychotic disorders can also present with symptoms mimicking PTSD; the key distinction between psychotic disorders and PTSD is that in the latter, symptoms are attributed to a prior traumatic experience. PTSD flashbacks, or reexperiencing, may resemble hallucinations as would be seen in a primary psychotic disorder. Common themes of reexperiencing in PTSD are the smells of artillery, the taste of dirt or blood, visions of the dead and wounded, and cries for help.

Depression. Individuals with PTSD may exhibit symptoms commonly seen in depression, including sleep disturbance, anhedonia, cognitive changes, and guilt. To distinguish depressive disorder from PTSD, the clinician should attempt to understand the time course of symptoms. For example, if the symptoms are present in the absence of low mood, they are more likely PTSD related. On the other hand, if symptoms are only present when the individual is depressed, or there is prominent anhedonia, the clinician should suspect depressive disorder. The presence of symptoms not commonly seen in depression, such as avoidance or intrusive thoughts, can also provide diagnostic clarity.

Interventions

Vignette *(continued)*

During his hospitalization, Mr. M was started on sertraline 50 mg daily and given daily psychotherapy, which provided modest relief for his symptoms. He was eventually discharged in a stable state with plans for outpatient psychiatric care.

The associated implicit agreement to begin healing may be therapeutic for the older adult with PTSD. Providers should discuss with the patient and family what is known about the patient's reactions to assist with developing strategies to minimize discomfort surrounding anticipated behaviors. Family members can be educated about the relationship between current stressors and triggering of past traumatic experiences; for example, if a patient is transitioning out of his home to go to a skilled nursing facility, this may trigger memories of being drafted and leaving his home to go to war. Collaboration with the patient and family and acknowledgment of their trepidations can enhance the clinician's understanding of the patient and family's unique experiences and best course of treatment.

Unfortunately, older adults with psychiatric illness are less likely to receive appropriate pharmacological treatments than younger adults (Bartels et al. 1997). The vast majority of pharmacotherapy trials for PTSD have not included older adults in their sample. Nonetheless, much of the general research likely applies to older adults, and there are data to support certain pharmacological interventions. These interventions can be initiated in the primary care setting.

Psychotherapy works in conjunction with pharmacotherapy. Psychotherapy is typically done by a licensed mental health provider (i.e., a licensed clinical social worker, psychologist, or, in some cases, psychiatrist) in an outpatient setting.

Pharmacotherapy

Selective serotonin reuptake inhibitors (SSRIs) are often recommended as first-line treatments for PTSD and have been associated with reduction in symptoms for some groups (Bernardy and Friedman 2015). Because elderly patients may be nonadherent to medications because of preconceived notions about addictive potential, concerns about side effects, or lack of understanding, it is important to be clear in communicating the risks and benefits with the patient. The patient should also receive clear communication about the importance of compliance and consistent dosing.

Choice of SSRI should consider the patient's other comorbidities. For example, paroxetine is among the most anticholinergic of the SSRIs and would be a poor choice in a patient taking bladder antispasmodics (e.g., oxybutynin), which are also anticholinergic. SSRIs shown to be most effective for PTSD are escitalopram, sertraline, and fluoxetine. In deciding among these, consider their side-effect profiles. Escitalopram is well tolerated in older adults but carries the risk of QTc prolongation. Sertraline is most effective in females but can be associated with gastrointestinal distress. Fluoxetine can potentiate anticoagulants and has many other drug-drug interactions.

Serotonin-norepinephrine reuptake inhibitors (SNRIs) are next-line treatments for PTSD symptoms. As with SSRIs, the main target of SNRIs is depressed mood. Certain SNRIs, such as venlafaxine, may be more activating and may help with PTSD-related avoidance behaviors but show no benefit for insomnia or hyperarousal. Mirtazapine, on the other hand, is helpful for hyperarousal and can promote sleep.

Because lack of sleep can exacerbate other PTSD symptoms, it is useful to treat insomnia. Prazosin, an α_1-adrenergic receptor antagonist traditionally used as an antihypertensive, is among the best-evidenced treatments for PTSD. It has been associated with a reduction in PTSD symptoms, nightmares, and sleep disturbance (Peskind et al. 2003). Starting at a low dosage can help mitigate risk of side effects, including dizziness and orthostatic hypotension. Blood pressure should be monitored in patients taking prazosin. Trazodone is an alternative to prazosin that is also useful for sleep onset in older adults with PTSD. This medication is also associated with risk of falls due to its sedative and alpha-blocking properties.

Benzodiazepines are widely prescribed for PTSD and can be effective in certain populations; however, these should not be considered drugs of choice and should especially be avoided in older adults because of increased risk for adverse drug effects, such as falls and delirium, as well as long-term increased risk of cognitive impairment (Billioti de Gage et al. 2014; Tune and Bylsma 1991). In the circumstance of patients who have not benefited from other PTSD treatments or who are unable to tolerate the first- and next-line agents (i.e., SSRI/SNRI, prazosin, trazodone), benzodiazepines with the shortest half-life and that avoid first-pass metabolism in the liver are preferable. These include lorazepam, temazepam, and oxazepam.

For patients with PTSD with comorbid major or mild neurocognitive disorder, psychotic symptoms can be prominent. In these individuals, low-dose antipsychotics such as quetiapine, risperidone, and aripiprazole can be useful.

Other antidepressants, anxiolytics, anticonvulsants, and mood stabilizers may benefit some patients. Medications should always be started at lower dosages and be increased slowly over time (Moye and Rouse 2015). Though geriatric patients may experience benefit at lower dosages compared with younger patients, they often require full dosages for therapeutic effect. With older age, variation in drug metabolism may alter the effectiveness of treatments and susceptibility to side effects. All medications used in the treatment of PTSD should be titrated to effect or to tolerability of side effects (Table 10–3).

Follow-up recommendations. The elderly patient starting pharmacological treatment for PTSD should be monitored closely for tolerability and adverse effects. This is especially important if the individual has other medical comorbidities that could be affected. For the first 3–4 weeks of treatment, and any time dosage adjustments are made, the patient should be followed closely with either weekly return visits or telephone encounters to monitor for falls, dizziness, hypotension, or other adverse effects. Once a satisfactory response has been achieved and the dosage is tolerable, the patient may begin to see the provider less frequently, such as

TABLE 10–3. Medications for the treatment of posttraumatic stress disorder in older adults

Medication	Starting dosage (po)	Titration schedule	Target dosage	Key considerations when treating older adults
Selective serotonin reuptake inhibitors				
Escitalopram	5 mg daily	5 mg weekly	5–10 mg daily	QTc prolongation
Sertraline	12.5 mg daily	12.5 mg weekly	12.5–100 mg daily	Gastrointestinal distress
Fluoxetine	5 mg daily	5 mg every other week	5–40 mg daily	CYP450 drug interactions
Serotonin-norepinephrine reuptake inhibitors				
Venlafaxine, sustained action	37.5 mg daily	37.5 mg weekly or every other week	37.5–150 mg daily	Hypertension; discontinuation syndrome if stopped abruptly
Mirtazapine	7.5 mg nightly	7.5 mg weekly	7.5–30 mg nightly	Weight gain
Other				
Prazosin	1 mg nightly	1 mg weekly	1–6 mg nightly	Hypotension, falls
Trazodone	12.5 mg nightly	12.5–25 mg weekly	12.5–100 mg nightly	Sedation

every 2–3 months. If the patient begins to feel the medication is not working, an office visit should be scheduled to discuss potential explanations, such as a recent stressor leading to worse symptoms, adverse effects of the medications, or inconsistent use. The provider may consider increasing the dosage or, if this is not feasible, switching to another agent.

Emergency situations: when to call 911. Providers should call 911 to facilitate transfer of the patient to the nearest emergency department for mental health evaluation in the following circumstances:

- Patient becomes acutely agitated or dangerous.
- Patient is thought to be at imminent suicide risk.
- Patient has expressed intent to harm others.
- Provider feels unsafe or uncomfortable.

Referral to mental health. Patients who are not imminently dangerous and who require additional diagnostic assessment should be referred for further evaluation by a mental health professional. Figure 10–4 demonstrates examples of common scenarios.

The patient should be referred to resources for psychotherapeutic support. If a patient remains symptomatic despite pharmacological treatment, or the patient's psychiatric presentation is complex, referral to psychiatry is appropriate. Referral to mental health specialists, including psychologists and social workers, who practice psychotherapy with PTSD and/or geriatric patients is also encouraged.

Psychotherapy

One of the major obstacles to psychotherapy in all patients with PTSD is the reticence to discuss the trauma story, and this may be even greater among older adults, many of whom rely on avoidance strategies (Macleod 1994). Nonetheless, the goal of psychotherapy is to reduce the stressful state by processing and integrating the trauma into the overall life experience (Buffum and Wolfe 1995). Primary care providers may consider referral to a therapist specializing in one of the following techniques based on the individual's personality and preferences.

Cognitive-Behavioral Therapies

Cognitive-behavioral therapy (CBT) aims to challenge negative thoughts and distortions. Trauma-focused CBTs, including prolonged exposure, cognitive processing therapy, and eye movement desensitization and

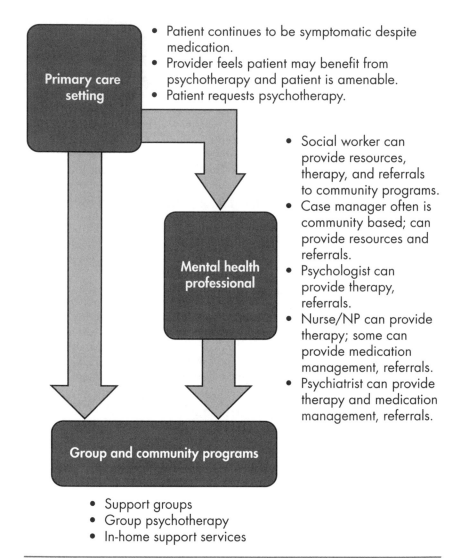

FIGURE 10–4. Common scenarios for referral of patients for further evaluation by a mental health professional.
Note. NP = nurse practitioner.

reprocessing, have been effectively used in the treatment of PTSD (Thomas and Gafner 1993). Among the most well-studied and effective in older adults is prolonged exposure (Clapp and Beck 2012; Cook et al. 2017; Dinnen et al. 2015; Thorp et al. 2012), which consists of 8–15 sessions of 90 minutes each, 1–2 times per week, and involves four key components: psychoeducation, breathing retraining, imaginal exposure, and in vivo exposure.

Trauma-Focused Group Therapy

Trauma-focused group therapy is another hallmark of PTSD treatment that can provide a unique arena for processing past experiences in a safe, cohesive environment. For veterans, the dynamic may mimic the "intense, symbiotic relationship of the combat unit" (Archibald anad Tuddenham 1965, p. 480). Group therapy for older adults is generally well tolerated but should be considered in the context of a patient's co-morbid respiratory or cardiovascular disease, because shared stories can lead to intense emotional states. To date, there is no evidence that modifications to therapy are universally necessary.

Supportive Therapy and Life Review

Life review is a technique modeled after Erikson's (1982) theory of developmental stages. In accord with Erikson's developmental stages, therapy may target *ego despair,* the sense that the individual's life has been insignificant in the context of aging. Extrapolating from this theory, the assessment of past experiences is a part of late life that can lead to successful processing of past trauma. Supportive therapy has also been used in older adults with PTSD (Hyer et al. 1995; Owens et al. 2005; Thorp et al. 2012).

Psychodynamic Psychotherapy

Psychodynamic/analytic therapies have also been suggested for the treatment of PTSD in older adults. One aspect of this work is based on the notion that coping mechanisms formerly used to escape distress, such as overcommitment to work or engagement in hobbies, become less accessible with changes in older age, such as retirement. Ego and self-worth are threatened with the loss of a professional identity, leading to unresolved psychic conflicts. The subsequent interpersonal conflicts and family dynamics have been major targets of therapy. Some have proposed a psychodynamic-supportive group therapy concept (Müller and Barash-Kishon 1998).

Behavioral Interventions

In addition to psychotherapy, there are several behavioral interventions for older adults with PTSD that can be provided in a typical office visit.

Sleep hygiene. Disturbances in sleep related to PTSD may contribute to maladaptive stress responses and may decrease the efficacy of first-line PTSD treatments (Germain 2013). As such, sleep is an integral part of treatment, and patients should be educated about sleep hygiene

(Bloom et al. 2009; Gooneratne and Vitiello 2014). The following are strategies to support sleep hygiene:

- Maintain a healthy sleep-wake cycle by getting enough sunlight exposure. Limit daytime naps.
- Exercise regularly during the daytime. Avoid vigorous exercise before bed.
- Limit caffeine, alcohol, and nicotine intake.
- Establish a nighttime routine. Try to go to sleep at the same time each night.
- Keep the sleep environment comfortable and relaxing. The bedroom should be cool and dark.
- Avoid watching television or reading in bed.
- Discontinue activities at least 1 hour before going to bed.

Meditation and mindfulness training. Mindfulness training may be useful in patients without cognitive impairment. Patients can be trained to shift attention from remembered fears to the present moment, thus permitting the perception of increased control over intrusive thoughts. This therapy is believed to reduce the level of arousal and contribute to improved emotional regulation.

Other behavioral interventions. Other interventions that can be provided in a primary care setting include the following:

- Educating the patient and caretaker/family about PTSD.
- Connecting the patient and caretaker/family to resources for social and financial support.
- Discussing psychiatric advance directives.

KEY POINTS

- Traumatic experiences occur at all stages of the life cycle, and psychological sequelae may differ based on the victim's age at the time of exposure.
- The most common symptoms of posttraumatic stress disorder (PTSD) are reexperiencing paralyzing fear from the trauma, hypervigilance, nightmares, and somatic symptoms such as tachycardia, diaphoresis, and insomnia.

- The presentation of PTSD in the elderly is unique and should be interpreted in the context of neuropsychiatric comorbidity and psychosocial stressors.
- Assessing posttraumatic stress in older adults is particularly challenging for several reasons:
    - Clinicians underestimate the prevalence of PTSD in older adults.
    - PTSD can manifest itself for the first time in older age.
    - Many older adults have learned to "live with" symptoms of PTSD, so they may not see it as a reason to seek medical attention.
- Older adults with PTSD often present with somatic symptoms.
- Many individuals have developed unhealthy coping strategies, such as substance use, to deal with their posttraumatic distress.

Resources

International Society for Traumatic Stress Studies: www.istss.org; (847) 480-9028; istss@istss.org
National Center for PTSD: www.ptsd.va.gov; (802) 296–6300; ncptsd@va.gov
National Clearinghouse on Abuse in Later Life (NCALL): http://ncall.us; (608) 255-0539; ncall@endabusewi.org
Posttraumatic Stress Disorder Alliance: www.ptsdalliance.org; (888) 436-6306; contact@ptsdalliance.org

References

Aldwin CM, Sutton KJ, Chiara G, et al: Age differences in stress, coping, and appraisal: findings from the Normative Aging Study. J Gerontol B Psychol Sci Soc Sci 51(4):179–188, 1996 8673639
American Psychiatric Association: Diagnostic and Statistical Manual of Mental Disorders, 5th Edition. Arlington, VA, American Psychiatric Association, 2013
Archibald HC, Tuddenham RD: Persistent Stress Reaction After Combat: A 20-Year Follow-Up. Arch Gen Psychiatry. 12(5):475–481, 1965
Averill PM, Beck JG: Posttraumatic stress disorder in older adults: a conceptual review. J Anxiety Disord 14(2):133–156, 2000 10864382
Bartels SJ, Horn S, Sharkey P, et al: Treatment of depression in older primary care patients in health maintenance organizations. Int J Psychiatry Med 27(3):215–231, 1997 9565725

Bernardy NC, Friedman MJ: Psychopharmacological strategies in the management of posttraumatic stress disorder (PTSD): what have we learned? Curr Psychiatry Rep 17(4):564, 2015 25749751

Billioti de Gage S, Moride Y, Ducruet T, et al: Benzodiazepine use and risk of Alzheimer's disease: case-control study. BMJ 349:g5205, 2014 25208536

Blake DD, Weathers FW, Nagy LM, et al: The development of a Clinician-Administered PTSD Scale. J Trauma Stress 8(1):75–90, 1995 7712061

Bloom HG, Ahmed I, Alessi CA, et al: Evidence-based recommendations for the assessment and management of sleep disorders in older persons. J Am Geriatr Soc 57(5):761–789, 2009 19484833

Breslau N, Peterson EL, Kessler RC, Schultz LR: Short screening scale for DSM-IV posttraumatic stress disorder. Am J Psychiatry 156(6):908–911, 1999 10360131

Buffum MD, Wolfe NS: Posttraumatic stress disorder and the World War II veteran. Geriatr Nurs 16(6):264–270, 1995 7498816

Clapp JD, Beck JG: Treatment of PTSD in older adults: do cognitive-behavioral interventions remain viable? Cognit Behav Pract 19(1):126–135, 2012 22383863

Cook JM: Post-traumatic stress disorder in older adults. PTSD Research Quarterly 12(3):1–7, 2011

Cook JM, Thompson R, Coyne JC, et al: Algorithm versus cut-point derived PTSD in ex-prisoners of war. J Psychopathol Behav Assess 25(4):267–271, 2003

Cook JM, McCarthy E, Thorp SR: Older Adults with PTSD: Brief State of Research and Evidence-Based Psychotherapy Case Illustration. Am J Geriatr Psychiatry 25(5):522–530, 2017 28214073

Davidson JR, Kudler HS, Saunders WB, et al: Symptom and comorbidity patterns in World War II and Vietnam veterans with posttraumatic stress disorder. Compr Psychiatry 31(2):162–170, 1990 2311383

Dinnen S, Simiola V, Cook JM: Post-traumatic stress disorder in older adults: a systematic review of the psychotherapy treatment literature. Aging Ment Health 19(2):144–150, 2015 24898218

Durai UNB, Chopra MP, Coakley E, et al: Exposure to trauma and posttraumatic stress disorder symptoms in older veterans attending primary care: comorbid conditions and self-rated health status. J Am Geriatr Soc 59(6):1087–1092, 2011 21649614

Erikson EH: The Life Cycle Completed. New York, WW Norton, 1982

Frueh BC, Elhai JD, Kaloupek DG: Unresolved issues in the assessment of trauma exposure and posttraumatic reactions, in Posttraumatic Stress Disorder: Issues and Controversies. Edited by Rosen GM. Hoboken, NJ, John Wiley and Sons, 2008, pp 63–84

Germain A: Sleep disturbances as the hallmark of PTSD: where are we now? Am J Psychiatry 170(4):372–382, 2013 23223954

Gooneratne NS, Vitiello MV: Sleep in older adults: normative changes, sleep disorders, and treatment options. Clin Geriatr Med 30(3):591–627, 2014 25037297

Higgins AB, Follette VM: Frequency and impact of interpersonal trauma in older women. Journal of Clinical Geropsychology 8(3):215–226, 2002

Hirschfeld RMA, Russell JM: Assessment and treatment of suicidal patients. N Engl J Med 337(13):910–915, 1997 9302306

Hyer L, Summers MN, Braswell L, et al: Posttraumatic stress disorder: silent problem among older combat veterans. Psychotherapy 32(2):348–364, 1995

Kang S, Aldwin CM, Choun S, et al: A life-span perspective on combat exposure and PTSD symptoms in later life: findings from the VA normative aging study. Gerontologist 56(1):22–32, 2016 26324040

Leskin G, Westrup D: PTSD Brief Screen: Posttraumatic Stress Disorder: Implications for Primary Care. Department of Defense/EES, 1999

Lohr JB, Palmer BW, Eidt CA, et al: Is post-traumatic stress disorder associated with premature senescence? A review of the literature. Am J Geriatr Psychiatry 23(7):709–725, 2015 25959921

Macleod AD: The reactivation of post-traumatic stress disorder in later life. Aust N Z J Psychiatry 28(4):625–634, 1994 7794206

Mota N, Tsai J, Kirwin PD, et al: Late-life exacerbation of PTSD symptoms in US veterans: results from the National Health and Resilience in Veterans Study. J Clin Psychiatry 77(3):348–354, 2016 27046308

Moye J, Rouse SJ: Posttraumatic stress in older adults: when medical diagnoses or treatments cause traumatic stress. Psychiatr Clin North Am 38(1):45–57, 2015 25725568

Müller U, Barash-Kishon R: Psychodynamic-supportive group therapy model for elderly Holocaust survivors. Int J Group Psychother 48(4):461–475, 1998 9766089

National Institute of Mental Health: Older Adults: Depression and Suicide Facts (NIH Publ No 99–4593). Bethesda, MD, National Institutes of Health, 2007

Norris FH: Epidemiology of trauma: frequency and impact of different potentially traumatic events on different demographic groups. J Consult Clin Psychol 60(3):409–418, 1992 1619095

Owens GP, Baker DG, Kasckow J, et al: Review of assessment and treatment of PTSD among elderly American armed forces veterans. Int J Geriatr Psychiatry 20(12):1118–1130, 2005 16315160

Peskind ER, Bonner LT, Hoff DJ, et al: Prazosin reduces trauma-related nightmares in older men with chronic posttraumatic stress disorder. J Geriatr Psychiatry Neurol 16(3):165–171, 2003 12967060

Pietrzak RH, Goldstein RB, Southwick SM, et al: Physical health conditions associated with posttraumatic stress disorder in U.S. older adults: results from wave 2 of the National Epidemiologic Survey on Alcohol and Related Conditions. J Am Geriatr Soc 60(2):296–303, 2012 22283516

Port CL, Engdahl B, Frazier P: A longitudinal and retrospective study of PTSD among older prisoners of war. Am J Psychiatry 158(9):1474–1479, 2001

Prins A, Ouimette P, Kimerling R, et al: The primary care PTSD screen (PC-PTSD): development and operating characteristics. Primary Care Psychiatry 9(1):9–14, 2003

Richmond JS, Beck JC: Posttraumatic stress disorder in a World War II veteran. Am J Psychiatry 143(11):1485–1486, 1986 3777252

Thomas R, Gafner G: PTSD in an elderly male: treatment with eye movement desensitization and reprocessing (EMDR). Clinical Gerontologist: The Journal of Aging and Mental Health 14(2):57–59, 1993

Thorp SR, Sones HM, Cook JM: Posttraumatic stress disorder among older adults, in Cognitive Behavior Therapy With Older Adults. Edited by Sorocco KH, Lauderdale S. New York, Springer, 2011, pp 189–217

Thorp SR, Stein MB, Jeste DV, et al: Prolonged exposure therapy for older veterans with posttraumatic stress disorder: a pilot study. Am J Geriatr Psychiatry 20(3):276–280, 2012 22273763

Tune LE, Bylsma FW: Benzodiazepine-induced and anticholinergic-induced delirium in the elderly. Int Psychogeriatr 3(2):397–408, 1991 1687445

Van Dyke C, Zilberg NJ, McKinnon JA: Posttraumatic stress disorder: a thirty-year delay in a World War II veteran. Am J Psychiatry 142(9):1070–1073, 1985 4025625

Weathers FW, Litz BT, Herman DS, et al: The PTSD Checklist (PCL): Reliability, Validity, and Diagnostic Utility. Paper Presented at the Annual Meeting of International Society for Traumatic Stress Studies, San Antonio, TX, September 1993

Yaffe K, Vittinghoff E, Lindquist K, et al: Posttraumatic stress disorder and risk of dementia among US veterans. Arch Gen Psychiatry 67(6):608–613, 2010 20530010

Evaluation and Treatment of Substance Use Disorders

"I Just Have One Drink With Dinner, Doc"

Karen Reimers, M.D., FRCPC
Ilse R. Wiechers, M.D., M.P.P., M.H.S.

Clinical Presentation

Chief Complaint

"I just have one drink with dinner, Doc."

Vignette

Mr. J is a 78-year-old man with atrial fibrillation, hyperlipidemia, hypertension, and gastroesophageal reflux disease who presents to his primary care provider with complaints of worsening depressive symptoms and memory problems. He reports almost a year of worsening financial and housing stressors along with very little interest in activities, low motivation, depressed mood, trouble sleeping, low energy, and poor appetite (with a 20-pound weight loss in the past 2 years, including 10 pounds in the past year), as well as thoughts of worthlessness. He denies thoughts of suicide and states that his children are his reason for living. He denies psychotic or manic symptoms. In addition, he reports problems remembering where he puts things and forgetting what he ate for dinner the night before. He also describes one occasion of getting lost on the way to his son's new house. He denies problems with activities of daily living or instrumental activities of daily living and has no observed language deficits. He thinks his symptoms have been worse in recent months. He is a nonsmoker and reports having a drink with dinner each evening.

His primary care physician considers that Mr. J is at risk for alcohol abuse and may be underreporting his intake and briefly counsels him about safe alcohol intake for older adults and starts him on citalopram 20 mg daily for depression.

Discussion

Increasing numbers of individuals are abusing drugs and alcohol in their later years. Substance abuse is common in primary care settings, and many patients seeking geriatric health services have risky alcohol or substance abuse (Draper et al. 2015). It is essential that all health care providers be aware of substance use disorders (SUDs) as well as their routine screening, assessment, and effective treatments in the older adult population. There is a need for additional training on addiction at all levels, including continuing education for psychiatrists and other mental health professionals. (De Jong et al. 2016).

SUDs in older people have many negative consequences, including physical and mental health problems, social and family strain, legal problems, and death from alcohol or drug overdose. The health effects of substance use in the geriatric population can be more dangerous than in younger substance abusers. Chronic health conditions and prescribed medications can increase the adverse effects of substance use in older people. Physical symptoms of substance abuse may include injuries, increased tolerance to medication, blackouts, and cognitive impairment, while psychiatric symptoms can include sleep disturbances, anxiety, depression, and mood swings (Mattson et al. 2017). Many problems associated with aging are risk factors for SUDs in older people, including bereavement, social isolation, lack of social support and financial difficulties, dementia (major or mild neurocognitive disorder), lack of mobility, and ill health (Gossop and Moos 2008).

Alcohol and drug use among older adults has received relatively little attention clinically and in terms of research initiatives. Evidence for best practices in the older population is lacking (Sullivan and Levin

TABLE 11–1.   Common stressors associated with late-onset substance use disorders

Death of spouse	Sleep problems
Retirement	Disability
Pain	

2016). Most clinical research trials specifically exclude older participants and thus have limited generalizability to this patient population.

SUDs in older individuals may stem from an early-onset pattern (i.e., the continuation of a lifelong pattern of ongoing substance abuse). Other individuals may have a late-onset pattern, initiating substance use for the first time in old age, commonly following a stressor such as medical illness or death of a spouse. Stress (Table 11–1), role/identity loss, and friends' approval of substance abuse are associated with an increased risk for late-onset SUD (Emiliussen et al. 2017).

Changing Patterns of Geriatric Substance Use Disorders

Historically, rates of SUDs in older cohorts have been lower than in younger cohorts (Arndt et al. 2011). Older adults have historically also been less likely to present for SUD treatment (Arndt et al. 2011). However, the number of Americans age 50 years and older with SUDs is projected to double from 2.8 million in 2006 to 5.7 million in 2020 (Wu and Blazer 2011).

Demographic changes with the aging of the baby boomer generation are leading to a rapid increase in SUDs in aging individuals. Baby boomers grew up in an era during the 1960s and 1970s with significant cultural changes in attitudes toward alcohol and drug use. They generally have more favorable attitudes toward substance use, and in their lifetimes, they have had easy access to and increased reliance on prescription medication (Moore et al. 2009).

Increasing evidence suggests that the current baby boomer cohort of aging adults, born from the mid-1940s to mid-1960s, abuses alcohol and psychoactive prescription medications at a much higher rate than previous generations did. Rates of abuse of alcohol, prescription drugs, marijuana, and other illicit drugs are rapidly increasing in the older adult population. SUDs are increasingly common among older adults as this generation ages (Kuerbis et al. 2014).

Challenges of Diagnosis: A Hidden Epidemic

Despite the known trends of increasing SUDs among older adults, geriatric addictions remain underidentified and undertreated. Identifying addictions in the elderly can be challenging, because substance abuse in older people is frequently hidden and difficult to detect in routine care settings. Clinicians may be unaware that their geriatric patients are abusing alcohol or other substances, including prescription medications.

Distinguishing between normal aging, polypharmacy, and SUD is often challenging because of symptom overlap. For example, problems such as neglecting responsibilities, problems in relationships, memory issues, changes in sleep patterns, or deterioration in physical appearance could all be signs of either normal aging, polypharmacy, or SUD. Symptoms of intoxication and withdrawal are often disguised in this population as geriatric syndromes such as falls, cognitive impairment, incontinence, and depression (Crome 2013).

Warning signs of a substance use problem in an older individual may include excessive preoccupation with having enough pills or timing of the doses, social withdrawal, unexplained injuries, sleep disturbances, and decline in functioning. One rule of thumb is that normal aging is generally quiet and slow, involving subtle changes over time, whereas sudden or dramatic changes are red flags that warrant further investigation (Haroutunian 2016).

Older adults are historically less likely to be screened for SUDs compared with younger cohorts (D'Amico et al. 2005). In general, primary care physicians and specialists do not routinely assess or screen older adults for SUDs despite the fact that older adults with multiple chronic health conditions and depression have an increased risk of problem drinking and SUD (Mowbray et al. 2017). Table 11–2 summarizes commonly used screening tests for SUDs in older adults.

Many health care professionals feel uncomfortable talking with older patients about their substance use (Kuerbis et al. 2014). Complicating the picture is the stigma these issues may have for older adults and their families, thus leading them to downplay or deflect questions about substance use. Ageism may contribute to a pattern of underdiagnosis; behavior considered a problem in younger adults often does not engender the same urgency for care in older adults.

Polypharmacy is a common problem among elderly people and can itself lead to addiction. Most older adults take prescription medications

TABLE 11–2. Screening tools for substance use disorders in older people

Brief intervention (as a clinical technique to express concern, advise, provide feedback, and offer referral; Le Roux et al. 2016)

CAGE (alcohol; see Table 11–7)

Michigan Alcohol Screening Test—Geriatric Version (MAST-G; alcohol)

Brown bag medication audit (polypharmacy; see Table 11–3)

Screener and Opioid Assessment for Patients with Pain (SOAPP; opioids)

Current Opioid Misuse Measure (COMM; opioids)

daily (National Institute on Drug Abuse 2018). Adverse reactions from polypharmacy are common and include confusion, falls, and death. Clinicians should carefully review medication regimens of their older patients and maintain accurate records of prescriptions. To help prevent and identify problems related to polypharmacy and prescription medication abuse in elderly patients, clinicians can consider a "brown bag" medication audit (Haroutunian 2016). This involves asking the patient to gather all home medications, including pill bottles, nasal spray, supplements, and over-the-counter drugs, into a brown paper bag. In the clinic, the clinician sorts through all the medications in the brown paper bag, eliminates all old and expired medications, and enters medication names into the database.

Discussing use of alcohol, illicit substances, and misuse of prescribed medications is best achieved through a supportive, nonconfrontational approach. Health care providers should approach this topic in the context of the overall health assessment, making an effort to relate it back to the presenting problem when possible, with a focus on health promotion. It is advised to start the discussion with nonjudgmental questions about alcohol use (e.g., "When was the last time you had a drink of alcohol?") and build up to more detailed questions about use patterns (e.g., "How often do you drink alcohol?"; "How much do you drink in a setting?"). Further questions about illicit substances and possible misuse of prescribed medications can follow, addressing, for example, recent and past use of alcohol, tobacco, illicit drugs, and prescription medications, including those the patient may have borrowed or otherwise diverted and over-the-counter medications. When needed, reassurances can be provided that asking these types of questions is something done with all patients (as it should be). If the screening questions elicit responses suggesting a specific SUD, further screening may include standardized instruments discussed later.

Vignette *(continued)*

Initially, Mr. J appears to be tolerating the new medication well. However, 3 weeks later, he is brought to the emergency department by his girlfriend, who is concerned about mental status changes, including confusion, slurred speech, and visual hallucinations (seeing people in the apartment who are not there). She reports that these symptoms have been occurring over the past week or two. Review of systems is also notable for a nonproductive paroxysmal cough over the past week, xerostomia, mild dyspnea on exertion, and fatigue.

In the emergency department, he is found to have mild nystagmus with vertical and lateral gaze, bibasilar crackles on lung examination, irregularly irregular heart rate, and 2+ pitting edema to knees bilaterally. His blood pressure is 127/81, and pulse is 91. Further workup is notable for a brain natriuretic peptide level of 600 pg/mL, new normocytic anemia, microhematuria, elevated alkaline phosphatase, and new small bilateral pleural effusions. Head computed tomography scan is unremarkable. He is offered 24-hour observation but refuses and goes home in the middle of the night with his girlfriend. He is told to stop his citalopram and follow up with primary care the next day.

When he is seen the next day in primary care, his blood pressure is in the 150s/80s and his heart rate is in the 120s on multiple repeats. He reports that he did not drink the night before because he was in the emergency department and reports that he has been cutting down his daily drinking since recent conversations with his primary care provider, although he cannot provide a clear report of his alcohol intake over the past week. Further history is gathered about his alcohol intake, and he endorses previously drinking two martinis every night over the past few years, which are best estimated to contain approximately 2–3 ounces of vodka in each drink.

Interdisciplinary Team Commentary

Primary care physician: I am worried about Mr. J's elevated blood pressure and heart rate, which I think may be related to poorly controlled atrial fibrillation and hypertension. I would like to gather more information from him about whether or not he is taking his medications as prescribed or whether he is missing doses. I am also concerned about his volume overload, and I would like to start some hydrochlorothiazide to address that and get more information about his nutrition and fluid intake. His newly identified hematuria has me worried enough that I am going to refer him to urology for further evaluation and workup. Finally, I think a referral to psychiatry is warranted now, because I am reluctant to restart another antidepressant given the altered mental status he has been exhibiting the past few weeks.

Psychiatrist: My biggest immediate concern for this patient is alcohol withdrawal, which is what I fear has tipped him over into the de-

TABLE 11–3.   Essential features of DSM-5 substance use disorder

Impaired control	Risky use
Craving	Tolerance
Social impairment	Withdrawal

Source.   Adapted from American Psychiatric Association 2013.

lirium that led to his emergency department visit. I am concerned he has been regularly drinking far more than he initially revealed and then has had a sudden decrease or possible cessation of drinking. I would want to talk in more detail with Mr. J about his alcohol use history and educate him more carefully about the risks of alcohol withdrawal. I would also want to get a better sense of where he is in terms of willingness to cut back on his use of alcohol. If he were willing to stop drinking entirely, I would need to have a better sense of his supports at home to determine whether outpatient detoxification would be safe, or whether he would need inpatient detoxification. I would also consider adding naltrexone to help reduce alcohol cravings. Once we have gotten past this immediate concern of active alcohol abuse, I would reevaluate his depressive and memory symptoms in the setting of sobriety. His mood and cognitive symptoms may improve or resolve after he stops drinking.

DSM-5 Criteria and Limitations for Older Adults

The DSM-5 (American Psychiatric Association 2013) diagnosis of SUD is based on a pathological pattern of behaviors related to use of the substance. Substance abuse produces intense direct activation of the brain reward system, leading to changes in behavior, motivation, and memory. Essential features of an SUD include cognitive, behavioral, and physiological symptoms and continuation of the abuse of the substance in spite of substance-related problems (Table 11–3). These criteria are applied, with minor variations, across 10 classes of drugs and also to the new diagnosis of gambling disorder. See Tables 11–4 and 11–5 for summaries of DSM-5 classes of drugs and intoxication, withdrawal, and other substance/medication-induced mental disorders.

Currently there is no gold standard for how to adapt the DSM-5 SUD diagnostic criteria for presentations in older individuals. Unfortunately, there are multiple difficulties in applying the standard DSM-5 SUD criteria to the aging population.

TABLE 11–4. DSM-5 classes of drugs in substance-related disorders

Alcohol	Opioids
Caffeine	Sedatives, hypnotics, and anxiolytics
Cannabis	Stimulants (amphetamine-type
Hallucinogens (includes phencyclidine	substances, cocaine, and others)
and other hallucinogens)	Tobacco
Inhalants	Other (or unknown) substances

Source.   Adapted from American Psychiatric Association 2013.

TABLE 11–5. DSM-5 intoxication, withdrawal, and other substance/medication-induced mental disorders

Psychotic disorders	Sleep disorders
Bipolar and related disorders	Sexual dysfunctions
Depressive disorders	Delirium
Anxiety disorders	Major or mild neurocognitive
Obsessive-compulsive and related	disorders
disorders	

Source.   Adapted from American Psychiatric Association 2013.

Older adults with medical problems or other age-related impairments may deny or not realize that symptoms are substance related. For example, the criterion that the individual takes more of a substance than intended is challenging to evaluate in a patient with cognitive impairment or lack of insight, because these conditions can interfere with self-monitoring. It can be difficult to assess older adults for recurrent hazardous use. Individuals may deny use because of stigma, or they may not realize that a previously safe level of use has become hazardous. The criterion of failure to fulfill role duties may not apply in individuals who are retired or out of the workforce. Older adults and their families frequently minimize their substance abuse after a role change, such as retirement. The criterion of unsuccessful efforts to cut down may not be met because these individuals may have a reduced incentive to decrease harmful use (Sullivan and Levin 2016).

Treatment

Geriatric SUDs are neglected but treatable illnesses. Increasing awareness of geriatric SUDs and referral to treatment can make a tremendous

TABLE 11–6.   Behavioral interventions to treat substance use disorders in older people

Cognitive-behavioral therapy

Helps individuals learn how to identify and correct problem behaviors

Involves both individual and group counseling

Focuses on relapse prevention, managing cravings, and coping skills

Contingency management

Includes monetary reward for desired behaviors

Offers tangible rewards to reinforce abstinence

Motivational enhancement therapy

Uses counseling to resolve ambivalence about change

Aims to increase commitment to making and maintaining healthy changes

Family and community-based treatment

Facilitates interactions and relationships

Optimizes support and involvement during substance use disorder treatment

Mutual-support 12-step approaches (e.g., Alcoholics Anonymous [AA])[a]

Note.   See the most recent edition of *Principles of Drug Addiction Treatment* (National Institute on Drug Abuse; see "Resources") for more information.
[a]Practical barriers may limit participation of older adults.

positive impact on the health and quality of life of older adults and their families (Le Roux et al. 2016).

Brief alcohol interventions can be learned by the broad array of clinicians working with older adults. These generally include an expression of concern, feedback to patients linking their drinking and health, and explicit advice to cut down. Brief interventions have value as a mechanism for dialogue between patient and provider and as an intervention that can be effective (Oslin 2005).

Treatment for SUDs in older people may consist of brief interventions and other behavioral therapies (Table 11–6). Programs for older people should consider special needs of the elderly, including medical and social service needs. Barriers to treatment for older people include lack of transportation, physical disabilities, reluctance to go out in the evening, and greater dependence on their spouse.

Older people are able to utilize offered treatments with positive effects on clinical outcomes. Many of the treatments can be offered in primary care settings, and this gives cause for hopefulness because many

TABLE 11-7. CAGE questionnaire

Have you ever felt you should **C**UT down on your drinking?

Have people **A**NNOYED you by criticizing your drinking?

Have you ever felt bad or **G**UILTY about your drinking?

Have you ever had a drink first thing in the morning to steady your nerves or get rid of a hangover (**E**YE-OPENER)?

Note. Two or more positive responses identify problem drinkers.

patients in this group consult with their primary care physician regularly (Bhatia et al. 2015).

Alcohol Abuse

Alcohol is the most commonly abused substance among older people, and misuse of alcohol is often a hidden phenomenon. Clinicians may underestimate the risk of alcohol use in older adults. However, alcohol use among older adults, including binge drinking, is increasing, and there are trends of increasing use among females. Screening tests for alcohol include the CAGE questionnaire (Mayfield et al. 1974; Table 11–7) and the Michigan Alcohol Screening Test—Geriatric version (MAST-G; Blow et al. 1992). Both are validated in older people, with sensitivity and specificity comparable to those in younger individuals.

Risk factors in older people include smoking, illicit drug use, and mental health problems (Han et al. 2017a). Late-onset alcohol abuse may be triggered by bereavement, medical illness, or retirement. Drinking in nursing home or assisted-living settings may provide older adults with a sense of continuity with life before retirement and preserve their identity and autonomy (Burruss et al. 2015).

Older adults are more sensitive to the effects of alcohol, and this increased sensitivity is due to multiple factors, including decreased lean body mass, diminished hepatic metabolism, medical comorbidities, and polypharmacy. Older people may experience marked intoxication symptoms following ingestion of amounts of alcohol that would be judged safe among younger adults, due to increased effects of alcohol on the central nervous system.

Guidelines for drinking limits in older people are evolving. There is controversy around exact drinking limits, and limits are generally lower for women than for men. The National Institute on Alcohol Abuse and Alcoholism currently recommends no more than one standard drink per day, or seven drinks per week, for those age 65 years or older (Table 11–8).

TABLE 11–8. Standard drink

One standard drink of "pure" alcohol in the United States is defined as 0.6 fluid ounce (fl. oz.) or 14 grams. This amount of alcohol is found in the following:

12 fl. oz. regular beer (~5% alcohol)

8–9 fl. oz. malt liquor (~7% alcohol)

5 fl. oz. wine (~12% alcohol)

1.5 fl. oz. distilled spirits, such as whiskey, vodka, rum (~40% alcohol)

Though it is controversial, many elderly people should probably avoid alcohol completely, including people taking prescription pain medications, sleeping pills, or psychotropic medicines; individuals with memory problems; and people with a history of falls or unsteady walking (Substance Abuse and Mental Health Services Administration 2017).

Detoxification is one of the first steps in treatment and should be carefully monitored. For older adults, detoxification is usually done in the inpatient setting because of the increased medical risks of withdrawal. Alcohol withdrawal can range from unnoticeable to mild to severe, with life-threatening symptoms such as autonomic hyperactivity, psychomotor agitation, tremors, hallucinations, delirium, seizures, and coma. Confusion may be the most prominent sign of early geriatric alcohol withdrawal syndrome. Alcohol withdrawal delirium usually occurs 2–10 days after the last drink (Hategan et al. 2016). Assessment can be done using a standardized tool such as the Clinical Institute Withdrawal Assessment for Alcohol–Revised (CIWA-Ar; Sullivan et al. 1989), which assesses for withdrawal symptoms, triggering administration of lorazepam or chlordiazepoxide according to symptom severity. Benzodiazepines remain the mainstay of alcohol withdrawal treatment and should be tapered rather than abruptly discontinued. Thiamine can prevent or treat Wernicke encephalopathy or Wernicke-Korsakoff syndrome. Naltrexone and acamprosate can be considered as pharmacological treatments to help the older patient stay sober longer term. Disulfiram is generally avoided because of the risk of liver problems and serious or lethal toxicity reactions. Naltrexone and acamprosate are approved by the U.S. Food and Drug Administration for treatment of alcohol use disorder and are effective in maintenance of abstinence. Naltrexone can also be helpful in reducing cravings and avoiding relapse (Table 11–9).

Alcohol interventions can work in older people. Specialized services and groups oriented toward older adults are under development but

TABLE 11–9. Medications for relapse prevention in alcohol use disorder

Naltrexone

  Opioid receptor antagonist that reduces pleasure of drinking and cravings

  Most well-studied substance use disorder pharmacotherapy treatment among older adults

  Relatively safe; small risk of hepatotoxicity

  50 mg taken daily or as needed (only daily treatment studied in older adults)

Acamprosate

  N-methyl-D-aspartate (NMDA) and γ-aminobutyric acid (GABA) receptor modulator that reduces pleasure of drinking and cravings

  Relatively safe; renal dosing required

  666 mg three times a day

Disulfiram

  An aldehyde dehydrogenase inhibitor that increases ill effects of alcohol ingestion by increasing acetaldehyde levels

  Generally avoid in older adults because of possible dangerous cardiovascular and hepatotoxic reactions

currently not widely available. Treatment strategies for alcohol use disorder can include personalized feedback, physician advice, educational materials and follow up, or simple interventions including brief interventions, leaflets, and alcohol assessments with advice to reduce drinking (Kelly et al. 2018). Connecting patients and families with community resources, including Alcoholics Anonymous and Al-Anon, can also help. Where it is available, residential substance rehabilitation treatment can be a valuable support.

Opioid Abuse

Opioids have high addictive potential, even in those who take their medication as prescribed, and abuse of these drugs has reached epidemic proportions in parts of the United States. Prescription opioid use may progress to heroin, which is increasingly common among older people (Mattson et al. 2017). In older people, opioids can cause breathing complications, confusion, drug interaction problems, and falls.

Chronic pain is a common reason for nonmedical use of prescription pain medications later in life. Older adults are more likely to have chronic pain and be prescribed prescription painkillers, and this can lead to negative consequences including physical and mental health issues, overdose, and death (Mattson et al. 2017). Baby boomers abuse prescription pain relievers at higher rates than older generations (Blazer and Wu 2009). Recent increases in rates of death and use of prescription opioids with suicidal intent are extremely concerning in the rapidly expanding elderly population (West et al. 2015). Opioids should be avoided for chronic noncancer pain management if possible (Munzing 2017).

Screening tests for opioids include the Screener and Opioid Assessment for Patients with Pain (SOAPP; Akbik et al. 2006) and Current Opioid Misuse Measure (COMM; Butler et al. 2007). Health care professionals should document and communicate findings and care needs of geriatric patients who misuse prescription opioids to the opioid prescriber and encourage follow-up with members of the patient's caregiver team.

Treatment for opioid use disorder should be offered to all patients, regardless of age. Detoxification should occur gradually with medical supervision and not be tapered precipitously due to risk of medical complications from withdrawal. Patients with opioid use disorder should be provided with harm reduction education and, ideally, the overdose reversal medication naloxone. Medication-assisted treatment (MAT) with agents such as methadone, buprenorphine/naloxone, and long-acting injectable naltrexone can be considered for older adults with opioid use disorder. Clinicians should start low and go slow when treating older adults with MAT, for example, using half the usual starting dosage and a lower maximum dosage of medications. Patients should be educated about the dangers of mixing MAT with other medications or substances, including alcohol and prescription drugs.

Benzodiazepine Abuse

Benzodiazepines, nonbenzodiazepine sleep medications, and (less commonly) barbiturates are often prescribed for sleep disturbances, which are highly prevalent in geriatric patients. Risk factors for abuse of prescription medications include female gender, social isolation, and a history of substance abuse (Culberson and Ziska 2008). Other factors that may be associated with benzodiazepine abuse in older adults include low self-control, depressive symptoms and negative emotionality, and poor health (Holtfreter et al. 2015).

Long-term use of benzodiazepines and other central nervous system depressants frequently leads to tolerance, requiring increasingly larger doses over time. Elderly people are particularly prone to adverse effects of benzodiazepines (Bogunovic and Greenfield 2004). Benzodiazepine use is associated with confusion, falls, and hip fractures in older people and is especially concerning because of the risk of fatal and nonfatal overdoses (Maree et al. 2016). Given this risk of harm, recent evidence-based clinical practice guidelines recommend that deprescribing (slow taper) of benzodiazepines be offered to adults age 65 and older who take benzodiazepines to treat insomnia, regardless of duration of use (Pottie et al. 2018).

Treatment of benzodiazepine dependence consists of a slow tapering of the medication. Benzodiazepine withdrawal symptoms in geriatric patients are similar to those of alcohol withdrawal, including confusion, disorientation, and potential for life-threatening delirium with seizures and coma. Detoxification should be carefully monitored and may need to occur slowly, often over weeks to months, and in some cases even years. Before a taper is begun, patients should be educated about the rationale for the taper, told that withdrawal symptoms may occur but will be mild and transient, and should be engaged in the taper planning, including decisions about the rate and duration of the taper.

No published evidence suggests that switching to long-acting benzodiazepines reduces incidence of withdrawal symptoms or is more effective than tapering with short-active benzodiazepines (Pottie et al. 2018). Thus, in older adults, who have increased risk of adverse events and toxicity with long-acting benzodiazepines, the risks of switching from short-acting to long-acting outweigh any potential benefit. Most studies involving benzodiazepine tapers include 25% dosage reduction every few weeks, with some switching to 12.5% dose reduction in the later part of the taper (Pottie et al. 2018). For patients who have been taking benzodiazepines chronically for prolonged periods (decades), the frequency for each step of dosage reduction may need to be lengthened (Table 11–10). The evidence suggests that a reduction in dosage is a reduction in harm, so while stopping entirely is ideal, any reduction in total daily dosage should be considered a good thing.

Cannabis Misuse

Epidemiological studies show that aging baby boomers embrace marijuana and illicit drugs in far greater numbers than previous generations did (Dinitto and Choi 2011). The prevalence of cannabis use has increased significantly in recent years among older adults in the United States, and the changing landscape toward normalized and legalized cannabis throughout the world underscores the need to understand the vulnerabilities, risks, and potential benefits of marijuana use in older people (Han et al. 2017b).

Seniors who dabbled with drugs in their youth may be more likely to turn to similar drugs, particularly marijuana, to treat ailments of old age

TABLE 11–10. **Example of benzodiazepine taper**

	Action	Dosage
	Starting dosage lorazepam 2 mg bid (4 mg total daily dosage)	
Step 1	Start	4 mg/day
Step 2	Total dosage reduction 25%	3 mg/day
Step 3	Total dosage reduction 50%	2 mg/day
Step 4	Hold dose	2 mg/day
Step 5	Current dosage reduction by ~25% at each step	1.5 mg/day
Step 6		1.25 mg/day
Step 7		1 mg/day
Step 8		0.75 mg/day
Step 9		0.5 mg/day
Step 10		0.25 mg/day
Step 11	Discontinue	

Note. Duration of time in between each step should be at least 2 weeks for chronic users, and up to 1–2 months. At lower dosages, exact 25% reductions may not be possible given available pill doses; round up or down based on previous experience with patient tolerating dosage reductions in earlier steps of the taper. For divided doses, engage patient in deciding which dose he or she wants to decrease at each step. Some patients may require three-times-daily rather than twice-daily dosing if interdose troughs result in breakthrough withdrawal symptoms.

including chronic pain. Modern breeds of cannabis are increasingly potent hybrid strains, with much higher levels of tetrahydrocannabinol (THC) than in the past. Older people may smoke marijuana or use cannabis concentrates, oils, or extracts topically, in edible preparations, or by vaporizer. Synthetic marijuana use is not limited to young people and often involves dangerous chemicals with unpredictable composition. It can be more potent than natural strains of cannabis and carries increased risk of psychiatric side effects (Kemp et al. 2016).

Stimulant Abuse

Abuse of cocaine, methamphetamine, and prescription stimulants is on the rise among older people and is associated with adverse medical and psychiatric consequences, including cardiovascular problems and cognitive impairment (Yarnell 2015). Cocaine-related admissions (i.e., where cocaine is the client's primary substance problem) are on the rise in the older adult population (Chhatre et al. 2017).

Vignette *(continued)*

Mr. J started to work with his primary care doctor to address his alcohol problem. He agreed to start taking naltrexone and began to cut back on his daily drinking as his cravings decreased. Mr. J was able to stay sober for 6 months, with improvement in his overall health and cognitive status, as well as reduction in depression symptoms.

Conclusion: Recovery Is Possible

As demographics change, cases of geriatric addictions are more frequently encountered in clinical practice. Substance abuse can complicate all aspects of the aging process. As clinicians increase their awareness of the scope of this problem and gain better understanding in this important area of practice, they can improve their skills at diagnosing and treating SUDs in older adults.

Older adults can recover from SUDs. Denial of addiction may be stronger in older adults than in younger people, but it is worth the effort to engage the patient and the patient's family in recovery efforts and learn new ways of communicating. Outcomes for older people are often as good as or better than for younger people (Sahker et al. 2015). Older adults are able to utilize offered treatments and benefit from the positive effects of brief interventions, education, counseling, and inpatient treatment.

Statements from older adults in recovery suggest that they are grateful for a new life free of substance abuse. Older adults in recovery express feeling relieved to find alternatives to prescription medications for chronic pain and anxiety, glad to contribute to society in meaningful ways, and happy to find new friends and relief from loneliness through engaging in treatment (Haroutunian 2016).

KEY POINTS

- Substance abuse is a growing public health problem among older adults.
- Health effects of substance abuse are even more dangerous for elderly people than for younger users.

- Substance use should be suspected if a patient is isolating himself or herself to hide drinking or drug use, is getting into legal trouble, or has an abrupt unexplained decline in functioning.
- Substance use disorders (SUDs) in older people remain underestimated, underdiagnosed, and undertreated. Ageism and complacency are common.
- Baby boomers have higher rates of SUDs compared with previous generations.
- Alcohol, marijuana, and prescription drug use are major areas of concern.
- The older patient should be referred to treatment after careful comprehensive evaluation, depending on patient preference and when outpatient detoxification and treatment efforts are unsuccessful or unacceptably high risk.
- Recovery is possible, and older adults can have good outcomes after treatment.

Resources

Readings

Bhatia U, Nadkarni A, Murthy P, et al: Recent advances in treatment for older people with substance use problems: an updated systematic and narrative review. Eur Geriatr Med 6(6):580–586, 2015

Elinson Z: Aging baby boomers bring drug habits into middle age. Wall Street Journal, March 16, 2015. Available at: www.wsj.com/articles/aging-baby-boomers-bring-drug-habits-into-middle-age-1426469057.

Haroutunian HL: Not as Prescribed: Recognizing and Facing Alcohol and Drug Misuse in Older Adults. Center City, MN, Hazelden, 2016

National Institute on Drug Abuse: Principles of Drug Addiction Treatment: A Research-Based Guide, 3rd Edition. Updated January 2018. Available at: www.drugabuse.gov/publications/principles-drug-addiction-treatment-research-based-guide-third-edition/preface.

Sullivan M, Levin FR: Addiction in the Older Patient. New York, Oxford University Press, 2016

Websites

Al-Anon: https://al-anon.org/

Alcoholics Anonymous: www.aa.org/

Deprescribing: https://deprescribing.org; Aims to share and exchange information about deprescribing approaches and deprescribing research with the public, health care providers, and researchers

Substance Abuse and Mental Health Services Administration national helpline for individuals and families facing mental and/or substance use disorders: www.samhsa.gov/find-help/national-helpline

References

Akbik H, Butler SF, Budman SH, et al: Validation and clinical application of the Screener and Opioid Assessment for Patients with Pain (SOAPP). J Pain Symptom Manage 32(3):287–293, 2006 16939853

American Psychiatric Association: Diagnostic and Statistical Manual of Mental Disorders, 5th Edition. Arlington, VA, American Psychiatric Association, 2013

Arndt S, Clayton R, Schultz SK: Trends in substance abuse treatment 1998–2008: increasing older adult first-time admissions for illicit drugs. Am J Geriatr Psychiatry 19(8):704–711, 2011 21785290

Bhatia U, Nadkarni A, Murthy P, et al: Recent advances in treatment for older people with substance use problems: an updated systematic and narrative review. Eur Geriatr Med 6(6):580–586, 2015

Blazer DG, Wu LT: Nonprescription use of pain relievers by middle-aged and elderly community-living adults: National Survey on Drug Use and Health. J Am Geriatr Soc 57(7):1252–1257, 2009 19486199

Blow F, Brower K, Schulenberg J, et al: The Michigan alcoholism screening test-geriatric version (MAST-G): a new elderly specific screening instrument. Alcohol Clin Exp Res 16(2):372, 1992

Bogunovic OJ, Greenfield SF: Practical geriatrics: use of benzodiazepines among elderly patients. Psychiatr Serv 55(3):233–235, 2004 15001721

Burruss K, Sacco P, Smith CA: Understanding older adults' attitudes and beliefs about drinking: perspectives of residents in congregate living. Ageing Soc 35(9):1889–1904, 2015

Butler SF, Budman SH, Fernandez KC, et al: Development and validation of the Current Opioid Misuse Measure. Pain 130(1–2):144–156, 2007 17493754

Chhatre S, Cook R, Mallik E, et al: Trends in substance use admissions among older adults. BMC Health Serv Res 17(1):584, 2017 28830504

Crome I: Substance misuse in the older person: setting higher standards. Clin Med (Lond) 13 (suppl 6):s46–s49, 2013 24298183

Culberson JW, Ziska M: Prescription drug misuse/abuse in the elderly. Geriatrics 63(9):22–31, 2008 18763848

D'Amico EJ, Paddock SM, Burnam A, et al: Identification of and guidance for problem drinking by general medical providers: results from a national survey. Med Care 43(3):229–236, 2005 15725979

De Jong CA, Goodair C, Crome I, et al: Substance misuse education for physicians: why older people are important. Yale J Biol Med 89(1):97–103, 2016 27505022

Dinitto DM, Choi NG: Marijuana use among older adults in the U.S.A.: user characteristics, patterns of use, and implications for intervention. Int Psychogeriatr 23(5):732–741, 2011 21108863

Draper B, Ridley N, Johnco C, et al: Screening for alcohol and substance use for older people in geriatric hospital and community health settings. Int Psychogeriatr 27(1):157–166, 2015 25247846

Emiliussen J, Nielsen AS, Andersen K: Identifying risk factors for late-onset (50+) alcohol use disorder and heavy drinking: a systematic review. Subst Use Misuse 52(12):1575–1588, 2017 28524740

Gossop M, Moos R: Substance misuse among older adults: a neglected but treatable problem. Addiction 103(3):347–348, 2008 18205895

Han BH, Moore AA, Sherman S, et al: Demographic trends of binge alcohol use and alcohol use disorders among older adults in the United States, 2005–2014. Drug Alcohol Depend 170:198–207, 2017a 27979428

Han BH, Sherman S, Mauro PM, et al: Demographic trends among older cannabis users in the United States, 2006–13. Addiction 112(3):516–525, 2017b 27767235

Haroutunian HL: Not as Prescribed: Recognizing and Facing Alcohol and Drug Misuse in Older Adults. Center City, MN, Hazelden, 2016

Hategan A, Bourgeois JA, Hirsch C: On-Call Geriatric Psychiatry: Handbook of Principles and Practice. New York, Springer International, 2016

Holtfreter K, Reisig MD, O'Neal EN: Prescription drug misuse in late adulthood: an empirical examination of competing explanations. J Drug Issues 45(4):351–367, 2015

Kelly S, Olanrewaju O, Cowan A, et al: Interventions to prevent and reduce excessive alcohol consumption in older people: a systematic review and meta-analysis. Age Ageing 47(2):175–184, 2018 28985250

Kemp AM, Clark MS, Dobbs T, et al: Top 10 facts you need to know about synthetic cannabinoids: not so nice spice. Am J Med 129(3):240–244, 2016 26522795

Kuerbis A, Sacco P, Blazer DG, et al: Substance abuse among older adults. Clin Geriatr Med 30(3):629–654, 2014 25037298

Le Roux C, Tang Y, Drexler K: Alcohol and opioid use disorder in older adults: neglected and treatable illnesses. Curr Psychiatry Rep 18(9):87, 2016 27488204

Maree RD, Marcum ZA, Saghafi E, et al: A systematic review of opioid and benzodiazepine misuse in older adults. Am J Geriatr Psychiatry 24(11):949–963, 2016 27567185

Mattson M, Lipari RN, Hays C, et al: A day in the life of older adults: substance use facts. The CBHSQ Report, May 11, 2017. Available at: https://www.samhsa.gov/data/sites/default/files/report_2792/ShortReport-2792.html. Accessed June 18, 2019.

Mayfield D, McLeod G, Hall P: The CAGE questionnaire: validation of a new alcoholism screening instrument. Am J Psychiatry 131(10):1121–1123, 1974 4416585

Moore AA, Karno MP, Grella CE, et al: Alcohol, tobacco, and nonmedical drug use in older U.S. adults: data from the 2001/02 national epidemiologic survey of alcohol and related conditions. J Am Geriatr Soc 57(12):2275–2281, 2009 19874409

Mowbray O, Washington T, Purser G, et al: Problem drinking and depression in older adults with multiple chronic health conditions. J Am Geriatr Soc 65(1):146–152, 2017 27748504

Munzing T: Physician guide to appropriate opioid prescribing for noncancer pain. Perm J 21:16–169, 2017

National Institute on Drug Abuse: Misuse of Prescription Drugs. Bethesda, MD, National Institutes of Health, 2018

Oslin DW: Evidence-based treatment of geriatric substance abuse. Psychiatr Clin North Am 28(4):897–911, ix, 2005 16325734

Pottie K, Thompson W, Davies S, et al: Deprescribing benzodiazepine receptor agonists: Evidence-based clinical practice guideline. Can Fam Physician 64(5):339-351, 2018 29760253

Sahker E, Schultz SK, Arndt S: Treatment of substance use disorders in older adults: implications for care delivery. J Am Geriatr Soc 63(11):2317–2323, 2015 26502741

Substance Abuse and Mental Health Services Administration: Get Connected: Linking Older Adults With Resources on Medication, Alcohol, and Mental Health. Rockville, MD, Substance Abuse and Mental Health Services Administration, 2017

Sullivan M, Levin FR: Addiction in the Older Patient. New York, Oxford University Press, 2016

Sullivan JT, Sykora K, Schneiderman J, et al: Assessment of alcohol withdrawal: the revised clinical institute withdrawal assessment for alcohol scale (CIWA-Ar). Br J Addict 84(11):1353–1357, 1989 2597811

West NA, Severtson SG, Green JL, et al: Trends in abuse and misuse of prescription opioids among older adults. Drug Alcohol Depend 149:117–121, 2015 25678441

Wu LT, Blazer DG: Illicit and nonmedical drug use among older adults: a review. J Aging Health 23(3):481–504, 2011 21084724

Yarnell SC: Cocaine abuse in later life: a case series and review of the literature. Prim Care Companion CNS Disord 17(2), 2015 26445694

Mild Cognitive Impairment

"I'm Forgetting Things. Is This Normal for My Age, or Do I Have Dementia?"

Iuliana Predescu, M.D.
Laura B. Dunn, M.D.

CHAPTER 12

Clinical Presentation

Chief Complaint

"I'm forgetting things. Is this normal for my age, or do I have dementia?"

Vignette

Ms. O is a 74-year-old widow who lives by herself. She presents to her primary care physician with a primary complaint of "forgetting things," which she says started more than 2 years ago. She reports that initially this happened only when she was tired or had a busy day, but recently she believes that it has been getting worse. In particular, she is afraid that she might be "getting dementia like my mother."

She reports that she is having difficulties remembering the names of people that she has known for a long time. Ms. O states that she can recognize their face, but "it's too embarrassing to ask people's names multiple times." She reports that she has always enjoyed cooking and has favorite recipes that she has been preparing for her family for years. Recently, she is having a hard time remembering all the ingredients and preparation steps; she says "this is very frustrating."

Ms. O reports that because of her memory concerns, about 6 months ago she began using a calendar, writing herself more reminders, and keeping a notebook to keep track of her activities. More concerning for her is "her bad concentration." For example, she reports that she "spent 3 hours just to pay a few bills in order to make sure that I am not making any mistakes."

She claims that she is able to independently perform all of her regular activities—shopping, preparing meals, housework, managing her medication, and taking care of personal hygiene—without any problems. She also reports that she is able to handle her finances without any help. She reports that she has had no problems with driving—that is, she has not had any accidents and has not gotten lost.

Ms. O worked as a chemistry teacher, and per her report, she enjoyed her profession very much. She was married for 47 years. She has two daughters, with whom she speaks daily, and they have lunch together almost every Sunday. Her husband passed away 5 years ago after he had a stroke. Losing her husband was hard, but her family and friends were very supportive. She reports that she still misses him but has learned to live without him. She likes staying active and walks daily for 30 minutes, volunteers at the hospital gift shop three times a week, and meets her friends for lunch or dinner almost daily.

Does Ms. O. have the first signs of dementia or something else?

Discussion

Some cognitive abilities, such as vocabulary and experiential skills, are well maintained until later in life, but other abilities such as processing speed, working memory, and executive function decline gradually over time. Structural and functional changes in the brain correlate with these age-related cognitive changes, including alterations in neuronal structure without neuronal death, loss of synapses, and dysfunction of neuronal networks. Age-related diseases accelerate the rate of neuronal dysfunction, neuronal loss, and cognitive decline, with many persons developing cognitive impairments severe enough to impair their everyday functional abilities (Harada et al. 2013). With the growth of the older adult population, it is important to distinguish among normal aging, mild cognitive impairment, and dementia (major neurocognitive disorder).

Mild cognitive impairment (MCI) is a term introduced in the late 1980s by Reisberg and colleagues to define subjects in the intermediate stage between normal aging and dementia (Reisberg 1988). In 1999, a group at the Mayo Clinic described subjects in their community aging study who had memory concerns beyond what was expected for age but whose overall cognitive functioning and abilities to perform daily life activities were preserved (Petersen et al. 2014). The first definition of MCI was focused on memory problems, and MCI was considered a prodrome to Alzheimer's disease (AD). However, it was later demonstrated that not all patients with MCI develop AD. In 2003, the first key symposium on MCI was held, and the Mayo Clinic's MCI criteria were expanded to include impairment in other areas of cognitive functioning except memory (Winblad et al. 2004). DSM-5 (American Psychiatric Association 2013) recognizes the predementia stage of cognitive impairment, using the term *mild neurocognitive disorder* (NCD), a condition that has many of the features of MCI (Box 12–1).

Box 12–1. Diagnostic Criteria for Mild Neurocognitive Disorder

---

A. Evidence of modest cognitive decline from a previous level of performance in one or more cognitive domains (complex attention, executive function, learning and memory, language, perceptual-motor, or social cognition) based on:
   1. Concern of the individual, a knowledgeable informant, or the clinician that there has been a mild decline in cognitive function; and
   2. A modest impairment in cognitive performance, preferably documented by standardized neuropsychological testing or, in its absence, another quantified clinical assessment.
B. The cognitive deficits do not interfere with capacity for independence in everyday activities (i.e., complex instrumental activities of daily living such as paying bills or managing medications are preserved, but greater effort, compensatory strategies, or accommodation may be required).
C. The cognitive deficits do not occur exclusively in the context of a delirium.
D. The cognitive deficits are not better explained by another mental disorder (e.g., major depressive disorder, schizophrenia).

Specify whether due to:
   Alzheimer's disease
   Frontotemporal lobar degeneration
   Lewy body disease
   Vascular disease
   Traumatic brain injury
   Substance/medication use
   HIV infection
   Prion disease

Parkinson's disease
Huntington's disease
Another medical condition
Multiple etiologies
Unspecified

Specify:

Without behavioral disturbance: If the cognitive disturbance is not accompanied by any clinically significant behavioral disturbance.

With behavioral disturbance *(specify disturbance):* If the cognitive disturbance is accompanied by a clinically significant behavioral disturbance (e.g., psychotic symptoms, mood disturbance, agitation, apathy, or other behavioral symptoms).

Source. Adapted from American Psychiatric Association: *Diagnostic and Statistical Manual of Mental Disorders,* 5th Edition. Arlington, VA, 2013, pp. 605–606. Copyright © 2013 American Psychiatric Association. Used with permission.

MCI or mild NCD is characterized by a discrete and distinct decline in one's usual cognitive abilities that is greater than expected for the patient's age and educational background but not severe enough to interfere with daily functioning.

Older adults with MCI are a heterogeneous group, and identification can be challenging for even the most experienced clinicians. Patients can present with a plethora of symptoms in addition to memory problems (Table 12–1). Impairment in one or more cognitive domains (Figure 12–1), in isolation or in conjunction with memory impairment, is crucial to note.

Classification

Current classification schemes divide MCI into two subtypes: *amnestic* type, characterized by impaired memory, and *nonamnestic* type, characterized by preserved memory in the presence of impairment in other cognitive domains, such as executive function, language, or visuospatial abilities. The impairment can be limited to one cognitive domain (MCI single domain) or to multiple domains (MCI multiple domains). MCI can thus be divided into four possible clinical subtypes (Petersen et al. 2014):

1. Amnestic MCI, single domain
2. Amnestic MCI, multiple domain
3. Nonamnestic MCI, single domain
4. Nonamnestic MCI, multiple domain

TABLE 12–1. **Mild cognitive impairment: most common symptoms**

Mild memory loss

Word finding difficulty

Having difficulty organizing, planning, or making decisions

Trouble with managing bills or accounts

Lack of initiative or motivation in the absence of depression

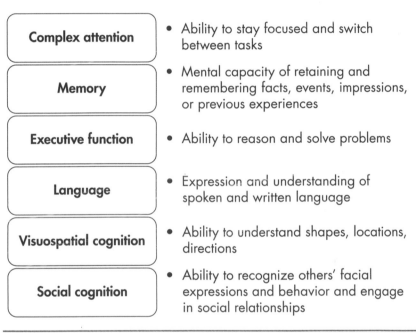

Complex attention
- Ability to stay focused and switch between tasks

Memory
- Mental capacity of retaining and remembering facts, events, impressions, or previous experiences

Executive function
- Ability to reason and solve problems

Language
- Expression and understanding of spoken and written language

Visuospatial cognition
- Ability to understand shapes, locations, directions

Social cognition
- Ability to recognize others' facial expressions and behavior and engage in social relationships

FIGURE 12–1. **Domains of cognitive functioning.**

Subcategorization of MCI is common in research endeavors but also has important implications for clinical prognosis and early intervention. For example, a patient with a decline in visuospatial functioning is more likely to have problems with driving and would benefit from a referral for a driving assessment test. A thorough neuropsychological assessment is not always available, and identifying the deficits in the context of a routine clinic visit can be challenging. Utilizing a global screening test such as the Montreal Cognitive Assessment (MoCA; Nasreddine et al. 2005) as part of the evaluation can provide important information about deficient domains.

Differential Diagnosis

Brain structural changes associated with cognitive decline typically begin a decade or more before clinical manifestations are noted; therefore, it is important to begin screening all individuals who are 65 years of age or older for cognitive impairment. In the presence of a medical or psychiatric condition that might accelerate cognitive decline, screening should be started earlier. The impairment can be very insidious and difficult for a patient to perceive. Frequently, the difficulties may be attributed to fatigue, insomnia, or other medical or psychiatric conditions. Initially, the symptoms might be noticed by the family; therefore, if possible, obtaining collateral information is strongly recommended.

The prevalence of MCI in people age 65 years and older is 10%–20% (Petersen 2016). The risk increases with age, especially for amnestic MCI (Luck et al. 2010); male gender for both amnestic and nonamnestic MCI; lower educational status for both amnestic and nonamnestic MCI (Luck et al. 2010, Roberts et al. 2012); vascular risk factors (Lopez et al. 2003) (e.g., diabetes and hypertension; Luck et al. 2010); presence of apolipoprotein E (APOE) E4 genotype; vitamin D deficiency; sleep-disordered breathing; and prior critical illness (e.g., sepsis) (Langa and Levine 2014).

Numerous other conditions need to be ruled out before making the diagnosis of MCI.

Depression, Anxiety, or Other Psychiatric Conditions

Even if a patient denies depressed mood, it is important to ask about other depressive symptoms: decrease or loss of interest in activities that he or she used to enjoy, isolation, guilty feelings, negative thoughts, hopelessness, and suicidal ideations or wish to be dead. In older adults, symptoms such as irritability and agitation could be the expression of depressed mood. On the other hand, "depression" reported by the patient or family can represent apathy and neurovegetative symptoms, both known to predict progression from amnestic MCI to dementia of AD (Andreescu et al. 2014). If possible, a screening tool such as the Geriatric Depression Scale (Yesavage et al. 1982–1983; score > 6 indicates depression on 15-item version) can provide important and immediate information.

Depression occurs in 20% of individuals with MCI (Lyketsos et al. 2002). It is important to note that depression itself is associated with cognitive impairment and can improve with successful treatment of the comorbid depression, but symptoms are less likely to completely remit if MCI is present. Also, depression co-occurring with MCI is more resistant to antidepressants. It is important to try to treat the depression as early as possible, because patients with both MCI and depression, especially those with poor response to antidepressants, are at more than twice the risk of developing dementia of Alzheimer's type compared with MCI patients without depression (Modrego and Ferrández 2004).

Anxiety in geriatric patients is very common; however, the relationship between anxiety and MCI is less understood. Studies indicate that anxiety symptoms in amnestic-type MCI predict conversion to AD, over and beyond the effects of depression, memory loss, or atrophy within AD neuroimaging biomarkers (Mah et al. 2015). Also, there is a complex association between anxiety and MCI, contingent on the onset and severity of anxiety symptoms and on the neuropsychological profile and functional consequences of the MCI (Andreescu et al. 2014). It is known that anxiety symptoms in older adults are associated with avoidance, decreased daily activities, increased isolation, dependency on family members, and overall decreased quality of life. The GAD-7 and GAD-2 are well-validated screening tools for generalized anxiety (see Chapter 4, "Diagnosis and Treatment of Generalized Anxiety Disorder"); however, they have not been validated in people with MCI. Among older adults in general, it has been recommended that the cutpoints be lowered for identification of clinically significant anxiety (Wild et al. 2014).

Alternatively, we recommend asking a few screening questions. Some examples would be "Would you describe yourself as a worrier?" or "Do you think that you easily become nervous or upset?" These questions are two of the generalized anxiety disorder screening questions from the Penn State Worry Questionnaire, a scale with good internal consistency, adequate test-retest reliability, and good convergent and divergent validity with samples consisting of older adults with generalized anxiety (Hopko et al. 2003).

Patients and family members should be educated about the effects of untreated depression and anxiety that may exacerbate the sequelae of MCI so that they are motivated to engage in proper treatment for ongoing psychiatric conditions.

Other psychiatric symptoms are rare; however, when they are present, this may suggest a different etiology, and therefore it is important to ask the patient about other symptoms. For example, the presence of recent personality changes might suggest frontotemporal dementia, or the presence of hallucinations might be an indicator of Lewy body dementia or depression with psychotic features.

To add to the clinical challenge, psychiatric symptoms can be present in 35%–75% of patients with MCI. Depression, apathy, anxiety, and irritability are more common (Apostolova and Cummings 2008). The Neuropsychiatric Inventory (Cummings et al. 1994) is the most widely used rating scale for neuropsychiatric symptoms in patients with dementias and other neurological disorders and can be used to assess the neuropsychiatric symptoms in MCI. To our knowledge, no scale specific for neuropsychiatric symptoms in MCI is available at this time.

Medical Problems

Multiple medical problems can contribute to cognitive impairment; hence, their early identification and treatment are critical. There are other situations, especially in the case of individuals older than 65 years, when the deficits persist longer than the expected duration of the illness. These might be explained by a delay in diagnosis or underlying irreversible cognitive impairment (Chari et al. 2015).

- *Hypothyroidism* can present as concentration problems and forgetfulness, but with the right treatment, it can be reversed. Subclinical hypothyroidism was found to produce significant impairment of cognition in elderly individuals, with thyroid-stimulating hormone level as a sensitive marker (Dugbartey 1998). Interestingly, older adults with subclinical hyperthyroidism had lower Mini Mental State Examination (MMSE) scores than euthyroid subjects (Ceresini et al. 2009).
- *Sleep apnea* is a very common condition in the elderly patient and is present not only in overweight patients but also in patients with a normal body mass index, especially if a family history of sleep apnea is present. The regular use of a continuous positive airway pressure machine can improve symptoms such as concentration and excessive daytime sleepiness.
- *Dehydration,* especially during warm months or in the presence of other illnesses that cause fluid loss, can present with cognitive impairment and even confusion in severe cases.
- *Malnutrition* occurs when people are not getting enough nutrients because of an inadequate or unbalanced diet or digestive problems that interfere with nutrient absorption. Vitamin B_{12} deficiency is one of the most common types of malnutrition, and confusion is the most common cognitive effect. Other vitamin deficiencies that can result in cognitive impairment in older patients are niacin and folic acid deficiency. Iron deficiency has been known to cause cognitive impairment in the elderly, independent of anemia (Chari et al. 2015). Recurrent episodes of hypoglycemia can cause cognitive im-

pairment, and in some cases this may lead to dementia (Whitmer et al. 2009).

- *Infections* can cause cognitive problems: confusion, difficulty concentrating, or forgetfulness. Urinary tract infections are a common cause of cognitive problems among older adults. Various central nervous system infections (such as chronic bacterial meningitis, neurosyphilis, tuberculous meningitis or tuberculoma, herpes encephalitis, AIDS dementia complex, and neurocysticercosis) can cause reversible cognitive impairment (Chari et al. 2015). HIV-associated neurological conditions can produce symptoms ranging from mild asymptomatic cognitive impairment to severe dementia. A few studies have documented that many of these conditions are reversible with highly active antiretroviral therapy treatment (Chari et al. 2015).

- *Strokes,* even minor ones, are a common cause of cognitive impairment. Other causes include head injuries with possible subdural hematoma, brain tumors, and chronic diseases, such as sickle cell disease or multiple sclerosis.

- *Sensory deficits* (hearing or vision problems) are very common in older adults and can appear as cognitive impairment. In time, MCI can worsen as a result of these deficits, due to the affected person becoming increasingly isolated and disengaged.

Medications

Geriatric populations are affected by multiple medication problems: taking a dose too high and developing side effects, taking the wrong medication, and drug-drug interactions. Polypharmacy is a real problem for geriatric populations, and cognitive impairment is a very common side effect of multiple medications. Benzodiazepines and nonbenzodiazepine hypnotics, valproic acid, opiates, anticholinergics, digoxin, atropine, carbamazepine, first-generation antihistamines, bladder antimuscarinics, muscle relaxants, and steroids are only a few medications that are known to cause cognitive impairment. Also, hypotension and hypoglycemia secondary to strict control of hypertension and diabetes mellitus may contribute to cognitive decline. A study done in Norway (2006–2008) indicated that 24% of the 206 patients included in the analysis had memory impairment that resulted as a side effect from a different medication (Tveito et al. 2016).

Substances (Drugs and Alcohol)

Alcohol, even in small amounts and when used for many years, can cause cognitive impairment. Chronic use of some recreational drugs may exacerbate normal age-related changes in the brain. For example, the natural decline in white matter volume observed after age 50 may be more dramatic in cocaine abusers than in the healthy aging population (Bartzokis et al. 2002). While it is known that marijuana has an impact on cognitive function for young people, currently there are no conclusive data regarding cognitive function of elderly patients using marijuana.

The number of older people with substance use problems or requiring treatment for a substance use disorder is estimated to more than double between 2001 and 2020. This is partly due to the size of the baby-boomer cohort (born between 1946 and 1964) and the higher rate of substance use among this group (Dowling et al. 2008). Therefore, it is important to always ask patients about the use of drugs and alcohol, regardless of their age.

Vignette *(continued)*

Ms. O denies any depressive or anxiety symptoms but admits to moments of irritability caused by her memory problem. She has hypertension, currently well managed with amlodipine and hydrochlorothiazide, hyperlipidemia treated with simvastatin, hypothyroidism managed with levothyroxine 100 µg daily, and a history of breast cancer (in remission for at least 10 years). She denies using any alcohol or drugs. She has a family history of dementia in both parents—her father was diagnosed in his 70s and her mother was diagnosed in her 80s—and a sister who had depression.

Her physical examination was unremarkable, with a body mass index of 20 kg/m² and a normal neurological examination.

Clinical Evaluation

Getting a good history of symptoms from the patient, family, or caregiver is very important, especially information about the onset, evolution, and specific circumstances of the observed changes (e.g., death in the family, retirement, onset of new illness, significant decline in physical health). It is critical to identify the type of onset of cognitive symptoms (e.g., insidious onset more characteristic of Alzheimer's-type MCI vs. abrupt onset following traumatic brain injury), as well as to establish the symptoms' evolution over time (e.g., gradual vs. stepwise, more characteristic of vascular-type MCI). Many times, it is very difficult to obtain a clear history of the debut of symptoms. Patients and family members tend to minimize the earliest signs of cognitive decline, con-

1. **History from patient and family**
   - Sleep apnea → Sleep medicine referral
   - Depression/anxiety → Treatment/psychiatry referral
   - Drug/alcohol use/misuse → Addiction treatment
   - Medication → Reconcile medication list/ deprescribe
2. **MMSE/MoCA**
3. **Physical examination**
   - Positive neurological finding → Neurology referral
   - Hearing/vision changes → Glasses/hearing aids
   - Infection → Example: urinary tract infection
4. **Laboratory tests**
   - CBC, CMP, TSH, vitamin B$_{12}$, vitamin D, RPR, HIV
5. **Brain imaging**—Dementia protocol
   - Rule out brain tumor, acute vestibular syndrome
6. **Neuropsychology**—Referral

Cognitive concerns

FIGURE 12–2. Algorithm for evaluation of mild cognitive impairment.

CBC=complete blood count; CMP=comprehensive metabolic panel; MMSE=Mini Mental State Examination; MoCA=Montreal Cognitive Assessment; RPR=rapid plasma reagin; TSH=thyroid-stimulating hormone.

sidering it a normal aging process or one explained by other medical or psychiatric conditions. It is more feasible to determine when the patient was last well, rather than when symptoms first started. An algorithm for the evaluation of MCI is presented in Figure 12–2.

A thorough interview with the patient and a family member is useful in clarifying the difference between MCI and dementia, because the symptoms and signs are overlapping. The main difference between the two conditions is the requirement for MCI cases to have preserved independence in functional abilities (Table 12–2). Gathering substantial subjective and objective information about activities of daily living (ADLs) and instrumental activities of daily living (IADLs) is very important. Because of the heterogeneity of cases, sometimes the distinction can be very challenging. As a general rule, very mild problems in IADLs are generally consistent with MCI, while basic ADLs should be preserved.

TABLE 12–2. Distinguishing among normal aging, mild cognitive impairment (MCI), and dementia

Normal aging	MCI (minor NCD)	Dementia (major NCD)
Longer time to process information	Problems with memory, usually short-term memory or another cognitive domain	Cognitive decline in one or more cognitive domains severe enough to disrupt daily life
Difficulty remembering names of new people, places, and other things	Problems are significant enough to be noticed by the patient or family, but not serious enough to interfere with daily life	
Normal MMSE and MoCA		

Note.   MMSE=Mini-Mental State Examination; MoCA=Montreal Cognitive Assessment; NCD=neurocognitive disorder.

Some of the following tests are absolutely recommended; others should be done only if indicated:

1. Blood tests (complete blood count, comprehensive metabolic panel, thyroid-stimulating hormone, vitamin B_{12}, vitamin D, rapid plasma reagin), HIV testing if necessary.
2. Magnetic resonance imaging (MRI) of the brain (rule out strokes or tumors). The classic gross neuroanatomical observation of a brain from a patient with AD is diffuse atrophy with flattened cortical sulci and enlarged cerebral ventricles. The classic and pathognomonic microscopic findings are senile plaques, neurofibrillary tangles, neuronal loss (particularly in the cortex and the hippocampus), synaptic loss, and granulovascular degeneration of the neurons (Sadock et al. 2005). One of the first signs of AD will be loss of hippocampal volume seen on MRI, and reduction of glucose metabolism or perfusion in temporoparietal cortex that may be detected with positron emission tomography (PET) or single-photon emission computed tomography scanning (Albert et al. 2011).
3. Fluorodeoxyglucose PET or PET for amyloid imaging along with a cerebrospinal fluid analysis in selected cases (e.g., suspicion of frontotemporal dementia).
4. Neurological examination to rule out other neurological conditions such as Parkinson's disease, stroke, and polyneuropathy.

5. Mental status examination, including MMSE, MoCA, or other standardized scales. The MMSE (Folstein et al. 1975) is brief, easy to use, and well known. However, it is less useful in evaluating patients with MCI because of ceiling effects, especially for well-educated individuals and those with high premorbid intelligence. It also has limitations in evaluating executive functions. The MoCA (Nasreddine et al. 2005) is a more reliable and comprehensive assessment of cognition and can assess abstract thinking, delayed recall, and verbal fluency better than the MMSE. The MoCA has been validated in various languages and has well-known population norms. In patients with transient ischemic attack or minor stroke, early cognitive impairment detected with the MoCA but not with the MMSE was independently associated with white matter damage on MRI, particularly reduced fractional anisotropy (Zamboni et al. 2017). The standardized scale should be repeated every 6 months to assess for changes over time. Different forms of the MoCA are available to prevent practice effects with repeated testing.

6. Functional assessment using the Functional Assessment Staging Test (FAST; Reisberg 1988), the Functional Activities Questionnaire (FAQ; Pfeffer et al. 1982), or the Alzheimer's Disease Cooperative Study/Activities of Daily Living Inventory adapted for patients with mild cognitive impairment (ADCS-MCI-ADL) (Pedrosa et al. 2010). The FAQ is a brief standardized instrument for clinicians to obtain IADL information from an informant. On the FAQ, individuals with MCI were reported to have more IADLs that "require assistance" compared with individuals with normal cognition (2.7 vs. 0.1; $P < 0.01$; Luck et al. 2010). Moreover, a cutpoint of 6 points or higher on the FAQ was 85% accurate in distinguishing patients with MCI from those with dementia (Widera et al. 2011).

7. Neuropsychological testing. Neuropsychological tests can detect subtle dysfunction in areas such as memory, language, visual-spatial skills, executive function, attention, psychomotor speed, and information processing, especially when the cognitive decline is very mild and would probably go undetected by the MMSE or even the MoCA. The tests are useful as a baseline and can assess the longitudinal evolution. See Chapter 13, "Neuropsychological Testing," for further discussion.

8. The Cambridge Neuropsychological Test Automated Battery (CANTAB) Mobile memory screening tool. CANTAB Mobile is designed to detect clinically relevant memory impairment in older adults. It is approved by the U.S. Food and Drug Administration (FDA) and in-

cludes Paired Associated Learning, a computerized test of visuospatial associative learning to assess episodic memory; the Geriatric Depression Scale; and the Activities of Daily Living scale. It can be administered by nonmedical staff in 10 minutes, is sensitive to MCI, and is available in more than 20 different languages (Cambridge Cognition website: www.cambridgecognition.com). The software can be ordered online (info@cantab.com).

9. Genetic testing. Rare families have genetic mutation that cause AD early in life in 50% of relatives: presenilin genes (*C1* and *C14*) and amyloid precursor protein *APP* gene (long arm of *C21*). *APOE-E4* is a common allele in 20% of population that increases risk; however, some people with *APOE-E4* never get AD and some without *APOE-E4* get AD, and therefore evaluation for this allele is *not* recommended as a predictive test (Avramopoulos 2009).

Vignette *(continued)*

Because Ms. O has hypothyroidism, the first step is to check her thyroid-stimulating hormone level, plus/minus free thyroxine (T_4). She also has a family history of depression, so she should definitely be screened for depression (e.g., using the Geriatric Depression Scale). She has hyperlipidemia, hypertension, and a history of cancer, which are risk factors for stroke. Her family history is positive for dementia in both parents, placing her at risk for developing dementia, especially of the Alzheimer's type.

Interventions

An overview of interventions for MCI is presented in Figure 12–3.

Family Education

Counseling patients and family on expectations is an important step. A survey done in 2012 by Home Instead Senior Care, the world's leading provider of home care services for seniors, revealed that Americans fear developing AD more than any other life-threatening disease, including cancer, stroke, heart disease, and diabetes. It is important to focus on their concerns and understanding of the disease and/or meaning of the test as well as address questions about prognosis, expectations, and treatment options.

Psychopharmacological Treatments

Currently, there is no pharmacological therapy approved by the FDA for MCI. Cholinesterase inhibitors have been proposed to slow the progres-

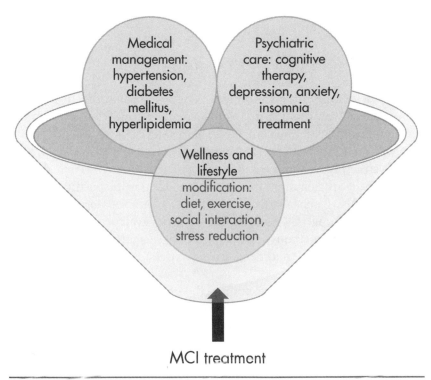

FIGURE 12–3. Treatment of mild cognitive impairment (MCI).

sion of MCI to AD, but data (Raschetti et al. 2007) show that the use of these agents in MCI was not associated with any delay in the onset of AD or dementia, and the risks associated with cholinesterase inhibitors are not negligible.

Other pharmacological treatments that have been studied for the treatment of MCI include vitamin E (Farina et al. 2012), metformin (Luchsinger et al. 2016), ginkgo biloba (Snitz et al. 2009), and testosterone (Emmelot-Vonk et al. 2008). No definitive evidence exists, however, to suggest that any of these treatments slow or prevent progression to dementia, or improve cognitive function, in people with MCI or dementia due to AD.

Prevention Strategies

The main recommendations that can be made at this time in terms of reducing the risk of MCI are stroke prevention by blood pressure control; smoking cessation; statin therapy; antiplatelet therapy; and anticoagulation or antithrombotic therapy for atrial fibrillation (Langa and Levine 2014).

Nonpharmacological Treatments

Cognitive rehabilitation therapies. Cognitive rehabilitation therapies are used to enhance or restore cognitive abilities, potentially through neuroplastic mechanisms. The results from various trials are promising but inconclusive (Huckans et al. 2013). A common approach utilizes structured and repeated practice of specific cognitive tasks and mental exercises as a means of improving abilities in specific cognitive domains. It also teaches individuals skills and compensatory strategies—for example, through the use of visual imagery, structured problem solving, and planning methods to compensate for executive dysfunction, and through the use of day planners, timers, and navigation devices (Huckans et al. 2013).

A spate of studies have examined the use of computer-based interventions and video games targeting cognitive deficits in MCI (Anguera et al. 2013; Barnes et al. 2009). Thus far, results are promising, but further work is clearly needed (Ben-Sadoun et al. 2018).

Behavioral interventions. Behavioral interventions, especially exercise and mental activity, may have small but beneficial effects on cognitive function in older adults with MCI (Langa and Levine 2014). Studies have brought new evidence that aerobic exercise significantly increased hippocampal volume in older women with probable MCI (ten Brinke et al. 2015); therefore, physical exercise should be recommended. Published studies suggest that greater adherence to a Mediterranean diet is associated with slower cognitive decline and lower risk of developing AD (Lourida et al. 2013). Weight loss strategies should be incorporated into treatment, because overweight and obesity at midlife independently increase the risk of dementia, AD, and vascular dementia (Xu et al. 2011).

Reducing stress by meditation and relaxation exercises is known to improve mood and memory, immune response, and life expectancy. Insomnia is a risk factor for worsening MCI; therefore, proper diagnosis and treatment are indicated. Socialization is an important protective factor for memory problems, and it is known that stimulating conversations increase both memory performance and mental speed. Observational studies suggest that social engagement may reduce the risk of cognitive decline and preserve memory, particularly in adults with fewer than 12 years of education or those with vascular disease (Ertel et al. 2008).

KEY POINTS

- Mild cognitive impairment (MCI) or mild neurocognitive disorder is characterized by a discrete and distinct decline in the patient's usual cognitive abilities that is greater than expected for the patient's age and educational background but not severe enough to interfere with daily functioning.
- Current classification schemes divide MCI into two subtypes: amnestic type, characterized by impaired memory; and nonamnestic type, characterized by preserved memory in the presence of impairment in other cognitive domains, such as executive function, language, or visuospatial abilities.
- Depression, which occurs in 20% of individuals with MCI, may be more resistant to antidepressants in people with MCI; depression treatment in these individuals should be initiated as early as possible. Other common symptoms include apathy, anxiety, and irritability.
- Medical conditions, medication side effects, and alcohol and substance use may be contributing factors to MCI and should be thoroughly evaluated.
- The Montreal Cognitive Assessment is a useful screening tool for the cognitive components of MCI. Useful assessments of functional activities include the Functional Assessment Staging Test and the Functional Activities Questionnaire.

Resources

Alzheimer's Association information about MCI: www.alz.org/alzheimers-dementia/what-is-dementia/related_conditions/mild-cognitive-impairment

Fact sheet for patients and families about MCI: www.alz.org/media/Documents/alzheimers-dementia-mild-cognitive-impairment-ts.pdf

Search tool for clinical trials: www.nia.nih.gov/alzheimers/clinical-trials

National Institute on Aging information portal: www.nia.nih.gov/health/alzheimers

Publications from National Institute on Aging: https://order.nia.nih.gov/view-all-publications

References

Albert MS, DeKosky ST, Dickson D, et al: The diagnosis of mild cognitive impairment due to Alzheimer's disease: recommendations from the National Institute on Aging–Alzheimer's Association workgroups on diagnostic guidelines for Alzheimer's disease. Alzheimers Dement 7(3):270–279, 2011 21514249

American Psychiatric Association: Diagnostic and Statistical Manual of Mental Disorders, 5th Edition, Arlington, VA, American Psychiatric Association, 2013

Andreescu C, Teverovsky E, Fu B, et al: Old worries and new anxieties: behavioral symptoms and mild cognitive impairment in a population study. Am J Geriatr Psychiatry 22(3):274–284, 2014 23759435

Anguera JA, Boccanfuso J, Rintoul JL, et al: Video game training enhances cognitive control in older adults. Nature 501(7465):97–101, 2013 24005416

Apostolova LG, Cummings JL: Neuropsychiatric manifestations in mild cognitive impairment: a systematic review of the literature. Dement Geriatr Cogn Disord 25(2):115–126, 2008 18087152

Avramopoulos D: Genetics of Alzheimer's disease: recent advances. Genome Med 1(3):34, 2009 19341505

Barnes DE, Yaffe K, Belfor N, et al: Computer-based cognitive training for mild cognitive impairment: results from a pilot randomized, controlled trial. Alzheimer Dis Assoc Disord 23(3):205–210, 2009 19812460

Bartzokis G, Beckson M, Lu PH, et al: Brain maturation may be arrested in chronic cocaine addicts. Biol Psychiatry 51(8):605–611, 2002 11955460

Ben-Sadoun G, Manera V, Alvarez J, et al: Recommendations for the design of serious games in neurodegenerative diseases. Front Aging Neurosci 10:13, 2018 29456501

Ceresini G, Lauretani F, Maggio M, et al: Thyroid function abnormalities and cognitive impairment in elderly people: results of the Invecchiare in Chianti study. J Am Geriatr Soc 57(1):89–93, 2009 19054181

Chari D, Ali R, Gupta R: Reversible dementia in elderly: really uncommon? Journal of Geriatric Mental Health 2(1):30, 2015

Cummings JL, Mega M, Gray K, et al: The Neuropsychiatric Inventory: comprehensive assessment of psychopathology in dementia. Neurology 44(12):2308-2314, 1994 7991117

Dowling GJ, Weiss SR, Condon TP: Drugs of abuse and the aging brain. Neuropsychopharmacology 33(2):209–218, 2008 17406645

Dugbartey AT: Neurocognitive aspects of hypothyroidism. Arch Intern Med 158(13):1413–1418, 1998 9665349

Emmelot-Vonk MH, Verhaar HJ, Nakhai Pour HR, et al: Effect of testosterone supplementation on functional mobility, cognition, and other parameters in older men: a randomized controlled trial. JAMA 299(1):39–52, 2008 18167405

Ertel KA, Glymour MM, Berkman LF: Effects of social integration on preserving memory function in a nationally representative US elderly population. Am J Public Health 98(7):1215–1220, 2008 18511736

Farina N, Isaac MG, Clark AR, et al: Vitamin E for Alzheimer's dementia and mild cognitive impairment. Cochrane Database Syst Rev 11:CD002854, 2012 23152215

Folstein MF, Folstein SE, McHugh PR: "Mini-mental state": a practical method for grading the cognitive state of patients for the clinician. J Psychiatr Res 12(3):189-198, 1975 1202204

Harada CN, Natelson Love MC, Triebel KL: Normal cognitive aging. Clin Geriatr Med 29(4):737–752, 2013 24094294

Hopko DR, Stanley MA, Reas DL, et al: Assessing worry in older adults: confirmatory factor analysis of the Penn State Worry Questionnaire and psychometric properties of an abbreviated model. Psychol Assess 15(2):173–183, 2003 12847777

Huckans M, Hutson L, Twamley E, et al: Efficacy of cognitive rehabilitation therapies for mild cognitive impairment (MCI) in older adults: working toward a theoretical model and evidence-based interventions. Neuropsychol Rev 23(1):63–80, 2013 23471631

Langa KM, Levine DA: The diagnosis and management of mild cognitive impairment: a clinical review. JAMA 312(23):2551–2561, 2014 5514304

Lopez OL, Jagust WJ, Dulberg C, et al: Risk factors for mild cognitive impairment in the Cardiovascular Health Study Cognition Study: part 2. Arch Neurol 60(10):1394–1399, 2003 14568809

Lourida I, Soni M, Thompson-Coon J, et al: Mediterranean diet, cognitive function, and dementia: a systematic review. Epidemiology 24(4):479–489, 2013 23680940

Luchsinger JA, Perez T, Chang H, et al: Metformin in Amnestic Mild Cognitive Impairment: Results of a Pilot Randomized Placebo Controlled Clinical Trial. J Alzheimers Dis 51(2):501–514, 2016 26890736

Luck T, Luppa M, Briel S, et al: Incidence of mild cognitive impairment: a systematic review. Dement Geriatr Cogn Disord 29(2):164–175, 2010 20150735

Lyketsos CG, Lopez O, Jones B, et al: Prevalence of neuropsychiatric symptoms in dementia and mild cognitive impairment: results from the cardiovascular health study. JAMA 288(12):1475–1483, 2002 12243634

Mah L, Binns MA, Steffens DC: Anxiety symptoms in amnestic mild cognitive impairment are associated with medial temporal atrophy and predict conversion to Alzheimer disease. Am J Geriatr Psychiatry 23(5):466–476, 2015 25500120

Modrego PJ, Ferrández J: Depression in patients with mild cognitive impairment increases the risk of developing dementia of Alzheimer type: a prospective cohort study. Arch Neurol 61(8):1290–1293, 2004 15313849

Nasreddine ZS, Phillips NA, Bédirian V, et al: The Montreal Cognitive Assessment, MoCA: a brief screening tool for mild cognitive impairment. J Am Geriatr Soc 53(4):695–699, 2005 15817019

Pedrosa H, De Sa A, Guerreiro M, et al: Functional evaluation distinguishes MCI patients from healthy elderly people—the ADCS/MCI/ADL scale. J Nutr Health Aging 14:703–709, 2010

Petersen RC: Mild cognitive impairment. Continuum (Minneap Minn) 22(2, Dementia):404–418, 2016 27042901

Petersen RC, Caracciolo B, Brayne C, et al: Mild cognitive impairment: a concept in evolution. J Intern Med 275(3):214–228, 2014 24605806

Pfeffer RI, Kurosaki TT, Harrah CH Jr, et al: Measurement of functional activities in older adults in the community. J Gerontol 37:323–329, 1982

Raschetti R, Albanese E, Vanacore N, et al: Cholinesterase inhibitors in mild cognitive impairment: a systematic review of randomised trials. PLoS Med 4(11):e338, 2007 18044984

Reisberg B: Functional Assessment Staging (FAST). Psychopharmacol Bull 24:653–659, 1988 3249767

Roberts RO, Geda YE, Knopman DS, et al: The incidence of MCI differs by sub-type and is higher in men: the Mayo Clinic Study of Aging. Neurology 78(5):342–351, 2012 22282647

Sadock BJ, Sadock VA, Kaplan HI: Kaplan and Sadock's Comprehensive Text-book of Psychiatry, Vol 2. Philadelphia, PA, Lippincott Williams and Wilkins, 2005

Snitz BE, O'Meara ES, Carlson MC, et al: Ginkgo biloba for preventing cognitive decline in older adults: a randomized trial. JAMA 302(24):2663–2670, 2009 20040554

ten Brinke LF, Bolandzadeh N, Nagamatsu LS, et al: Aerobic exercise increases hippocampal volume in older women with probable mild cognitive impair-ment: a 6-month randomised controlled trial. Br J Sports Med 49(4):248–254, 2015 24711660

Tveito M, Correll CU, Bramness JG, et al: Correlates of major medication side effects interfering with daily performance: results from a cross-sectional cohort study of older psychiatric patients. Int Psychogeriatr 28(2):331–340, 2016 26412479

Whitmer RA, Karter AJ, Yaffe K, et al: Hypoglycemic episodes and risk of de-mentia in older patients with type 2 diabetes mellitus. JAMA 301(15):1565–1572, 2009 19366776

Widera E, Steenpass V, Marson D, et al: Finances in the older patient with cog-nitive impairment: "He didn't want me to take over." JAMA 305(7):698–706, 2011 21325186

Wild B, Eckl A, Herzog W, et al: Assessing generalized anxiety disorder in el-derly people using the GAD-7 and GAD-2 scales: results of a validation study. Am J Geriatr Psychiatry 22(10):1029–1038, 2014 23768681

Winblad B, Palmer K, Kivipelto M, et al: Mild cognitive impairment—beyond controversies, towards a consensus: report of the International Working Group on Mild Cognitive Impairment. J Intern Med 256(3):240–246, 2004 15324367

Xu WL, Atti AR, Gatz M, et al: Midlife overweight and obesity increase late-life dementia risk: a population-based twin study. Neurology 76(18):1568–1574, 2011 21536637

Yesavage JA, Brink TL, Rose TL, et al: Development and validation of a geriatric depression screening scale: a preliminary report. J Psychiatr Res 17(1):37-49, 1982–1983 7183759

Zamboni G, Griffanti L, Jenkinson M, et al: White matter imaging correlates of early cognitive impairment detected by the Montreal Cognitive Assessment after transient ischemic attack and minor stroke. Stroke 48(6):1539–1547, 2017 28487328

Neuropsychological Testing

"I Sometimes Forget Things"

Tonita E. Wroolie, Ph.D., ABPP
Erin L. Cassidy-Eagle, Ph.D., CBSM, DBSM
Laura B. Dunn, M.D.

CHAPTER 13

Clinical Presentation

Chief Complaint

"I sometimes forget things."

Vignette

Mr. G is a 76-year-old married man who presents to his primary care provider for his annual physical. Accompanying him is his second wife, to whom he has been married for 15 years. Mr. G is his usual pleasant self and denies any significant concerns about his mood or memory other than occasional forgetfulness ("I sometimes forget things"). His wife agrees that he sometimes forgets things that she asks him to do (such as getting certain items from the grocery store), but she says that otherwise he "is doing great." Mr. G is being treated for mild hypertension, hyperlipidemia, and benign prostatic hypertrophy. His current medications include aspirin, amlodipine, simvastatin, and sildenafil. His physician notes that he appears to be walking slower and more cautiously than he did at his visit a year ago. Mr. G denies current alcohol or substance use, although he was a heavy drinker for approximately 10 years while in his forties.

The primary care physician refills Mr. G's medications but does not perform a cognitive screening test at this time given the minimal concerns of both Mr. G and his wife. Of note, when the physician casually asks Mr. G how his kids are doing, Mr. G's expression changes. He looks slightly upset and, glancing at his wife, says that his son and his daughter "are trying to control my life." His wife says, "They're just having some issues right now, but I'm sure it will pass." Pressed for time, the physician does not pursue this statement further, assuming there is just some transitory underlying family tension or discord, because on previous visits Mr. G always enjoyed talking about his adult children's lives and accomplishments.

Eight months later, the physician learns from an inpatient hospitalist that Mr. G was admitted overnight for observation after an unwitnessed fall that resulted in a laceration to his left cheek and a bruised shoulder. He was home alone at the time and was unable to recall what happened leading up to the fall. His wife brought him to the emergency department after finding him lying on the kitchen floor in a confused state. A head computed tomography (CT) scan performed in the emergency department was negative for hemorrhage but showed "generalized volume loss without lobar predominance." The inpatient team noted that on the morning after his admission to the hospital, Mr. G, despite denying significant memory problems other than mild forgetfulness, obtained a score of 20 out of 30 on the Montreal Cognitive Assessment (MoCA), suggesting a cognitive impairment. The team noted that Mr. G's wife does not believe that Mr. G has cognitive impairment and that she appeared to dismiss the team's concerns, stating that he has just been "tired lately." The team noted that when the wife was not present in the room, Mr. G was unable to provide even basic medical information about himself, stating, "I do have some medical problems; you can ask my wife what they are." Additionally, he was unable to say what medications he takes and stated, "My wife manages all of that." The team suggested to his primary care physician that Mr. G should receive more comprehensive neuropsychological testing after his discharge from the hospital to better understand his deficits and abilities.

Following this advice, the physician places a referral for neuropsychological testing and schedules Mr. G for a follow-up visit. At the follow-up visit, the physician interviews Mr. G alone for the first time in several years, even though his wife is displeased when asked to leave the exam room. The physician is surprised to note that Mr. G appears significantly more confused than at his visit 8 months ago. He continues to show minimal concern about his memory and states that everyone is "making a mountain out of a molehill" regarding his fall. The physician highly suspects that Mr. G has a neurocognitive disorder (NCD) and suggests that the patient undergo amyloid positron emission tomography imaging to help clarify whether he has Alzheimer's disease or another NCD. The patient defers this decision to his wife, who states, "He doesn't want that test. They already did a brain scan when he was in the hospital, so he doesn't need another one."

Discussion

Interdisciplinary Team Commentary

Geriatric psychiatrist: The first concern I have based on this vignette is the accuracy of the patient's and his wife's report of Mr. G's cognitive and functional status. For a variety of reasons, one or both parties in a marriage may either deny or not recognize the existence of a cognitive impairment, and the primary care physician should conduct an interview with the patient alone during annual visits to obtain an unbiased view of the patient's cognitive status. A spouse may minimize their partner's symptoms while in the same room, whether out of a desire to help the patient "save face" or out of actual lack of awareness that the patient is experiencing a decline.

Mr. G's MoCA score of 20 out of 30 raises serious concern of an underlying NCD. Conducting an independent interview with his adult children (collateral informants) will help obtain a more thorough history of his cognitive and functional abilities. Because family members often have differing opinions of a patient's abilities and needs, it is imperative that a formal neuropsychological assessment of cognition be conducted to help clarify specific deficits and provide recommendations.

Finally, Mr. G's statement that his kids have "turned against him" should alert the physician to changes in family dynamics and possible risk of abuse (elders are at particular risk of financial abuse). Conflicts regarding who has control over a patient's finances or decision making can cause family disruption or even legal disputes. If abuse is suspected, a report to Adult Protective Services is mandated.

Neuropsychologist: Mr. G was referred for a neuropsychological evaluation to clarify his cognitive deficits and an initial appointment was made. His wife subsequently canceled the appointment, and when the primary care physician inquired as to why the appointment was canceled, Mr. G's wife stated, "Oh, he doesn't need that testing, and it will just upset him." The physician stressed to the wife that an evaluation was necessary, and she reluctantly brought him to the rescheduled appointment. Because of concerns about Mr. G's care and safety, the evaluation was to also assess his capacity to choose his durable power of attorney (DPOA) for financial and health care decisions, to manage his finances, and to be left alone without supervision. More typically, assessments are used to just clarify deficits and suggest possible or probable neurocognitive diagnoses. Mr. G had several risk factors for cognitive decline (i.e., advanced age, hyperlipidemia, impaired fasting glucose, and hypertension). There was also magnetic resonance imaging (MRI) evidence of possible vascular changes as well as a general volume loss. Mr. G also displayed motor signs in addition to suspected small vessel disease in the subcortical and periventricular regions, putting him at risk for falls.

Multiple concerning issues are present in this case, and because there was evidence that Mr. G had significant cognitive decline, a battery specifically designed to assess dementia was chosen along with other measures to make sure all cognitive domains were assessed.

Cognitive Assessment

Cognitive Screening

Having a baseline and yearly measure of cognition that can be used as a point of comparison with current status will assist in the understanding of the extent and course of cognitive decline. Per Medicare guidelines (Cordell et al. 2013), physicians are required to conduct baseline and annual cognitive impairment screening during annual wellness visits. Although there are no established measure guidelines, several screening tools are currently available, including the MoCA (Nasreddine et al. 2005), Mini-Cog (Borson et al. 2003), Memory Impairment Screen (MIS; Buschke et al. 1999), General Practitioner Assessment of Cognition (GPCOG; Brodaty et al. 2002), and the Mini-Mental Status Exam (MMSE; Folstein et al. 1975). (For other dementia assessment scales used in primary care, see Sheehan 2012.)

Neuropsychological Assessment

Neuropsychology is defined as the study of the structures and functions of the brain and their relationship to behavior. A neuropsychological assessment is a lengthy process consisting of a clinical interview, a mental status examination, a review of medical records, patient's psychiatric history, patient's family of origin medical and psychiatric history, and feedback of the testing results to the patient (and family members, given the patient's consent/assent) (Table 13–1). Cognitive and psychological testing provides information about specific cognitive domains and psychological functioning. After the testing is completed, the patient's performance on each neuropsychological measure is scored and compared with normative data for the patient's age range and sometimes his or her educational level and/or gender. A report is then generated from the results with diagnostic impressions and recommendations.

Cognitive Domains

Usually a measure or estimate of intellectual (global) abilities thought to "hold" or maintain in spite of cognitive decline is used to provide a level of baseline premorbid functioning. For clarity, cognitive domains

TABLE 13–1. Components of a neuropsychological assessment

Clinical interview
  Character, severity, and progress of presenting problem
  Psychosocial history (includes developmental milestones, problems)

Review of medical records
  Medical history
    Medical conditions and surgeries
    Medications
    Brain imaging
  Psychiatric history
    Age at onset
    Psychiatric hospitalizations

Family medical and psychiatric history

Collateral interviews (family and caregivers) if patient is a poor historian

Mental status examination

Neuropsychological assessment
  Cognitive testing
  Psychological testing

Generation of a report
  Findings
  Diagnostic impressions
  Recommendations

are reported as separate entities; however, cognitive abilities do not occur in a vacuum. For instance, when a patient complains of a "memory problem," it is better to consider the acquisition and retrieval of information as a dynamic process, such as follows:

- Input of information first starts with *attention,* that is, the ability to notice or attend to information.
- The next step is *learning,* which often requires rehearsal of the information to be learned.
- *Encoding* is laying information down into memory stores.
- *Memory,* or output, is when information is pulled out of memory stores either freely or with cues. Often patients will complain of memory problems when there may in fact be a problem with one of the stages of input, particularly with advancing age.

- *Processing speed* is how efficiently or quickly information can be understood and manipulated. If processing is slowed, it becomes more difficult to input information, especially with larger amounts of material.
- Brain-based *language abilities* entail both the ability to express (e.g., naming and verbal fluency) and understand language.
- *Executive functions* are higher-order abilities that include cognitive flexibility (also called set-shifting or divided attention), inhibition, organization, planning, and judgment.
- *Gross motor* symptoms are typically observed, and fine motor, strength, and graphomotor speed are measured.
- Finally, *psychiatric symptoms* such as depression, anxiety, and personality factors are assessed. Depression and anxiety have a negative impact on cognition, but cognitive complaints should not be dismissed as solely due to affective states.

Although cognitive domains are organized into distinct categories (Table 13–2), assessment measures often utilize multiple cognitive processes. For instance, a task in which a patient is asked to draw a line connecting alternating numbers and letters not only requires cognitive flexibility but also taps into other cognitive processes such as visual scanning, processing, and graphomotor speed and number and letter sequencing knowledge. Although screening tools are useful in primary care to detect cognitive impairment or measure progression over time, they are limited in specifying which cognitive domains are impaired. They also do not allow for practice to make sure a patient fully understands the instructions. Additionally, screening tools also typically use cutoff scores and do not take education level or premorbid functioning into account, putting some patients at risk for false-positive diagnoses and missing early detection of cognitive decline in other patients. Dementia batteries that measure multiple cognitive domains are sometimes utilized. Some of the more common batteries include the following:

- Repeatable Battery for the Assessment of Neuropsychological Status
- Dementia Rating Scale
- Modified Mini-Mental State Examination

Referral for Neuropsychological Assessment

Normal aging is commonly accompanied by declines in sensory perception, processing speed, working memory, visuospatial processing and constructional praxis, complex attention/executive function (e.g., inhi-

TABLE 13–2. Cognitive domains and selected assessment measures

Cognitive domain	Commonly used assessment measure[a]
Intellectual functioning	Wechsler Adult Scale of Intelligence National Adult Reading Test
Attention	Digit Span Arithmetic
Processing speed	Coding Symbol Search
Language	Boston Naming Test Verbal fluency tests Multilingual Aphasia Examination
Visuospatial/Constructions	Rey Complex Figure Test Block Design
Learning and memory	California Verbal Learning Test Rey Complex Figure Test
Executive functions	Trail Making Test Stroop Delis-Kaplan Executive Function System
Motor	Pegboard tests Finger tapping tests Hand dynamometer
Psychiatric symptoms	Geriatric Depression Scale Beck Depression Inventory Symptom Checklist–90 Minnesota Multiphasic Personality Inventory Millon Clinical Multiaxial Inventory

[a]Not an exhaustive list.

bition of an overlearned response), learning and retrieval of newly learned material, word finding (i.e., naming people or items), and motor abilities (Murman 2015). Because of the numerous and normal age-related cognitive changes, pathological changes may be hard to detect during a routine physical examination, particularly during early stages. In pathological aging, declines and deficits are dependent on but not always specific to the underlying disease process. Therefore, distinguishing between normal and abnormal cognitive changes is crucial for both diagnostic and treatment purposes. A neuropsychological assessment is an important component of a comprehensive evaluation of cognitive impairment. It is important to note that even when structural brain imaging (MRI, CT) findings are normal or normal for age, it does not rule out functional problems or pathological processes.

Cognitive decline may not always be obvious, especially when time is limited during a physician appointment. One possible sign of cognitive decline is short-term memory loss. Does the patient forget what he or she has just been told, or does he or she repeat comments or questions within a short period of time? Communication or comprehension problems might indicate a brain-based language impairment exhibited by significant word finding, paraphasia errors, or difficulty comprehending instructions. Calculation difficulties that are not premorbid may raise concerns about managing finances, so asking whether a patient is having difficulty managing his or her bills may reveal cognitive issues. Reduced self-awareness of the individual's own deficits is often a sign of advanced cognitive decline such that the patient may deny any problems; therefore, obtaining collateral information may be necessary. Other observable behavioral signs of cognitive decline include perseveration (i.e., lack of mental flexibility), disinhibition, new onset of delusions or hallucinations, and poor grooming and hygiene. Emotional signs of possible cognitive decline include late onset of depression or anxiety, significant emotional distress, and emotional lability or inappropriateness. Finally, development of problems in functional abilities that are needed to live independently (i.e., instrumental activities of daily living), such as the ability to shop and prepare food, housekeeping, doing laundry, using transportation, or managing money, is a cause for concern.

Dementia Versus Major Neurocognitive Disorder

Dementia is defined as having memory impairment in addition to impairment in at least one other cognitive domain. Because this definition was problematic in diagnosing some significant cognitive disorders, the term *major neurocognitive disorder* was introduced in DSM-5 (Box 13–1; American Psychiatric Association 2013).

Box 13–1.   Diagnostic Criteria for Major Neurocognitive Disorder

---

A. Evidence of significant cognitive decline from a previous level of performance in one or more cognitive domains (complex attention, executive function, learning and memory, language, perceptual-motor, or social cognition) based on:

1. Concern of the individual, a knowledgeable informant, or the clinician that there has been a significant decline in cognitive function; and
2. A substantial impairment in cognitive performance, preferably documented by standardized neuropsychological testing or, in its absence, another quantified clinical assessment.

B. The cognitive deficits interfere with independence in everyday activities (i.e., at a minimum, requiring assistance with complex instrumental activities of daily living such as paying bills or managing medications).
C. The cognitive deficits do not occur exclusively in the context of a delirium.
D. The cognitive deficits are not better explained by another mental disorder (e.g., major depressive disorder, schizophrenia).

Specify whether due to:
Alzheimer's disease
Frontotemporal lobar degeneration
Lewy body disease
Vascular disease
Traumatic brain injury
Substance/medication use
HIV infection
Prion disease
Parkinson's disease
Huntington's disease
Another medical condition
Multiple etiologies
Unspecified

Specify:
Without behavioral disturbance: If the cognitive disturbance is not accompanied by any clinically significant behavioral disturbance.
With behavioral disturbance *(specify disturbance)*: If the cognitive disturbance is accompanied by a clinically significant behavioral disturbance (e.g., psychotic symptoms, mood disturbance, agitation, apathy, or other behavioral symptoms).

Specify current severity:
Mild: Difficulties with instrumental activities of daily living (e.g., housework, managing money).
Moderate: Difficulties with basic activities of daily living (e.g., feeding, dressing).
Severe: Fully dependent.

NCD is classified as major or mild depending on the level of cognitive decline (Table 13–3), with a probable or possible cause as part of the diagnosis.

Vignette *(continued)*

Mr. G's neuropsychological evaluation revealed the following: The mental status examination showed that Mr. G was oriented to person, place, month, and day of the month but disoriented to the day of the week and year. His spontaneous speech was reduced, and he mostly spoke only in response to questions. Affect was blunted, and he reported his mood as "afraid." He denied any sleep or appetite changes or problems. He denied current but reported past suicidal ideation. He also denied current or past hallucinations, and there did not appear to be any evidence of overt psychosis. Although he was able to follow simple testing instructions with reminders and clarifications, he appeared confused by more difficult tasks. He also perseverated on prior test instructions during subsequent tasks. A left-handed tremor was observed, facial expression was reduced, and lip-smacking throughout the testing session was noted.

The cognitive testing results showed that on a global dementia scale overall, Mr. G scored in the severely impaired range. He also had significant impairment on most cognitive domains, with the most significant and severe deficits found in learning and memory, executive function, processing speed, verbal fluency, and visuospatial and constructional abilities. He displayed milder deficits in his ability to comprehend and execute verbal commands, simple reasoning, and judgment for hypothetical problems. His attention abilities were in the average range for simple verbal attention but declined when information became increasingly complex, sometimes to the point of his becoming confused. Given the results of testing, Mr. G's presentation met the criteria for a major NCD.

It was concluded that given Mr. G's significant cognitive deficits, he lacked the capacity to appoint a DPOA; he required 24-hour supervision; and he should not be left unattended because he would not be able to provide adequate care for himself or manage emergency situations. Because of his brain-based language deficits, he would not be able to express his needs adequately or be able to thoroughly understand what was being said. He also lacked the capacity to make sound health care decisions. However, it was suggested that when health care issues and decisions arose, they should be explained to him using simple language to aid his understanding. It was also concluded that he lacked the capacity to manage his finances. Finally, if family members could or would not adequately provide for his needs and safety, appointment of a court-appointed conservator was warranted.

The Neuropsychological Report

Unfortunately, there is no consistency across reports, and some contain more details than others. What is in a report depends on the referral

TABLE 13–3. Major and mild neurocognitive disorders

Major neurocognitive disorder	Mild neurocognitive disorder
Significant cognitive decline	Modest cognitive decline
Deficits interfere with independence	Deficits do not interfere with independence
Not due to delirium	Not due to delirium
Not due to other mental disorder	Not due to other mental disorder

question, and this can vary widely from specific (i.e., assess memory problems) to general (i.e., assess cognitive functioning or obtain a baseline). At minimum, there should be reporting on the levels of functioning within each cognitive domain assessed. Therefore, understanding the different cognitive domains will help the physician better understand the impact of deficits on a patient's functional abilities, inform further diagnostic tests, and inform treatment.

Neuropsychological reports usually contain medical and psychosocial history, subjective cognitive complaints, tests utilized, objective findings, summary of findings, potential cause of impairments and/or diagnostic impressions, and recommendations. If questions arise, the physician should not hesitate to contact the psychologist who conducted the assessment to help clarify the findings and how they relate to a patient's difficulties.

Talking to Families About Neuropsychological Testing

Professionals of all stripes who work with older patients and their families may need to introduce the idea of neuropsychological testing, as well as help patients and families understand the meaning of the results (Table 13–4). The best approach is to explain how a neuropsychological assessment is a useful tool for helping characterize deficits and informing a diagnosis. More often than not, patients and their families feel a sense of validation when provided an explanation of cognitive difficulties or noticed changes in behavior or function. A neuropsychological assessment also provides evidence of preserved abilities, which can be reassuring. After meeting with a neuropsychologist to review the results of an evaluation, patients (especially those with cognitive impairment) and families may continue to have questions. Therefore, it is important for the

TABLE 13–4. Neuropsychological testing: key points to make with patients and families

Neuropsychological testing

  Is part of a comprehensive assessment to aid in making a diagnosis

  Can help explain cognitive difficulties and behaviors

  May result in additional recommendations, such as the following:

    Strategies to improve functioning

    Treatment considerations

    Consultations with other services

    Complementary evaluations

  Can suggest ways to address safety issues

physician to have a basic understanding of the relationship between cognitive deficits and behaviors. Furthermore, providing education and resources will assist patients and families to better cope with cognitive impairment and make decisions and arrangements for the future.

Safety Concerns

Several issues pose a risk to those with cognitive decline, such as the following:

- Individuals with memory impairment may forget to take medication or take more medication than prescribed.
- Observed gait and balance problems put a person at risk for falls, and physical therapy referrals should be made along with safety measures implemented in the home.
- It is extremely important for the safety of the patient and the community to ask about driving. For the safety of patients and the community, patients should be questioned about recent scratches, dents, or accidents, and if there is concern, a report to the Department of Motor Vehicles should be made for a driving evaluation.
- A patient who appears overly dependent on someone else may be the victim of abuse.
- Older adults in general, and those with cognitive decline in particular, are at risk for financial abuse.

KEY POINTS

- Cognitive screening is useful but not sufficient for detection of cognitive decline.
- Distinguishing between normal age-related and pathological cognitive changes can be difficult.
- Neuropsychological assessments provide information about a patient's functional abilities.
- A neuropsychological assessment aids diagnosis and helps to inform treatment.
- Family members do not always agree on or notice cognitive changes.
- Cognitive decline may pose serious safety issues.

Resources

Resources for Families: Organizations

Alzheimer's Association: 225 N. Michigan Ave., Floor 17, Chicago, IL 60601; (800) 272-3900; www.alz.org

Alzheimer's Association: Facts and Figures, 2018. Available at: www.alz.org/alzheimers-dementia/facts-figures

Alzheimer's Association: 10 Early Signs and Symptoms of Alzheimer's. Chicago, IL, Alzheimer's Association, 2018. Available at: www.alz.org/alzheimers-dementia/10_signs (Provides a useful summary for families and a form to fill out and bring to medical appointment.)

American Psychological Association: Cognitive Aging Efforts: Recent Publications, Webinars, and Activities Related to APA Cognitive Aging Efforts. Available at: www.apa.org/pi/aging/resources/cognitive-aging-efforts.aspx

American Psychological Association: Memory and Aging. Available at: www.apa.org/pi/aging/memory-and-aging.pdf.

World Health Organization: Fact File: 10 Facts on Dementia. Available at: www.who.int/features/factfiles/dementia/dementia_facts/en

Resources for Clinicians

Alzheimer's Association: Cognitive Assessment Toolkit: A Guide to Detect Cognitive Impairment Quickly and Efficiently During the Medicare Annual Wellness Visit. Chicago, IL, Alzheimer's Association, n.d. Available at: www.alz.org/getmedia/9687d51e-641a-43a1-a96b-b29eb00e72bb/cognitive-assessment-toolkit

Nasreddine M: Montreal Cognitive Assessment (website), 2018. Available at: www.mocatest.org (Includes translations into many languages.)

References

American Psychiatric Association: Diagnostic and Statistical Manual of Mental Disorders, 5th Edition. Arlington, VA, American Psychiatric Association, 2013

Borson S, Scanlan JM, Chen P, et al: The Mini-Cog as a screen for dementia: validation in a population-based sample. J Am Geriatr Soc 51(10):1451–1454, 2003 14511167

Brodaty H, Pond D, Kemp NM, et al: The GPCOG: a new screening test for dementia designed for general practice. J Am Geriatr Soc 50(3):530–534, 2002 11943052

Buschke H, Kuslansky G, Katz M, et al: Screening for dementia with the memory impairment screen. Neurology 52(2):231–238, 1999 9932936

Cordell CB, Borson S, Boustani M, et al: Alzheimer's Association recommendations for operationalizing the detection of cognitive impairment during the Medicare Annual Wellness Visit in a primary care setting. Alzheimers Dement 9(2):141–150, 2013 23265826

Folstein MF, Folstein SE, McHugh PR: "Mini-mental state." A practical method for grading the cognitive state of patients for the clinician. J Psychiatr Res 12(3):189–198, 1975 1202204

Murman DL: The impact of age on cognition. Semin Hear 36(3):111–121, 2015 27516712

Nasreddine ZS, Phillips NA, Bédirian V, et al: The Montreal Cognitive Assessment, MoCA: a brief screening tool for mild cognitive impairment. J Am Geriatr Soc 53(4):695–699, 2005 15817019

Sheehan B: Assessment scales in dementia. Ther Adv Neurol Disorder 5(6):349–358, 2012 23139705

Behavioral and Psychological Symptoms of Dementia

"Little Soldiers Are Invading My Backyard"

Awais Aftab, M.D.
Daniel Kim, M.D.

CHAPTER 14

Clinical Presentation

Chief Complaint

"Little soldiers are invading my backyard."

Vignette

Mr. P was a 76-year-old married white man who presented to a geriatric psychiatry clinic for visual hallucinations that had emerged several months prior to his initial evaluation. He was an affable bear of a man who required a walker to ambulate because of ongoing symptoms of Parkinson's disease, diagnosed 2 years ago. He had experienced limited response to his Parkinson's medications of carbidopa-levodopa, entacapone, amantadine, and pramipexole. On initial interview, he acknowledged that "little Asian soldiers are invading my backyard." His wife reported that he had initially had fair insight regarding these hallucinations but that they were now causing him increased anxiety and distress, as well as increased irritability when his fears were challenged by his wife. On interview, Mr. P acknowledged that the hallucinations were "most likely a figment of my imagination," but when pressed he stated, "The other possibility I'd like you to consider is that my home *is* being invaded."

These symptoms of hallucinations, anxiety, and irritability were entirely new. He had been, and remained, a successful businessman who owned a company that was now primarily managed by his son, but in which Mr. P remained heavily involved. Before this he had been an officer in the U.S. Marine Corps for more than 10 years, including combat service in Vietnam, with an honorable discharge as a captain. He had no history of psychiatric illness, although he acknowledged worsening appetite and sleep disruption over the year before his initial evaluation. His wife also noted the family's increased concerns about his business decisions, which were increasingly monitored by his son, as well as his financial acumen, because he was frequently making multiple—at times conflicting—investment decisions a day. His initial score on the Montreal Cognitive Assessment (MoCA) was 22, with deficits in delayed recall, construction, and executive functioning. Other than his previous diagnosis of Parkinson's disease, his only other medical issues were benign prostatic hypertrophy and hypercholesterolemia. A workup for potentially reversible causes of dementia, including brain magnetic resonance imaging, was completed, with unremarkable findings.

Discussion

The global prevalence of dementia, estimated at 44 million in 2013, is predicted to increase to 76 million by the year 2030, indicative of the dire current and future need for care (Prince et al. 2013). Dementia, one of the three costliest diseases in the United States (Hurd et al. 2013), is a disease defined by cognitive deficits. The *Diagnostic and Statistical Manual of Mental Disorders*, Fifth Edition (DSM-5) replaces *dementia* with the preferred nomenclature of *major neurocognitive disorder*, but also permits the continued use of the term dementia because it is widely accepted by physicians and patients. Given the extensive reliance on the term dementia in existing literature, we will use "dementia" and "major neurocognitive disorder" interchangeably in this chapter.

The most challenging and distressing symptoms for patients and caregivers are the behavioral and psychological symptoms of dementia (BPSD). These symptoms (also referred to as neuropsychiatric symptoms, or NPS) include psychosis (delusions, hallucinations), agitation, aggression, depression, anxiety, apathy, disinhibition, and wandering (see Table 14–1) (Zhao et al. 2016).

TABLE 14–1. Behavioral and psychological symptoms of dementia

Agitation (contextually inappropriate and excessive psychomotor activity)	Delusions
	Hallucinations
Aggression	Sleep problems
Depression	Hoarding
Apathy	Wandering
Anxiety	Disinhibition (sexually and socially
Repetitive questioning	inappropriate behaviors)

These behavioral manifestations are among the most difficult clinical aspects of major neurocognitive disorder to manage. Frequently, however, responsibility for managing BPSD falls primarily on the shoulders of family members or other loved ones. Overwhelmed, and all too often facing limited resources in the community, family caregivers in turn commonly experience anxiety, depression, and burnout as well as the stress of reduced income from sacrificed careers. Moreover, BPSD can cause tremendous distress to patients and caregivers, lead to increased hospitalizations and cost of care, and are associated with worse outcomes, such as earlier placement in a residential care facility, increased morbidity, and earlier mortality (Kales et al. 2015).

Prevalence of BPSD

A host of studies suggest that BPSD are nearly universal, and symptoms frequently co-occur, with higher prevalence rates reported among patients with more severe dementia (Lyketsos et al. 2000, 2002). In the Cache County Study, 97% of subjects with dementia had one or more BPSD when followed over 5 years (Steinberg et al. 2008). The most commonly experienced symptoms were apathy, depression, and anxiety. In a systematic review of 28 studies of prevalence of NPS in nursing home patients with dementia, the mean prevalence of having at least one neuropsychiatric symptom was 82%, with agitation and apathy being the most prevalent (Selbæk et al. 2013). In a meta-analysis of NPS in Alzheimer's disease, the most prevalent neuropsychiatric symptom was apathy (49%), followed by depression (42%), aggression (40%), anxiety (39%), and sleep disorder (39%). Prevalence of delusions and hallucinations was 31% and 16%, respectively (Zhao et al. 2016). Although any NPS may be experienced in any type of major neurocognitive disorder, certain symptoms are more common in some types. For instance, depression tends to be more commonly experienced in vascular dementia, hallucinations are a hallmark feature of Lewy body dementia, and disinhibition is often observed earlier in frontotemporal dementia.

Delusions are more prevalent than hallucinations in Alzheimer's dementia, but both are common (Bassiony and Lyketsos 2003; Ropacki and Jeste 2005). Delusions of theft are the most commonly experienced delusions. Other delusional themes include phantom boarder syndrome (in which the patient believes that someone uninvited is living in his or her home); misidentification syndromes (delusional beliefs that the identity of a person has been replaced or altered) such as Capgras syndrome (delusional belief that a spouse or another close relative has been replaced by an identical-looking impostor); persecutory delusions; and delusions of infidelity.

Assessment of BPSD

Evaluation of BPSD should include assessment of the following elements:

- Type, frequency, severity, pattern, context, and timing of symptoms
- Risk of harm to self and others

    - If the patient poses an elevated risk of harm to self or others, a higher level of treatment, such as an inpatient unit, may be needed.

- Presence of delirium

    - Subjects with dementia are predisposed to delirium, and agitation and psychosis may be secondary to delirium rather than dementia by itself. The hallmark of delirium is an acute confusional state marked by impairments in attention and orientation developing over a short period of time. Since delirium is the result of an underlying medical illness (e.g., urinary tract infection, pneumonia) and affects long-term prognosis and mortality, it is vital to look for and rule out delirium in new onset of BPSD.

- Precipitating factors

    - Other clinical factors, such as pain, constipation, chronic medical illness, medication side effects, sensory deficits, and sleep disturbances, may contribute to BPSD. Particular emphasis should be placed on assessing and identifying potentially modifiable contributory factors. Common modifiable factors are outlined in Table 14–2 (Kales et al. 2015).

TABLE 14–2. Modifiable factors in management of behavioral and psychological symptoms of dementia (BPSD)

Patient factors
Unmet needs and resulting effects, such as sleep, rest, thirst, hunger, urinary retention, constipation, fear
Acute medical problems: pain, discomfort, infection (e.g., urinary tract), medication side effect or interaction
Sensory deficits
Boredom

Caregiver factors
Caregiver stress, depression, and burnout
Poor understanding of dementia and BPSD
Poor communication with the patient
Unrealistic expectations

Environmental factors
Overstimulating or understimulating environment
Unsafe environment
Lack of activity
Lack of established routine

Rating Scales for NPS

It is a standard of care to assess and monitor NPS using rating scales as part of clinical assessment; this is also a recommendation in the American Psychiatric Association guidelines on the use of antipsychotics in dementia (Reus et al. 2016). Table 14–3 describes several available tools for assessment of NPS in research and clinical practice (Forester and Oxman 2003).

DICE Approach

In recent years, a multidisciplinary national expert panel recommended a comprehensive DICE approach to BPSD (Kales et al. 2015). DICE is an acronym for "Describe, Investigate, Create, and Evaluate." The DICE approach emanates directly from successful caregiver research interventions. The approach comprises four steps:

TABLE 14–3. Available tools for assessment of behavioral and psychological symptoms of dementia

Scale name	Authors	Informant and administration method	Items	Completion time[a], minutes	Neuropsychiatric symptoms assessed	Validation
Alzheimer's Disease Assessment Scale (ADAS)	Rosen et al. 1984	Patient and caregiver; administered usually in research setting by trained professionals	21	45	Depression, agitation, psychosis, vegetative symptoms; does not assess anxiety, aggression, apathy	Interrater and test-retest reliability, concurrent validity, outpatient setting
Behavioral Pathology in Alzheimer's Disease Rating Scale (BEHAVE-AD)	Reisberg et al. 1989	Caregiver; clinician interview	26	20	Paranoid and delusional ideation, hallucinations, aggressiveness, activity disturbances, diurnal rhythm disturbances, affective disturbances and anxieties, phobias	Interrater reliability; outpatient setting

TABLE 14–3. Available tools for assessment of behavioral and psychological symptoms of dementia *(continued)*

Scale name	Authors	Informant and administration method	Items	Completion time[a], minutes	Neuropsychiatric symptoms assessed	Validation
Consortium to Establish a Registry for Alzheimer's Disease (CERAD) Behavior Rating Scale for Dementia (C-BRSD)	Tariot et al. 1995	Caregiver administered, usually in research setting by trained professionals	46	20–30	Agitation, aggression, affect, psychosis, apathy, irritability	Interrater reliability; outpatient setting
Cohen-Mansfield Agitation Inventory (CMAI)	Cohen-Mansfield 1986	Nursing staff/caregiver administered, usually in research setting by trained professionals	29	15	Agitation and aggression	Interrater reliability; construct, content, convergent validity; nursing home setting
The Neuropsychiatric Inventory (NPI)	Cummings et al. 1994	Caregiver; clinician interview	12	10	Agitation, aggression, affect, psychosis, apathy, disinhibition, irritability, psychomotor, eating	Content, concurrent validity; outpatient setting

TABLE 14–3. Available tools for assessment of behavioral and psychological symptoms of dementia (continued)

Scale name	Authors	Informant and administration method	Items	Completion time[a], minutes	Neuropsychiatric symptoms assessed	Validation
Neuropsychiatric Inventory—Questionnaire (NPI-Q)	Kaufer et al. 2000	Caregiver; self-administered	12	5	Agitation, aggression, affect, psychosis, apathy, disinhibition, irritability, psychomotor, eating	Cross-validated with NPI; outpatient setting (a version for nursing homes is also available)
Pittsburgh Agitation Scale (PAS)	Rosen et al. 1994	Nursing staff; direct observation of behavior	4	1	Agitation, aggression, aberrant vocalizations, psychomotor, resistance to care	Interrater reliability; inpatient or nursing home setting
Psychogeriatric Dependency Rating Scale (PGDRS)	Wilkinson and Graham-White 1980	Nursing staff; direct observation of behavior	16	20	Developed to assess dependency (nursing time demanded by patient); agitation, aggression, psychosis, orientation, physical problems	Interrater reliability; inpatient setting

[a]Average.

- *Step 1: Describe.* The clinician should obtain accurate descriptions of the symptoms and the context in which they occur, along with any identifiable antecedents or triggers.
- *Step 2: Investigate.* The clinician should examine and identify all possible contributing factors.
- *Step 3: Create.* The clinician, caregiver, and patient (if able) should collaborate to create and implement a treatment plan. The treatment plan should target the problems and modifiable factors identified in step 2. Behavioral interventions are first-line, followed by pharmacological interventions in cases in which the symptoms do not respond to behavioral strategies or pose significant risk of harm.
- *Step 4: Evaluate.* The clinician should assess whether recommended strategies were attempted and implemented effectively. A trial of dosage reduction or discontinuation of psychotropic medications, if they were used, should be considered.

Management of BPSD

Agitation and Psychosis

Nonpharmacological Management

Nonpharmacological interventions are universally recommended as first-line management for BPSD (Kales et al. 2015). Nonpharmacological strategies can be divided into two groups:

1. *Individualized strategies designed to target modifiable factors of BPSD identified during assessment.* These strategies are individually tailored to the patient on the basis of problem areas identified during evaluation of modifiable factors. In addition, the following generalized strategies are relatively easy to implement and are of potential benefit in most cases (Kales et al. 2015):

   - Providing education for the caregiver
   - Enhancing effective communication between the caregiver and the person with dementia
   - Creating meaningful activities for the person with dementia
   - Simplifying tasks and establishing structured routines
   - Ensuring safety and simplifying and enhancing the environment

2. *Standardized nonpharmacological interventions.* Person-centered care, communication skills training, and adapted dementia care mapping were shown to reduce agitation immediately and for up to

6 months in a systematic review of 33 randomized controlled trials (Livingston et al. 2014). All three involve improving the caregiver's understanding of, communication with, and care of dementia patients. Group activities and music therapy decreased agitation in the short term but did not demonstrate sustained long-term benefit. Aroma therapy and light therapy were ineffective in controlled trials. Brodaty and Arasaratnam (2012), in a meta-analysis of 23 randomized controlled trials regarding the effectiveness of community-based nonpharmacological interventions delivered through family caregivers, reported that family caregiver interventions were effective in reducing BPSD (overall effect size, 0.34) and in ameliorating caregiver reactions. Of note, the effect size of 0.34 is greater than what has been reported for antipsychotic medications.

Overall, nonpharmacological interventions with the greatest evidence of benefit are those based on family caregiver interventions. These interventions include skills training for caregivers, education for caregivers, planning activities with caregiver for care recipient, environmental redesign, enhanced support for caregivers, and self-care techniques for caregivers, among others.

Pharmacological Management

Pharmacological treatment is recommended when behavioral interventions have failed to treat symptoms that are severe or cause significant distress, and for the management of acute situations in which the safety of the patient or caregiver is in jeopardy. No medication has approval from the U.S. Food and Drug Administration (FDA) for the treatment of BPSD in dementia in United States, and therefore all treatment with medications is off-label. (Of note, risperidone is licensed in Britain for short-term treatment of persistent aggression in patients with moderate to severe Alzheimer's dementia unresponsive to nonpharmacological approaches and when there is risk of harm to self or others; risperidone use for BPSD is also approved in Canada.) Although off-label prescribing is accompanied by an increased risk of liability, evidence-based use is justified when risks and benefits have been carefully weighed and appropriate consent has been obtained.

- **Antipsychotics.** Among pharmacological agents, atypical antipsychotics have the best evidence of efficacy (albeit modest). Unfortunately, they are also linked with evidence of serious harm in the form of increased risk of mortality.

Efficacy.   Efficacy of typical antipsychotics in the treatment of agitation and psychosis is small at best (Sink et al. 2005). One early meta-analysis published in 1990 demonstrated that typical antipsychotics were effective, although the effect size was small: if 100 patients are treated with typical antipsychotics, 18 patients would be expected to experience some benefit (beyond that of placebo). In a Cochrane review and meta-analysis of five randomized controlled trials using haloperidol, haloperidol was of some benefit in reducing aggression but was not effective in the treatment of agitation (Lonergan et al. 2002).

Efficacy of atypical antipsychotics for BPSD has been demonstrated in multiple systematic reviews and a meta-analysis. In a 2011 meta-analysis (Maher et al. 2011) of data from 14 randomized controlled trials reporting a total global outcome score for BPSD (including symptoms such as psychosis, mood alterations, and aggression), small but statistically significant effects sizes, ranging from 0.12 to 0.20, were observed for aripiprazole, olanzapine, and risperidone (Table 14–4). These three medications were also found to be superior to placebo specifically in the treatment of agitation, whereas only risperidone was found to be superior to placebo specifically in treating psychosis. Quetiapine was not found to be superior to placebo for any of the three symptom domains (i.e., overall BPSD, agitation, psychosis).

Mortality and other serious risks.   In 2003, the FDA updated the prescribing information for risperidone with a warning for increased cerebrovascular adverse events, including stroke, in elderly patients with dementia. In 2005 the FDA issued a black box warning for the entire class of atypical antipsychotics, with a reported 1.6- to 1.7-fold increase in mortality in placebo-controlled trials with olanzapine, aripiprazole, risperidone, and quetiapine. Most of the causes of death were heart-related events (e.g., heart failure, sudden death) or infections (mostly pneumonia). In 2008, the black box warning was also applied to typical antipsychotics (Shah and Aftab 2016).

The increased risk of mortality with the use of atypical antipsychotics has consistently been reproduced in subsequent studies. A meta-analysis of randomized controlled trials by Schneider et al. (2005) reported increased mortality in dementia patients treated with atypical antipsychotics with an odds ratio of 1.54. The mortality risk increased with the duration of treatment (Ballard et al. 2009). Higher dosages of antipsychotic are associated with a higher mortality risk.

TABLE 14–4. **Efficacy of atypical antipsychotics in the treatment of behavioral and psychological symptoms of dementia**

Medication	Symptom domain	Number of RCTs	Effect size	SMD (95% CI)[a]
Risperidone	BPSD (global)	6	Small	0.19 (0.00–0.38)
	Agitation	6	Small	0.22 (0.009–0.35)
	Psychosis	5	Small	0.20 (0.05–0.36)
Olanzapine	BPSD (global)	4	Very small	0.12 (0.00–0.25)
	Agitation	5	Very small	0.10 (0.07–0.31)
	Psychosis	5	Nonsignificant	0.05 (−0.07–0.17)
Aripiprazole	BPSD (global)	3	Small	0.20 (0.04–0.35)
	Agitation	2	Small	0.30 (0.05–0.55)[b]
	Psychosis	3	Nonsignificant	0.14 (−0.02–0.29)
Quetiapine	BPSD (global)	3	Nonsignificant	0.13 (−0.03–0.28)
	Agitation	5	Nonsignificant	0.06 (−0.14–0.25)
	Psychosis	3	Nonsignificant	0.04 (−0.11–0.19)

Note. BPSD = behavioral and psychological symptoms of dementia; RCT = randomized controlled trial; SMD = standardized mean difference.
[a]Meta-analysis conducted by Maher et al. (2011).
[b]Aripiprazole only had two trials with agitation data in the systematic review, and although the results were not pooled, the calculated SMDs from the two studies were very similar: 0.31 (0.10–0.52) and 0.30 (0.05–0.55).

The risks noted in atypical antipsychotics are not lessened in typical antipsychotics; they are significantly *higher* (Wang et al. 2005). Several studies (Gerhard et al. 2014; Huybrechts et al. 2012; Kales et al. 2012) have reported a higher risk of mortality with haloperidol (hazard ratio ~1.5) and a lower risk of mortality with quetiapine (hazard ratio ~0.8) compared with risperidone. Aripiprazole and olanzapine appear to have a risk similar to risperidone. Again, higher dosages of antipsychotic are associated with a higher mortality risk, irrespective of class.

Among atypical antipsychotics, risperidone has been associated with increased risk of stroke (number needed to harm [NNH] = 53) in pooled data from randomized controlled trials. Risk of cardiovascular events other than stroke also appears to be increased with use of risperidone

TABLE 14–5. Antipsychotic use in management of behavioral and psychological symptoms of dementia (BPSD): practical considerations

Antipsychotic dosing for adults with BPSD is substantially lower than dosing for adults with psychotic disorders.[a] Start at a low dosage and titrate to minimum effective dosage as tolerated.

Typical daily dosage ranges for atypical antipsychotics for BPSD are as follows:

Risperidone: 0.5–2 mg/day

Olanzapine: 2.5–10 mg/day

Aripiprazole: 2.5–15 mg/day

Quetiapine: 12.5–200 mg/day

Taper and discontinue if no clinically significant response is seen after a 4-week trial.

If adequate response is seen with an antipsychotic, consider tapering and discontinuing the agent within 4 months of behavioral stability while monitoring closely for recurrence; if there is prior history of symptom recurrence with tapering, the antipsychotic should be continued.

Haloperidol and other first-generation antipsychotics should not be used as first-line medication for nonemergency treatment of BPSD.

[a]Although dosage of antipsychotic medications is generally lower in older adults, older adults with primary psychotic disorder or bipolar disorder may require doses higher than are typically used for BPSD.

and olanzapine (NNH=34 and 48, respectively) compared with placebo, whereas an association has not been shown with quetiapine and aripiprazole (Reus et al. 2016). Other potential serious risks of antipsychotic therapy in subjects with major neurocognitive disorder include myocardial infarction, cognitive changes, sedation/fatigue, extrapyramidal side effects, tardive dyskinesia, falls and hip fractures, weight gain, and metabolic side effects (Reus et al. 2016). Table 14–5 outlines some practical considerations related to antipsychotic use in BPSD.

• **Cholinesterase inhibitors and memantine.** Evidence regarding the use of cholinesterase inhibitors for agitation and psychosis is limited. A systematic review found that 11 out of 14 studies demonstrated no efficacy compared with placebo (Rodda et al. 2009). A subsequent meta-analysis showed a small benefit for BPSD, with a standardized mean difference of 0.12, which is of unclear clinical significance (Wang et al. 2015). Memantine's benefit for agitation in dementia was suggested by post hoc data from earlier studies; however, a randomized trial designed to investigate its efficacy for agitation in Alzheimer's found no benefit compared with placebo, and lack of efficacy was also demonstrated in a subsequent meta-analysis (Wang et al. 2015). In practice, most patients with BPSD will likely already be taking cholinesterase inhibitors and/or memantine as a treatment for cognitive symptoms of dementia.

- **Anticonvulsants.** Anticonvulsants have no proven efficacy for BPSD. A Cochrane review concluded that valproate is ineffective for treatment of agitation in dementia (Lonergan and Luxenberg 2009), and it has subsequently been reported that valproate may have a mortality risk similar to that of antipsychotics. There is some small and limited evidence for use of carbamazepine (Gallagher and Herrmann 2014).

- **Antidepressants.** Antidepressants have been investigated as treatment options for agitation and psychosis in dementia, and there is some evidence of benefit with sertraline and citalopram compared with placebo (Seitz et al. 2011). Citalopram has been better studied among antidepressants. Citalopram (mean maximum dose = 31 mg) was of comparable efficacy to risperidone in a 12-week randomized controlled trial in nondepressed patients with dementia for the treatment of agitation and psychotic symptoms (Pollock et al. 2007). In the Citalopram for Agitation in Alzheimer Disease (CITAD) study, citalopram (30 mg/day) was compared with placebo for a treatment period of 9 weeks. Citalopram at 30 mg/day significantly reduced agitation and caregiver distress in study subjects (Porsteinsson et al. 2014). However, in 2011 the FDA recommended curtailing citalopram's maximum dosage in individuals older than 60 years to 20 mg/day because of concern of QT interval prolongation at higher dosages. Dosages of citalopram greater than 20 mg/day should only be used after potential risks and benefits for the patient are carefully considered and informed consent is obtained.

- **Benzodiazepines.** In cross-sectional and cohort studies, benzodiazepines show some short-term benefit in the treatment of agitation (Defrancesco et al. 2015); however, randomized, placebo-controlled studies are lacking. Current recommendation is to avoid nonemergency use of benzodiazepines in subjects with dementia. Benzodiazepines are associated with cognitive decline and contribute to increased falls and hip fractures. Multiple studies have demonstrated negative effects of benzodiazepines on cognitive function in dementia, but despite recommendations against it, the use of benzodiazepines in dementia remains prevalent (Defrancesco et al. 2015).

Vignette *(continued)*

Mr. P's symptoms improved initially with streamlining of his parkinsonian medications (i.e., amantadine and pramipexole were discontinued) and addition of a selective serotonin reuptake inhibitor (SSRI) (i.e., citalopram) as well as a cholinesterase inhibitor (i.e., donepezil). Mr. P was also started on physical therapy, with his wife actively encouraging daily exercise; he declined participation in a senior day program. With these interventions, his irritability resolved and sleep improved, as did his insight into the visual hallucinations. However, this improvement was not long-lasting; within 6 months, his complaints of an Asian military home invasion had resurfaced. He was also increasingly having nightmares, apparently of his combat experience in Vietnam, though this was frequently intermixed with his visual hallucinations. The addition of scheduled gabapentin was of limited benefit for sleep and nocturnal agitation, and he consequently was started on low-dose quetiapine. He subsequently had a fall in the middle of the night during a physical altercation with his wife and was admitted to an inpatient geriatric psychiatry unit for further evaluation.

Depression

Depression is often a complicated diagnosis in the setting of neurocognitive impairment because of overlapping symptoms; each disorder can cause a syndrome similar to the other, and each can serve as a risk factor for the development of the other. Placebo-controlled, randomized trials have produced conflicting results (Sepehry et al. 2012), and although there is no definitive evidence of superior efficacy over placebo for depression in the setting of dementia, antidepressants remain the first-line treatment option in practice. Psychotherapy is also a treatment option in patients with mild to moderate dementia. Tricyclic antidepressants should be avoided given their anticholinergic properties. Paroxetine is also typically avoided because of its anticholinergic effects, and fluoxetine is considered undesirable because of its long half-life and drug interactions. Sertraline, citalopram, and escitalopram are commonly used agents (citalopram and escitalopram have maximum dosages of 20 mg/day and 10 mg/day, respectively, in the geriatric population). Finally, electroconvulsive therapy should be actively considered if pharmacological interventions are ineffective, despite the challenges of obtaining informed consent from a patient with dementia or having a proxy-conservator appointed if the patient lacks the capacity to make informed decisions, and despite the cognitive side effects that remain largely transient even in the presence of preexisting dementia (Meyer et al. 2018).

Sleep Disturbances and Insomnia

An estimated one-quarter to one-third of patients with Alzheimer's dementia experience sleep disturbances (Deschenes and McCurry 2009; McCurry et al. 1999). Sleeping difficulties in patients with dementia typically fall into one of three categories:

1. Insomnia (difficulty falling and/or staying asleep; most common sleep disturbance)
2. Excessive daytime sleepiness
3. Unusual sleep-related behaviors and movements (restless legs syndrome and rapid eye movement sleep behavior disorders are particularly common in dementia with Lewy bodies/Parkinson's disease dementia)

These sleep difficulties may be secondary to other psychiatric syndromes (depression, anxiety, psychosis, agitation), due to medication side effects, or due to other factors such as a decrease in daytime physical activity. Behavioral interventions to promote sleep hygiene are preferred strategies. Ensuring adequate activity and physical exercise during waking hours, increasing natural light exposure during the day, and restricting caffeine later in the day can all be helpful (Deschenes and McCurry 2009; McCurry et al. 1999). Efficacy and safety of medications for insomnia are poorly studied in patients with dementia, and none can be unequivocally recommended (McCleery et al. 2014). A Cochrane review found randomized controlled trials for only three drugs: melatonin, ramelteon, and trazodone; melatonin and ramelteon had no evidence of efficacy, whereas low-dose trazodone (50 mg) had some evidence of benefit in one small study (McCleery et al. 2014).

Apathy

Apathy can occur in the setting of depression, but also independently. In many cases, it may be impossible to distinguish between the two. Cholinesterase inhibitors may have some positive benefit. Antidepressants and methylphenidate are common pharmacological strategies. Some randomized, placebo-controlled evidence supports the use of methylphenidate as a treatment for apathy, with and without comorbid depression (Lavretsky et al. 2015; Padala et al. 2018). In clinical practice, it is advisable to start with a low dosage (5 mg daily), which may then be titrated up to 10 mg twice daily.

Sexually Inappropriate Behavior

Verbal (using sexually explicit language) as well as physical (e.g., exposing genitalia, grabbing, masturbating in public) sexually inappropriate behavior can be seen in dementia of any type and severity. Very limited research evidence is available to guide management, and it is mostly restricted to case reports or small case series. SSRIs are preferred pharmacological agents on the basis of anecdotal evidence. Cyproterone acetate and medroxyprogesterone acetate (antiandrogens), leuprolide (luteinizing hormone–releasing hormone agonist), and estrogen (oral or transdermal) can also be considered (Guay 2008). Hormonal agents should be utilized with great caution given their side-effect profiles. Antipsychotics, mood stabilizers, cimetidine, and pindolol also have some anecdotal evidence in support of their use (Ozkan et al. 2008).

Vignette *(continued)*

During his hospitalization, Mr. P was taken off quetiapine, because of the orthostatic hypotension that likely contributed to his fall, and started on aripiprazole. Entacapone was also discontinued because of persistent hallucinations and agitation despite aripiprazole titration, and then low-dose prazosin was started to target persistent nocturnal restlessness and agitation associated with nightmares with combat-related themes. Though he experienced initial resurgence of orthostatic hypotension, this resolved with the use of compression stockings as well as initiation of fludrocortisone, enabling continued use of this medication regimen, eventual reduction in nocturnal agitation, and near resolution of visual hallucinations.

Following his inpatient hospitalization, the patient moved into an assisted living facility along with his wife. There he was actively engaged in a memory day program that included exercise groups, music therapy, morning bright-light exposure, and reminiscence groups. With the medication adjustments and the establishment of a daily schedule of activities, the patient's hallucinations were minimally intrusive, behavioral lability more responsive to redirection, and sleep largely consolidated to the nighttime hours.

KEY POINTS

- Behavioral and psychological symptoms of dementia (BPSD)—such as agitation, apathy, disinhibition, psychosis—are nearly universal *at some point in the course* of dementia, with higher prevalence in later stages.

- Evaluation of BPSD should include a comprehensive history, risk assessment, delirium assessment, and identification of precipitating factors (such as pain, constipation, medication side effects, medical illness) and contributing factors (such as caregiver stress).
- Nonpharmacological interventions are universally recommended as first-line management for BPSD, with family and caregiver interventions demonstrating the greatest evidence of benefit.
- Among pharmacological agents, atypical antipsychotics have the best (albeit modest) evidence of efficacy in the treatment of BPSD; their use is, however, associated with an increased risk of mortality. Antidepressants such as citalopram may also be helpful for agitation in patients.

Resources

Resources for Patients and Families

Alzheimer's Association caregiving page: "Stages and Behaviors." Available at: www.alz.org/care/alzheimers-dementia-stages-behaviors.asp
Alzheimer's Association: "I Have Alzheimer's." Available at: www.alz.org/help-support/i-have-alz
Alzheimer's Foundation of America: Caregiving Resources: https://alzfdn.org/caregiving-resources
National Institute on Aging: www.nia.nih.gov/health/topics/dementia

Resources for Clinicians

American Psychiatric Association: The American Psychiatric Association Practice Guideline on the Use of Antipsychotics to Treat Agitation or Psychosis in Patients With Dementia. Arlington, VA, American Psychiatric Association, 2016. Available at: https://psychiatryonline.org/doi/pdf/10.1176/appi.books.9780890426807
Cochrane Library: Dementia and Cognitive Improvement Group: https://dementia.cochrane.org
International Psychogeriatric Association: IPA Complete Guides to Behavioral and Psychological Symptoms of Dementia (BPSD). Cambridge, United Kingdom, Cambridge University Press, 2015. Available at: www.ipa-online.org/publications/guides-to-bpsd.
Kales HC, Gitlin LN, Lyketsos CG: Management of neuropsychiatric symptoms of dementia in clinical settings: recommendations from a multidisciplinary expert panel. J Am Geriatr Soc 62:762–769, 2014

References

Ballard C, Hanney ML, Theodoulou M, et al: The dementia antipsychotic withdrawal trial (DART-AD): long-term follow-up of a randomised placebo-controlled trial. Lancet Neurol 8(2):151–157, 2009 19138567

Bassiony MM, Lyketsos CG: Delusions and hallucinations in Alzheimer's disease: review of the brain decade. Psychosomatics 44(5):388–401, 2003 12954913

Brodaty H, Arasaratnam C: Meta-analysis of nonpharmacological interventions for neuropsychiatric symptoms of dementia. Am J Psychiatry 169(9):946–953, 2012 22952073

Cohen-Mansfield J: Agitated behaviors in the elderly, II: preliminary results in the cognitively deteriorated. J Am Geriatr Soc 34(10):722–727, 1986 3760436

Cummings JL, Mega M, Gray K, et al: The Neuropsychiatric Inventory: comprehensive assessment of psychopathology in dementia. Neurology 44(12):2308–2314, 1994 7991117

Defrancesco M, Marksteiner J, Fleischhacker WW, et al: Use of benzodiazepines in Alzheimer's disease: a systematic review of literature. Int J Neuropsychopharmacol 18(10):pyv055, 2015 25991652

Deschenes CL, McCurry SM: Current treatments for sleep disturbances in individuals with dementia. Curr Psychiatry Rep 11(1):20–26, 2009 19187704

Forester BP, Oxman TE: Measures to assess the noncognitive symptoms of dementia in the primary care setting. Prim Care Companion J Clin Psychiatry 5(4):158–163, 2003 15213777

Gallagher D, Herrmann N: Antiepileptic drugs for the treatment of agitation and aggression in dementia: do they have a place in therapy? Drugs 74(15):1747–1755, 2014 25239267

Gerhard T, Huybrechts K, Olfson M, et al: Comparative mortality risks of antipsychotic medications in community-dwelling older adults. Br J Psychiatry 205(1):44–51, 2014 23929443

Guay DR: Inappropriate sexual behaviors in cognitively impaired older individuals. Am J Geriatr Pharmacother 6(5):269–288, 2008 19161930

Hurd MD, Martorell P, Delavande A, et al: Monetary costs of dementia in the United States. N Engl J Med 368(14):1326–1334, 2013 23550670

Huybrechts KF, Gerhard T, Crystal S, et al: Differential risk of death in older residents in nursing homes prescribed specific antipsychotic drugs: population based cohort study. BMJ 344:e977, 2012 22362541

Kales HC, Kim HM, Zivin K, et al: Risk of mortality among individual antipsychotics in patients with dementia. Am J Psychiatry 169(1):71–79, 2012 22193526

Kales HC, Gitlin LN, Lyketsos CG: Assessment and management of behavioral and psychological symptoms of dementia. BMJ 350:h369, 2015 25731881

Kaufer DI, Cummings JL, Ketchel P, et al: Validation of the NPI-Q, a brief clinical form of the Neuropsychiatric Inventory. J Neuropsychiatry Clin Neurosci 12(2):233–239, 2000 11001602

Lavretsky H, Reinlieb M, St Cyr N, et al: Citalopram, methylphenidate, or their combination in geriatric depression: a randomized, double-blind, placebo-controlled trial. Am J Psychiatry 172(6):561–569, 2015 25677354

Livingston G, Kelly L, Lewis-Holmes E, et al: Non-pharmacological interventions for agitation in dementia: systematic review of randomised controlled trials. Br J Psychiatry 205(6):436–442, 2014 25452601

Lonergan E, Luxenberg J: Valproate preparations for agitation in dementia. Cochrane Database Syst Rev (3):CD003945, 2009 19588348

Lonergan E, Luxenberg J, Colford J: Haloperidol for agitation in dementia. Cochrane Database Syst Rev (2):CD002852, 2002 12076456

Lyketsos CG, Steinberg M, Tschanz JT, et al: Mental and behavioral disturbances in dementia: findings from the Cache County Study on Memory in Aging. Am J Psychiatry 157(5):708–714, 2000 10784462

Lyketsos CG, Lopez O, Jones B, et al: Prevalence of neuropsychiatric symptoms in dementia and mild cognitive impairment: results from the cardiovascular health study. JAMA 288(12):1475–1483, 2002 12243634

Maher AR, Maglione M, Bagley S, et al: Efficacy and comparative effectiveness of atypical antipsychotic medications for off-label uses in adults: a systematic review and meta-analysis. JAMA 306(12):1359–1369, 2011 21954480

McCleery J, Cohen DA, Sharpley AL: Pharmacotherapies for sleep disturbances in Alzheimer's disease. Cochrane Database Syst Rev (3):CD009178, 2014 24659320

McCurry SM, Logsdon RG, Teri L, et al: Characteristics of sleep disturbance in community-dwelling Alzheimer's disease patients. J Geriatr Psychiatry Neurol 12(2):53–59, 1999 10483925

Meyer JP, Swetter SK, Kellner CH: Electroconvulsive therapy in geriatric psychiatry: a selective review. Psychiatr Clin North Am 41(1):79–93, 2018 29412850

Ozkan B, Wilkins K, Muralee S, et al: Pharmacotherapy for inappropriate sexual behaviors in dementia: a systematic review of literature. Am J Alzheimers Dis Other Demen 23(4):344–354, 2008 18509106

Padala PR, Padala KP, Lensing SY, et al: Methylphenidate for apathy in community-dwelling older veterans with mild Alzheimer's disease: a double-blind, randomized, placebo-controlled trial. Am J Psychiatry 175(2):159–168, 2018 28945120

Pollock BG, Mulsant BH, Rosen J, et al: A double-blind comparison of citalopram and risperidone for the treatment of behavioral and psychotic symptoms associated with dementia. Am J Geriatr Psychiatry 15(11):942–952, 2007 17846102

Porsteinsson AP, Drye LT, Pollock BG, et al: Effect of citalopram on agitation in Alzheimer disease: the CitAD randomized clinical trial. JAMA 311(7):682–691, 2014 24549548

Prince M, Guerchet M, Prina M: Policy Brief for Heads of Government: The Global Impact of Dementia 2013–2050. London, Alzheimer's Disease International, 2013. Available at: https://www.alz.co.uk/research/GlobalImpactDementia2013.pdf. Accessed August 5, 2018.

Reisberg B, Franssen E, Scalan RS, et al: Stage specific incidence of potentially remediable behavioral symptoms in aging and Alzheimer disease: a study of 120 patients using BEHAVE-AD. Bull Clin Neurosci 54:95–112, 1989

Reus VI, Fochtmann LJ, Eyler AE, et al: The American Psychiatric Association practice guideline on the use of antipsychotics to treat agitation or psychosis in patients with dementia. Am J Psychiatry 173(5):543–546, 2016 27133416

Rodda J, Morgan S, Walker Z: Are cholinesterase inhibitors effective in the management of the behavioral and psychological symptoms of dementia in Alzheimer's disease? A systematic review of randomized, placebo-controlled trials of donepezil, rivastigmine and galantamine. Int Psychogeriatr 21(5):813–824, 2009 19538824

Ropacki SA, Jeste DV: Epidemiology of and risk factors for psychosis of Alzheimer's disease: a review of 55 studies published from 1990 to 2003. Am J Psychiatry 162(11):2022–2030, 2005 16263838

Rosen WG, Mohs RC, Davis KL: A new rating scale for Alzheimer's disease. Am J Psychiatry 141(11):1356–1364, 1984 6496779

Rosen J, Burgio L, Kollar M, et al: A user-friendly instrument for rating agitation in dementia patients. Am J Geriatr Psychiatry 2(1):52–59, 1994 21629007

Schneider LS, Dagerman KS, Insel P: Risk of death with atypical antipsychotic drug treatment for dementia: meta-analysis of randomized placebo-controlled trials. JAMA 294(15):1934–1943, 2005 16234500

Seitz DP, Adunuri N, Gill SS, et al: Antidepressants for agitation and psychosis in dementia. Cochrane Database Syst Rev (2):CD008191, 2011 21328305

Selbæk G, Engedal K, Bergh S: The prevalence and course of neuropsychiatric symptoms in nursing home patients with dementia: a systematic review. J Am Med Dir Assoc 14(3):161–169, 2013 23168112

Sepehry AA, Lee PE, Hsiung GY, et al: Effect of selective serotonin reuptake inhibitors in Alzheimer's disease with comorbid depression: a meta-analysis of depression and cognitive outcomes. Drugs Aging 29(10):793–806, 2012 23079957

Shah AA, Aftab A: Should physicians prescribe antipsychotics in dementia? Psychiatr Ann 46(2):97–102, 2016

Sink KM, Holden KF, Yaffe K: Pharmacological treatment of neuropsychiatric symptoms of dementia: a review of the evidence. JAMA 293(5):596–608, 2005 15687315

Steinberg M, Shao H, Zandi P, et al: Point and 5-year period prevalence of neuropsychiatric symptoms in dementia: the Cache County Study. Int J Geriatr Psychiatry 23(2):170–177, 2008 17607801

Tariot PN, Mack JL, Patterson MB, et al: The Behavior Rating Scale for Dementia of the Consortium to Establish a Registry for Alzheimer's Disease. The Behavioral Pathology Committee of the Consortium to Establish a Registry for Alzheimer's Disease. Am J Psychiatry 152(9):1349–1357, 1995 7653692

Wang J, Yu JT, Wang HF, et al: Pharmacological treatment of neuropsychiatric symptoms in Alzheimer's disease: a systematic review and meta-analysis. J Neurol Neurosurg Psychiatry 86(1):101–109, 2015 24876182

Wang PS, Schneeweiss S, Avorn J, et al: Risk of death in elderly users of conventional vs. atypical antipsychotic medications. N Engl J Med 353(22):2335–2341, 2005 16319382

Wilkinson IM, Graham-White J: Psychogeriatric dependency rating scales (PG-DRS): a method of assessment for use by nurses. Br J Psychiatry 137:558–565, 1980 6452189

Zhao QF, Tan L, Wang HF, et al: The prevalence of neuropsychiatric symptoms in Alzheimer's disease: systematic review and meta-analysis. J Affect Disord 190:264–271, 2016 26540080

Delirium

"My Mother Is Not Herself"

Patricia Serrano, M.D.
Elizabeth Hathaway, M.D.
Ajita Mathur, M.D.

CHAPTER 15

Clinical Presentation

Chief Complaint

"My mother is not herself."

Vignette

Ms. N, an 81-year-old woman, presents to the emergency department accompanied by her daughter, who noticed that in the past 2 days her mother has become less talkative, sleeps all day, and has stopped eating. In the emergency department, Ms. N appears confused and yells incoherently when awakened.

Ms. N's past medical history is significant for diabetes, hypertension, deep venous thrombosis, glaucoma, and obesity. She also has a past psychiatric history of depression and Alzheimer's disease that was diagnosed 5 years ago. During the past year she has usually been disoriented to time and place but could carry on a conversation about events that happened in the past. She gets lost in her apartment complex, so her daughter lives with her in a two-bedroom apartment and supervises her at all times as her primary caregiver. Ms. N is able to walk but loses her balance easily and is prone to falls. She needs assistance with all her activities of daily living.

Ms. N's daughter reports that her mother was discharged home from the hospital 10 days ago. At the time of admission, she presented with similar complaints and was admitted for "altered mental status." During that admission, she was diagnosed with a urinary tract infection and treated with antibiotics. After a short hospitalization, she became alert, was able to answer questions, and was discharged home with oral antibiotics.

A few days after discharge she visited her primary care physician in the company of her daughter. At that visit, her daughter expressed concerns that her mother appeared anxious, especially at night, and had had difficulty sleeping since she got home from the hospital. Her doctor prescribed clonazepam 0.5 mg three times a day.

At the time of the current visit, Ms. N's vital signs, comprehensive metabolic panel, blood count, and urinalysis are unremarkable. Her head computed tomography (CT) scan shows no changes from prior scans or acute pathology.

Interdisciplinary Team Commentary

Internal medicine physician: We're concerned Ms. N has an infection or another medical cause that has triggered this episode of confusion, but all the imaging and basic laboratory values are within normal limits. I would like the psychiatrist to comment on the possibility of the symptoms being related to the patient's diagnosis of Alzheimer's disease, as well as the appropriate course of treatment.

Psychiatrist: It's highly likely that Ms. N had an episode of delirium at the time of her first hospitalization secondary to a urinary tract infection. Delirium at that time improved once the underlying infection was treated with antibiotics, but it's likely that the delirium was not fully resolved. It manifested in the anxiety and poor sleep she is experiencing at night. It is understandable to think this could be secondary to "sundowning" that many patients with Alzheimer's disease experience as their disease progresses, but it appears Ms. N didn't have this symptom prior to the urinary tract infection, which makes delirium a more likely diagnosis. At the time the primary care physician met the patient, it's possible he did not find documentation in the chart that Ms. N had had recent delirium and wasn't aware that benzodiazepines in older adults can exacerbate or trigger delirium. Given that her symptoms worsened after the start of this medication, it's likely to be the primary cause of her current presentation.

Clinical social worker: Ms. N's daughter is the primary and sole caregiver of her mother. She would benefit from assistance at home so she has time to rest and take care of herself. It's important to educate her on what delirium is and what she can do to help her mother, and provide her with resources, such as information about the local Alzheimer's Association.

Discussion

Definition of Delirium

Delirium is a common clinical syndrome characterized by acute fluctuation in attention and cognition (Oh et al. 2017). The prevalence of delirium in the community setting is low (1%–2%; Inouye et al. 2014b), but the syndrome usually prompts patients to seek care. In the acute care setting, 10.5%–39% of older adults present with delirium at hospital admission (Yeo et al. 2017).

Delirium is an independent risk factor for increased length of stay in the hospital, higher risk of complications from hospitalization, and higher rates of discharge to long-term care (Inouye 2006). Moreover, delirium increases the risk of mortality (Marcantonio 2017) and can also accelerate the trajectory of cognitive decline in patients with Alzheimer's disease (Inouye et al. 2014b; Marcantonio 2017).

Unfortunately, delirium commonly goes unrecognized and is often managed inappropriately, despite its devastating, long-term consequences for patients and their families (Oh et al. 2017). It also places a high economic burden on the health care system. A study published in *JAMA* in 2008 estimated that the cost attributable to delirium ranges from $38 billion to $152 billion each year in the United States (Leslie et al. 2008). Given the high incidence of delirium in older adults and the high rates of associated adverse outcomes and mortality, a suspected case should be managed as delirium until proven otherwise (Inouye et al. 2014b).

Diagnostic Criteria

The diagnosis of delirium is made clinically by using information provided by the history, an informed observer, physical examination, mental status examination, and review of laboratory and radiological testing (American Geriatrics Society Expert Panel on Postoperative Delirium in Older Adults 2015b).

The core features of delirium (Figure 15–1) include acute and fluctuating onset of inattention, disorganized thinking, and altered level of consciousness.

Per DSM-5 criteria (American Psychiatric Association 2013), the disturbance represents a change from baseline attention and awareness that is not better explained by a preexisting, established, or evolving neurocognitive disorder.

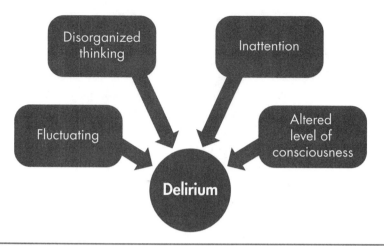

FIGURE 15–1.   Core features of delirium.

Source.   Modeled after the Confusion Assessment Method (Inouye et al. 1990).

Clinical Features

- Presentation is often varied.
- Sleep-wake cycle disturbances include excessive sleepiness, napping, fragmentation, or reversal of the sleep cycle (Caplan 2018). Sleep disturbance is one of the most frequent symptoms, seen in 92%–97% of patients with delirium (Gupta et al. 2008).
- "Sundowning" is used to describe confusion at the end of the day that is common in patients with Alzheimer's disease, but it is also seen in patients with delirium.
- Mood symptoms such as lability, irritability, withdrawn affect, or depressive features may be present (Meagher et al. 2011).
- Psychotic symptoms, including hallucinations, delusions, or paranoia, are present in approximately 50% of cases, with visual hallucinations being the most common (Gupta et al. 2008).
- Motor disturbances such as hyper- or hypoactivity are present.

Subtypes of Delirium

Three types of delirium are commonly described: hypoactive, hyperactive, and mixed (Morandi et al. 2017) (Figure 15–2).

1. Patients with the hyperactive type present with restlessness, agitation, hypervigilance, and hallucinations. This type is often confused with a primary psychotic process such as schizophrenia.

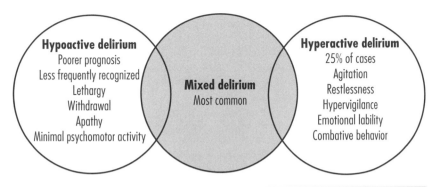

FIGURE 15–2. Delirium subtypes.

2. Patients with hypoactive delirium present with lethargy, sedation, and slow motor and verbal responses. This presentation can be mistaken for catatonia or depression. Hypoactive delirium is often missed because the symptoms are less disruptive to caregivers.
3. Patients with the mixed type present with characteristics of both hyperactive and hypoactive subtypes.

Pathophysiology

The pathophysiology of delirium is not fully understood. Evidence suggests that drug toxicity, inflammation, and acute stress responses can all contribute markedly to disruption of neurotransmission and, ultimately, to the development of delirium (Fong et al. 2009). Increased dopamine, decreased acetylcholine, and either increased or low γ-aminobutyric acid and serotonin are commonly described changes in the development of delirium (Calvo-Ayala and Khan 2013; Maldonado 2017).

Impaired acetylcholine neurotransmission fits with the concept of decreased cognitive reserve (as with Alzheimer's disease or multiple clinical comorbidities) as a risk factor for delirium, but the concept has not been firmly demonstrated (Brown and Douglas 2015), nor have cholinesterase inhibitors shown a strong effect for delirium prevention (Gamberini et al. 2009; Liptzin et al. 2005; Sampson et al. 2007).

Given that delirium is found in patients with a high inflammatory burden, associated inflammatory markers have been examined (Fong et al. 2009; Khan et al. 2011). Studies have documented significant associations between proinflammatory cytokines and delirium (Khan et al. 2011). Acetylcholine may inhibit the release of interleukin-6 and thereby help in controlling brain inflammation (Khan et al. 2011). In processes in which acetylcholine is depleted, it is possible that the inflammatory cascade is less controlled in the brain. Also, cytokines may induce a reduction in cholinergic activity, which would result in a repetitive cycle of inadequate regulation of inflammation due to cholinergic depletion (Calvo-Ayala and Khan 2013).

Causes

Delirium has a wide range of potential etiologies and is often multifactorial, with interacting predisposing and precipitating conditions. Patient factors that increase the risk for delirium include older age; increased comorbidity burden; and baseline impairment in cognition, functional capacity, vision, or hearing (Inouye et al. 2014b). Certain clinical situations, such as surgery or hospitalization, especially in the intensive care unit, are particularly associated with delirium.

Medications, whether prescribed or illicit, are important to consider as a common cause of delirium. Opioids, benzodiazepines, and anticholinergic medications are commonly known to be deliriogenic.

Withdrawal from alcohol, illicit drugs, or medications can also trigger delirium. This can occur after medications are stopped, when patients are transferred between services or institutions, or in the context of surgery or hospitalization. In the case of withdrawal from alcohol or benzodiazepines, benzodiazepines may be beneficial (Alagiakrishnan and Wiens 2004).

Similarly, judicious utilization of opioids may have a role in delirium prevention because uncontrolled pain is a delirium risk factor; however, nonopioid management is preferred whenever possible (American Geriatrics Society Expert Panel on Postoperative Delirium in Older Adults 2015a).

Limited or lower-quality evidence suggests that antihistamines, tricyclic antidepressants, and nifedipine may also be associated with delirium (Brown and Douglas 2015). In cases of polypharmacy, the temporal relation of a medication change to delirium onset may be a key clue to etiology.

Any form of infection and the associated inflammatory response can trigger delirium; urinary or respiratory tract infections are common culprits. Metabolic abnormalities such as hypoglycemia, hypoxia, and hypercarbia may also contribute.

Other medical causes of acute mental status change may raise concern for delirium and should be considered in the differential diagnosis.

Differential Diagnosis

Cognitive impairment is a risk factor, and delirium can be superimposed with Alzheimer's disease. The fluctuating course and acute change from baseline, characteristics of delirium, are the keys to differentiating it from Alzheimer's disease.

Stroke or hemorrhage might manifest as delirium (Maldonado 2017). Focal neurological signs (e.g., hemiparesis) should raise suspicion. Hemiparesis or hemispatial neglect might be subtle on examination. Focal atrophy or microvascular ischemic changes in imaging may suggest predisposition to delirium.

Postictal states or partial seizures may also manifest as delirium (Caplan 2018). In such cases, an electroencephalogram (EEG) can aid in differentiating the diagnosis (Inouye et al. 2014b).

Assessment Scales

Several validated tools can identify, screen, diagnose, and assess the severity of delirium (Grover and Kate 2012).

- The Confusion Assessment Method (CAM), published in 1990, is the most widely used instrument to screen for and diagnose delirium. It is based on the presence of the core features of delirium mentioned in Figure 15–1. It has a sensitivity of 94%, a specificity of 89%, and high inter-rater reliability (Inouye et al. 2014b). Training for administering staff is recommended for best performance (Inouye et al. 2014b).
- The Delirium Rating Scale—Revised–98 (Trzepacz et al. 2001) is the most appropriate tool for measuring delirium severity (Inouye et al. 2014b). It has scale items that include language, thought processes, motor symptoms, and cognition that are designed to capture symptom severity (Oh et al. 2017).
- The Nursing Delirium Symptom Checklist is a behavioral checklist that has a sensitivity of 72% and specificity of 80% (Oh et al. 2017). Limitations include the potential for overweighting of hyperactive or agitation symptoms and the risk of missing hypoactive delirium (Oh et al. 2017).
- The Intensive Care Delirium Screening Checklist has a sensitivity of 74% and specificity of 82% (Gusmao-Flores et al. 2012). It is an eight-item screening tool based on DSM criteria and applied to data that can be collected through medical records or to information obtained from the multidisciplinary team (Gusmao-Flores et al. 2012).

Inattention, a cardinal symptom of delirium, should be routinely tested. Serial sevens or months of the year backward are appropriate options in evaluating attention (Meagher et al. 2011).

Workup of Delirium

Many causes of delirium are treatable and reversible, meaning that a thorough workup can help prevent morbidity and mortality from both delirium and the underlying medical causes. Prior medical records should be reviewed, with particular attention to the medication list and any recent changes (O'Mahony et al. 2011). Collateral information from an informed observer such as a family member or caregiver is critical to establish the patient's baseline and degree of mental status change. A thorough physical examination should include vital signs, neurological assessment, and mental status exam.

Laboratory studies to consider include a complete blood count with differential, an electrolyte panel, liver function tests, calcium, magnesium, and phosphorus. Potential sources of infection can be evaluated with a chest X ray, blood cultures, urinalysis, and urine cultures. Ammonia, thyroid-stimulating hormone, HIV, arterial blood gas, rapid plasma reagin, and vitamin B_{12} can also be considered (Brown and Douglas 2015). In patients who are immunosuppressed or have undergone a recent neurological procedure, lumbar puncture may be pursued.

An EEG can also aid in identifying the etiology, particularly in those with a prior history of or suspicion for seizure or a known intracranial mass (Brown and Douglas 2015). Regardless of the cause, generalized slowing to the theta-delta range is consistently found (Caplan 2018; Inouye et al. 2014b; Meagher et al. 2011).

Clinical history and neurological examination will guide whether to pursue imaging such as noncontrast head CT or brain magnetic resonance imaging; in an inpatient setting the clinician may also consider neurology consultation. Toxicology screening may also be informative if there is concern for intoxication or withdrawal. Consulting psychiatry is helpful to confirm diagnosis and guide workup and management.

Older patients risk functional decline with hospitalization (Covinsky et al. 2003); thus, while a change in mental status in the outpatient setting should prompt consideration of transfer to an emergency department, in facilities such as nursing homes that may have sufficient resources on-site for a thorough workup and treatment of the underlying cause, transfer to a higher level of care may carry more risks than benefits to an older adult.

Management

There are multiple clinical practice guidelines regarding the management of delirium (American Psychiatric Association 1999; Young et al.

2010), including focused guidelines for specific populations such as intensive care unit patients (Barr et al. 2013) and postoperative patients (American Geriatrics Society Expert Panel on Postoperative Delirium in Older Adults 2015b). However, the quality of guidelines is limited by constraints of the supporting literature and newer findings that may not be included; thus, whenever possible, the underlying evidence base rather than practice guidelines alone will steer recommendations in this text. Broadly speaking, there is stronger evidence for nonpharmacological interventions than for pharmacological management of delirium.

Given the morbidity, mortality, and cost associated with delirium, primary prevention is a cornerstone of delirium management and can reduce the incidence of this issue (Inouye et al. 1999; Kratz et al. 2015). Nonpharmacological prevention strategies have the strongest evidence base; one meta-analysis found that multicomponent nonpharmacological interventions utilizing various combinations of hearing, vision, hydration, sleep-wake cycle preservation, early mobility, and cognition/orientation interventions lowered the odds of delirium by 44% among participants in four randomized or matched trials (Hshieh et al. 2015).

For prevention of postoperative delirium in particular, formal guidelines include educational programs for health care professionals, multicomponent nonpharmacological interventions, optimization of postoperative analgesia, and avoidance of deliriogenic medications (American Geriatrics Society Expert Panel on Postoperative Delirium in Older Adults 2015a). Other studies also suggest that bispectral index monitoring, an EEG analysis, to monitor depth of anesthesia may help reduce postoperative delirium (Chan et al. 2013; Radtke et al. 2013; Sieber et al. 2010; Whitlock et al. 2014).

When prevention efforts are unsuccessful, underlying medical causes precipitating the delirium should be identified and managed (Oh et al. 2017). Nonpharmacological options for management, such as reorientation, avoidance of restraints (including tethers such as catheters), early mobilization, and sensory aids, have generally been studied in multicomponent interventions and have been shown to reduce duration of delirium (Brown and Douglas 2015), although the evidence base is stronger for prevention than management (American Geriatrics Society Expert Panel on Postoperative Delirium in Older Adults 2015a).

There is insufficient evidence to support pharmacological approaches for the prevention or treatment of delirium (Inouye et al. 2014b; Neufeld et al. 2016), and providers should be mindful of deliriogenic agents such as anticholinergics, opioids, and benzodiazepines. Prophylactic use of antipsychotics is not recommended (American Geriatrics Society Expert Panel on Postoperative Delirium in Older Adults 2015b; Barr et al. 2013; Neufeld et al. 2016).

Neither antipsychotics nor benzodiazepines are recommended except in cases where severe agitation risks harm to self or others (American Geriatrics Society Expert Panel on Postoperative Delirium in Older Adults 2015b; Barr et al. 2013). In such cases, antipsychotics are the first-line therapy (Brown and Douglas 2015), although there are no U.S. Food and Drug Administration (FDA)–approved medications for the treatment of delirium.

Data to guide the selection of particular antipsychotic agents are heterogeneous and inconclusive, with larger-scale randomized controlled trials "urgently required" to better evaluate atypical antipsychotic options versus haloperidol and placebo (Rivière et al. 2019). Benzodiazepines should be avoided except when indicated for alcohol or benzodiazepine withdrawal (Clegg and Young 2011; Oh et al. 2017).

At present, haloperidol, with its multiple routes of administration, is the most widely used and studied antipsychotic option; potential risks include extrapyramidal symptoms and QTc prolongation, particularly with the intravenous formulation (Lacasse et al. 2006; Maldonado 2017). Prior to haloperidol being used, cardiac conditions and electrolyte abnormalities must be assessed. If a patient's QTc interval is greater than 25% of his or her baseline or more than 500 msec, haloperidol should be avoided (Marcantonio 2017). When haloperidol is being administered, it is important to remember that the oral dose has half the potency of the parenteral dose (Caplan 2018). In older adults, starting doses should range from 0.25 mg to 0.5 mg orally (Maldonado 2017; Marcantonio 2017). If one dose fails to calm an agitated patient, a higher dose 30 minutes later should be considered (Oh et al. 2017).

Although Maldonado (2017) noted that there is no evidence that another agent is clinically superior or safer and named haloperidol as the treatment of choice, barring cardiac problems or electrolyte abnormalities, use of atypical antipsychotics is increasing. A recent review tentatively concluded that the evidence does not show atypical antipsychotics to be less efficacious than haloperidol, with olanzapine and quetiapine as the best-supported alternative options (Rivière et al. 2019); risperidone and ziprasidone have also been studied in randomized controlled trials.

Limited evidence supports the use of melatonin (Al-Aama et al. 2011) or ramelteon (Hatta et al. 2014) for delirium prevention, with pooled analysis finding no benefit among hospitalized non–intensive care unit patients (Siddiqi et al. 2016). In spite of this, some researchers recommend melatonin 6 mg or ramelteon 8 mg at night to promote a more natural sleep (Al-Aama et al. 2011; Choy et al. 2018; Maldonado 2017).

Symptom severity should be tracked to monitor the clinical course and treatment response. A variety of tools are available for this purpose, including the Delirium Rating Scale—Revised–98, Memorial Delirium Assessment Scale (Breitbart et al. 1997), and the newer CAM–Severity Scale (Inouye et al. 2014a).

Vignette *(continued)*

In Ms. N's case, it is very likely that she had delirium during and after her first hospitalization and that the evening anxiety referenced by her daughter was a symptom of this syndrome. An appropriate workup on arrival to the hospital ruled out infection and exacerbation of other medical issues as precipitating factors for her more recent decline. Recent initiation of a benzodiazepine exacerbated Ms. N's delirium, leading to rehospitalization.

Clonazepam was tapered and discontinued as appropriate. Non-pharmacological management tools were also implemented to improve resolution of the syndrome, with Ms. N's daughter encouraged to reorient the patient often, foster a good sleep-wake cycle with daytime mobilization and avoidance of naps, and help keep Ms. N's glasses and hearing aids on. At the time of discharge, appropriate medication reconciliation was done, and the team spoke to Ms. N's primary care physician for proper continuity of care.

Ms. N was discharged home with arrangements to have physical therapy at home three times per week. The social worker arranged home health aide services so Ms. N's daughter can have help taking care of her mother.

KEY POINTS

- Delirium is multifactorial.
- The incidence of delirium is higher in patients with Alzheimer's disease than in other patients.
- It is important to screen for delirium and maintain a high index of suspicion to prevent and treat possible cases.
- Early recognition and treatment of underlying causes can minimize negative outcomes.
- It is important to assess current and recent medications and, whenever possible, stop the medications that increase risk, such as anticholinergics, antihistamines, opioids, and benzodiazepines.
- Medications should be changed to a safer alternative when possible.

- There is no U.S. Food and Drug Administration–approved medication for delirium. Antipsychotic medication is the first-line therapy when resulting agitation endangers the patient or others.

Resources

American Delirium Society: www.americandeliriumsociety.org (Has information for patients, families, and medical professionals.)

HealthinAging.org: Tips for Managing Delirium in Older Adults. New York, Health in Aging Foundation, 2014. Available at: www.healthinaging.org/tools-and-tips/tips-managing-delirium-older-adults (Includes tips and tools for family and caregivers, as well as a printer-friendly PDF)

Hospital Elder Life Program: What You Can Do (website). Boston, MA, Hospital Elder Life Program, 2018. Available at: https://www.hospitalelderlifeprogram.org/for-family-members/what-you-can-do (Ten tips for family and caregivers to avoid confusion in the hospital.)

Hospital Elder Life Program: www.hospitalelderlifeprogram.org. (Has explanations about what delirium is and why it is so important. It also has a bibliography and useful links.)

References

Al-Aama T, Brymer C, Gutmanis I, et al: Melatonin decreases delirium in elderly patients: a randomized, placebo-controlled trial. Int J Geriatr Psychiatry 26(7):687–694, 2011 20845391

Alagiakrishnan K, Wiens CA: An approach to drug induced delirium in the elderly. Postgrad Med J 80(945):388–393, 2004 15254302

American Geriatrics Society Expert Panel on Postoperative Delirium in Older Adults: American Geriatrics Society abstracted clinical practice guideline for postoperative delirium in older adults. J Am Geriatr Soc 63(1):142–150, 2015a 25495432

American Geriatrics Society Expert Panel on Postoperative Delirium in Older Adults: Postoperative delirium in older adults: best practice statement from the American Geriatrics Society. J Am Coll Surg 220(2):136–148, 2015b 25535170

American Psychiatric Association: Practice guideline for the treatment of patients with delirium. Am J Psychiatry 156 (5 suppl):1–20, 1999 10327941

American Psychiatric Association: Diagnostic and Statistical Manual of Mental Disorders, 5th Edition. Arlington, VA, American Psychiatric Association, 2013

Barr J, Fraser GL, Puntillo K, et al: Clinical practice guidelines for the management of pain, agitation, and delirium in adult patients in the intensive care unit. Crit Care Med 41(1):263–306, 2013 23269131

Breitbart W, Rosenfeld B, Roth A, et al: The Memorial Delirium Assessment Scale. J Pain Symptom Manage 13(3):128–137, 1997 9114631

Brown EG, Douglas VC: Moving beyond metabolic encephalopathy: an update on delirium prevention, workup, and management. Semin Neurol 35(6):646–655, 2015 26595865

Calvo-Ayala E, Khan B: Delirium management in critically ill patients. J Symptoms Signs 2(1):23–32, 2013 25383387

Caplan JP: Delirious patients, in Massachusetts General Hospital Handbook of General Hospital Psychiatry, 7th Edition. Edited by Stern TA, Freudenreich O, Smith FA, et al. Philadelphia, PA, Elsevier, 2018, pp 83–93

Chan MTV, Cheng BCP, Lee TMC, et al: BIS-guided anesthesia decreases postoperative delirium and cognitive decline. J Neurosurg Anesthesiol 25(1):33–42, 2013 23027226

Choy SW, Yeoh AC, Lee ZZ, et al: Melatonin and the prevention and management of delirium: a scoping study. Front Med (Lausanne) 4(Jan):242, 2018 29376051

Clegg A, Young JB: Which medications to avoid in people at risk of delirium: a systematic review. Age Ageing 40(1):23–29, 2011 21068014

Covinsky KE, Palmer RM, Fortinsky RH, et al: Loss of independence in activities of daily living in older adults hospitalized with medical illnesses: increased vulnerability with age. J Am Geriatr Soc 51(4):451–458, 2003 12657063

Fong TG, Tulebaev SR, Inouye SK: Delirium in elderly adults: diagnosis, prevention and treatment. Nat Rev Neurol 5(4):210–220, 2009 19347026

Gamberini M, Bolliger D, Lurati Buse GA, et al: Rivastigmine for the prevention of postoperative delirium in elderly patients undergoing elective cardiac surgery—a randomized controlled trial. Crit Care Med 37(5):1762–1768, 2009 19325490

Grover S, Kate N: Assessment scales for delirium: a review. World J Psychiatry 2(4):58–70, 2012 24175169

Gupta N, de Jonghe J, Schieveld J, et al: Delirium phenomenology: what can we learn from the symptoms of delirium? J Psychosom Res 65(3):215–222, 2008 18707943

Gusmao-Flores D, Salluh JIF, Chalhub RÁ, et al: The Confusion Assessment Method for the Intensive Care Unit (CAM-ICU) and Intensive Care Delirium Screening Checklist (ICDSC) for the diagnosis of delirium: a systematic review and meta-analysis of clinical studies. Crit Care 16(4):R115, 2012 22759376

Hatta K, Kishi Y, Wada K, et al: Preventive effects of ramelteon on delirium: a randomized placebo-controlled trial. JAMA Psychiatry 71(4):397–403, 2014 24554232

Hshieh TT, Yue J, Oh E, et al: Effectiveness of multicomponent nonpharmacological delirium interventions: a meta-analysis. JAMA Intern Med 175(4):512–520, 2015 25643002

Inouye SK: Delirium in older persons. N Engl J Med 354(11):1157–1165, 2006 16540616

Inouye SK, van Dyck CH, Alessi CA, et al: Clarifying confusion: the confusion assessment method. A new method for detection of delirium. Ann Intern Med 113(12):941–948, 1990 2240918

Inouye SK, Bogardus ST Jr, Charpentier PA, et al: A multicomponent intervention to prevent delirium in hospitalized older patients. N Engl J Med 340(9):669–676, 1999 10053175

Inouye SK, Kosar CM, Tommet D, et al: The CAM-S: development and validation of a new scoring system for delirium severity in 2 cohorts. Ann Intern Med 160(8):526–533, 2014a 24733193

Inouye SK, Westendorp RGJ, Saczynski JS: Delirium in elderly people. Lancet 383(9920):911–922, 2014b 23992774

Khan BA, Zawahiri M, Campbell NL, et al: Biomarkers for delirium—a review. J Am Geriatr Soc 59 (suppl 2):S256–S261, 2011 22091570

Kratz T, Heinrich M, Schlauß E, et al: Preventing postoperative delirium. Dtsch Arztebl Int 112(17):289–296, 2015 26008890

Lacasse H, Perreault MM, Williamson DR: Systematic review of antipsychotics for the treatment of hospital-associated delirium in medically or surgically ill patients. Ann Pharmacother 40(11):1966–1973, 2006 17047137

Leslie DL, Marcantonio ER, Zhang Y, et al: One-year health care costs associated with delirium in the elderly population. Arch Intern Med 168(1):27–32, 2008 18195192

Liptzin B, Laki A, Garb JL, et al: Donepezil in the prevention and treatment of post-surgical delirium. Am J Geriatr Psychiatry 13(12):1100–1106, 2005 16319303

Maldonado JR: Acute brain failure: pathophysiology, diagnosis, management, and sequelae of delirium. Crit Care Clin 33(3):461–519, 2017 28601132

Marcantonio ER: Delirium in hospitalized older adults. N Engl J Med 377(15):1456–1466, 2017 29020579

Meagher DJ, Norton JW, Trzepacz PT: Delirium in the elderly, in Principles and Practice of Geriatric Psychiatry, 2nd Edition. Edited by Agronin ME, Maletta GJ. Philadelphia, PA, Lippincott Williams and Wilkins, 2011, pp 383–403

Morandi A, Di Santo SG, Cherubini A, et al: Clinical features associated with delirium motor subtypes in older inpatients: results of a multicenter study. Am J Geriatr Psychiatry 25(10):1064–1071, 2017 28579352

Neufeld KJ, Yue J, Robinson TN, et al: Antipsychotic medication for prevention and treatment of delirium in hospitalized adults: a systematic review and meta-analysis. J Am Geriatr Soc 64(4):705–714, 2016 27004732

O'Mahony R, Murthy L, Akunne A, et al: Synopsis of the National Institute for Health and Clinical Excellence guideline for prevention of delirium. Ann Intern Med 154(11):746–751, 2011 21646557

Oh ES, Fong TG, Hshieh TT, et al: Delirium in older persons: advances in diagnosis and treatment. JAMA 318(12):1161–1174, 2017 28973626

Radtke FM, Franck M, Lendner J, et al: Monitoring depth of anaesthesia in a randomized trial decreases the rate of postoperative delirium but not postoperative cognitive dysfunction. Br J Anaesth 110 (suppl 1):i98–i105, 2013 23539235

Rivière J, van der Mast RC, Vandenberghe J, et al: Efficacy and tolerability of atypical antipsychotics in the treatment of delirium: a systematic review of the literature. Psychosomatics 60(1):18–26, 2019

Sampson EL, Raven PR, Ndhlovu PN, et al: A randomized, double-blind, placebo-controlled trial of donepezil hydrochloride (Aricept) for reducing the incidence of postoperative delirium after elective total hip replacement. Int J Geriatr Psychiatry 22(4):343–349, 2007 17006875

Siddiqi N, Harrison JK, Clegg A, et al: Interventions for preventing delirium in hospitalised non-ICU patients. Cochrane Database Syst Rev 3:CD005563, 2016 26967259

Sieber FE, Zakriya KJ, Gottschalk A, et al: Sedation depth during spinal anesthesia and the development of postoperative delirium in elderly patients undergoing hip fracture repair. Mayo Clin Proc 85(1):18–26, 2010 20042557

Trzepacz PT, Mittal D, Torres R, et al: Validation of the Delirium Rating Scale–revised-98: comparison with the delirium rating scale and the cognitive test for delirium. J Neuropsychiatry Clin Neurosci 13(2):229–242, 2001 11449030

Whitlock EL, Torres BA, Lin N, et al: Postoperative delirium in a substudy of cardiothoracic surgical patients in the BAG-RECALL clinical trial. Anesth Analg 118(4):809–817, 2014 24413548

Yeo QM, Wiley TL, Smith MN, et al: Oral agents for the management of agitation and agitated delirium in critically ill patients. Crit Care Nurs Q 40(4):344–362, 2017 28834857

Young J, Murthy L, Westby M, et al: Diagnosis, prevention, and management of delirium: summary of NICE guidance. BMJ 341:c3704, 2010 20667955

Inpatient Issues: Behavioral and Pharmacological Interventions

"He Tried to Kick a Staff Member and Fell"

Nishina A. Thomas, M.D.
Monica Mathys, Pharm.D.
Mary (Molly) E. Camp, M.D.

CHAPTER 16

Clinical Presentation

Chief Complaint

"He tried to kick a staff member and fell."

Vignette

Mr. R is an 83-year-old man with Alzheimer's disease (severe) who was admitted to the inpatient psychiatry unit due to agitation at his nursing home. Over the past few weeks, he has become increasingly aggressive during activities such as bathing, dressing, or toileting. During one particularly severe episode of agitation that was not amenable to redirection, he fell while trying to kick a staff member. The nursing home called 911, and he was brought to the emergency department for evaluation.

In the emergency department, Mr. R's lab results and vital signs were unremarkable. A computed tomography scan of the head and hip X rays were negative for any acute findings or fracture. Mr. R resisted a full physical examination, including musculoskeletal and neurological, but gross observations did not reveal any apparent injuries or acute illnesses. He was admitted to the psychiatry inpatient unit for treatment of behavioral disturbances.

On the inpatient unit, Mr. R frequently paced the halls, and he became aggressive during perineal care. He was given as-needed olanzapine 2.5 mg orally and was placed on 1:1 observation because of his high activity level, aggressive behavior, and risk of falls. On day 2, a staff member observed him briefly gripping his right side and grimacing. He would not allow her to examine or assist him at that time. On day 3 of admission, Mr. R refused breakfast and stood in the hallway holding his lower right abdomen and groin. With the assistance of a staff member with whom Mr. R had especially good rapport, physical examination was repeated, and he was found to have a reducible right inguinal hernia.

Surgery was consulted immediately. Since Mr. R lacked capacity for medical decision making, his wife was present as his surrogate decision maker. With explanation of risks and benefits of surgical correction, his wife and surgical team agreed that surgery would be avoided if possible. Occupational therapy was consulted, and they worked with the hospital's prosthetics department to order a truss that the patient could wear for comfort. After several tries, he eventually allowed the staff to help him put on the garment, at which time he appeared more comfortable, and his agitation greatly improved.

Discussion

The Agitated Older Adult Inpatient

Mr. R's case raises many important points about the care of older adults in an inpatient setting. Mr. R experienced increasing neuropsychiatric symptoms of dementia (major neurocognitive disorder), namely, agitation and aggression, over a subacute timeframe. His symptoms eventually progressed to the point that he required emergent evaluation for two reasons: 1) aggression that was preventing caregivers from meeting his needs outside of the hospital and 2) physical injury sustained as a result of these behaviors. Acute inpatient care presents both opportunities and challenges in the care of older adults. On one hand, diagnostic tests, specialized treatments, and consultations from specialty services are more readily available than in the outpatient setting. On the other hand, acute care by definition involves a change in the patient's environment, which can present unfamiliar (and often unpleasant) stimuli that can exacerbate behavioral symptoms and complicate treatment. In this chapter, we outline salient points related to the evaluation and treatment of older adults with dementia in this specific treatment setting.

This chapter also follows the popular "DICE" (Describe, Investigate, Create, and Evaluate) approach (Kales et al. 2014) endorsed by the Detroit Expert Panel in 2011 (Table 16–1).

Evaluation and Differential Diagnosis

When an older adult patient presents with agitation, it is important to consider medical etiologies if the agitation occurs in an acute or subacute timeframe (Thakur and Gwyther 2015). Physiological illness or injury often results in delirium in an older adult. Mr. R has three important risk factors for delirium: residence in a long-term care facility or hospital, age (65 years or older), and history of cognitive impairment or dementia (National Institute for Health and Clinical Excellence 2010). Timely recognition of delirium can expedite treatment and improve long-term mortality (Witlox et al. 2010). (For additional information about delirium in older adults, see Chapter 15, "Delirium.") Aside from delirium, other reversible etiologies of agitation, such as pain, may be present; such causes can be treated to provide relief to the patient (Husebo et al. 2011). It is prudent to take an organized, stepwise approach to ensure a thorough evaluation. The following has been adapted from Denise Nassisi's "The Evaluation and Management of the Acutely Agitated Elderly Patient" (Nassisi et al. 2006):

1. *History.* Obtain a detailed medical history from as many sources as possible—this includes the patient, witnesses, staff at the nursing home or inpatient unit, family, caregivers, and primary care providers.

   - Inquire about the patient's baseline behavior and level of functioning.
   - Review all medications and recent changes, because these are common precipitants of delirium in the elderly (Fick et al. 2003).
   - Focus the interview on causal factors related to the presentation, such as history of injury (trauma or fall), lack of oral intake, presence of systemic disease including metabolic and cardiopulmonary disorders, symptoms of infection, and substance use or withdrawal (American College of Emergency Physicians 1999).
   - Take advantage of the observations that can be made in the inpatient setting and note different times of day or other triggers associated with behavioral disturbances.

TABLE 16–1. "DICE" approach to neuropsychiatric symptoms of dementia

Describe the problematic behavior's context, as well as the social and physical environment; obtain the patient's perspective; and identify the degree of distress to the patient and caregiver.

Investigate possible causes of problem behavior.

Create a treatment plan.

Evaluate the effect of the treatment plan on the problematic behavior.

- Request that nursing staff utilize rating scales for the patient's behavior, such as the Cohen-Mansfield Agitation Inventory (Cohen-Mansfield and Libin 2004).
- Gather data from multiple informants to address various aspects of the patient's unmet needs. For instance, nurse aides may ascertain unmet physical needs such as constipation, whereas an activity therapist may assess social needs (Cohen-Mansfield et al. 2015).

2. *Cognitive screening.* Complete a mental status evaluation with the patient such as a Montreal Cognitive Assessment (Nasreddine et al. 2005), Mini Mental State Examination (Folstein et al. 1975), or Mini-Cog (Borson et al. 2003). If possible, compare these findings with prior examinations that used the same screening tool. Also, screen for delirium with tools such as the Confusion Assessment Method (Inouye et al. 1990).

3. *Vital signs.* Check vital signs, including temperature, heart rate, blood pressure, and oxygen saturation, on a routine basis. Take a baseline weight and compare it with prior readings if possible. Consider orthostatic vital signs in patients who have a high fall risk or who are taking medications that may cause orthostasis. Monitor blood glucose in patients at risk for hypo- or hyperglycemia.

4. *Physical examination:* A complete physical examination is an important part of the initial evaluation. As with Mr. R, agitation may prevent a thorough evaluation on the first try. In these cases, the examination may need to be repeated at a later time. If a complete examination is not possible, target areas of patient complaint, searching for evidence of medical causes for the patient's presentation, such as infection, trauma, or focal neurological deficits.

5. *Laboratory workup:* Consider a laboratory workup to rule out medical contributors (Table 16–2).

6. *Imaging:* Radiology services may be more readily available in inpatient settings than outpatient ones (Table 16–2).
7. *Other procedures:* Consider electroencephalography if seizures are suspected. Also consider a lumbar puncture to evaluate for an infectious etiology or suspected normal pressure hydrocephalus signs and symptoms. Because agitation in the elderly is often associated with sensory impairment, particularly visual and auditory deficits, audiometric and visual testing may identify potential areas for further intervention (Steffens et al. 2015).
8. *Consultations:* When the patient's condition warrants consultation from other services, the input of these interdisciplinary providers can be invaluable. Compared with an outpatient consultation, an inpatient consult may provide more opportunity for timely evaluation and in-person collaboration between providers.

When working with a patient in a higher level of care such as an intensive care unit (ICU), medical floor, or psychiatric inpatient unit in a medical hospital, health care providers can optimize diagnostic evaluation by utilizing the various laboratory, imaging, procedural, and consultation services (e.g., medical subspecialists, pharmacists) accessible within the facility. (For additional information regarding geriatric psychiatry care across various treatment settings, see Hategan et al. 2016.) Once the etiology of the agitation has been narrowed down using the strategy described, appropriate interventions can be implemented.

Nonpharmacological Interventions

Nonpharmacological interventions include a wide variety of approaches involving either the patient or the patient's environment—or both (Gitlin et al. 2012). As an important part of the comprehensive treatment plan, these interventions should be implemented early and reevaluated often during the care of the patient (Salzman et al. 2008). Following the initial evaluation of the agitation, the next appropriate question is often "What behavioral interventions have been tried, and what has been the response?" (Yohanna and Cifu 2017).

Despite the importance of these interventions, there is a scarcity of literature on nonpharmacological interventions on acute psychiatric or medical inpatient units specifically. In the existing body of research (primarily conducted in nursing homes or residential settings), evi-

TABLE 16–2. Inpatient evaluation of behavioral changes in older adults

Contributing factors	Evaluation
Pharmacological	
Drug-drug interactions Adverse effects Addition or change to medications Accidental misuse	Medication reconciliation to identify anticholinergic properties, excessive dosing, or regimens that are not easily administered
Medical comorbidities	
Cardiovascular (e.g., chest pain, shortness of breath, diaphoresis)	ECG; serum troponin and myoglobin levels; D-dimer test
Endocrine (e.g., unintentional weight change, temperature intolerance, anxiety/depression, unexplained diaphoresis, dysphagia, palpitations, hypo- or hyperglycemia)	TSH and serum glucose levels; serum cortisol level or ACTH stimulation test
Gastrointestinal (e.g., abdominal discomfort or abnormal bowel movements, cirrhosis)	Abdominal physical exam; LFTs; lipase and ammonia levels
Infectious disease	Blood cultures, CBC, urinalysis with culture, skin examination In some cases, imaging (chest X ray or other radiological examination) or lumbar puncture may be warranted
Neurological: focal neurological deficits, fall, seizures	Neurological examination, head CT, EEG
Nutritional deficits, volume depletion (dehydration or blood loss)	Intake and output; fluids and meals If malnutrition suspected: B_{12}, folate, albumin, prealbumin, CBC, urine-specific gravity, serum osmolarity, BUN/Cr ratio

Pain
  Exacerbation of chronic or acute pain
  Recent surgery
	Physical examination for signs of recent injury, nonverbal signs of pain, pain assessment scale, review of analgesic regimen

Renal: impaired kidney function or electrolyte disturbance	Serum chemistries, BUN/Cr ratio

TABLE 16–2. Inpatient evaluation of behavioral changes in older adults *(continued)*

Contributing factors	Evaluation
Medical comorbidities *(continued)*	
Respiratory distress, hypoxia	Pulse oximetry, arterial blood gas measurement
Rheumatological: fatigue, intermittent fevers, myalgias, arthralgias	ESR, CRP
Sleep interruptions	Observations by nighttime staff for parasomnias of LBD or RLS
Sensory deficits	Audiology testing, vision testing
Psychiatric comorbidities	
Paranoia, perceptual distortions (e.g., hallucinations, delusions)	Assessment for new onset, quality, frequency of symptoms as noted by caregivers
Substance use or withdrawal, ingestions	Review of social history and occupational or other exposures; urine drug screen; serum alcohol, salicylate, and acetaminophen levels

Note. ACTH=adrenocorticotropin hormone; BUN=blood urea nitrogen; CBC=complete blood count; Cr=creatinine; CRP=C-reactive protein; CT=computed tomography; ECG=electrocardiography; EEG=electroencephalography; ESR=erythrocyte sedimentation rate; LBD=Lewy body dementia; LFT=liver function test; RLS=restless legs syndrome; TSH=thyroid-stimulating hormone.
Source. Adapted from American College of Emergency Physicians 1999; Hategan et al. 2016; Kalish et al. 2014; Steffens et al. 2015.

dence does not definitely indicate which nonpharmacological interventions are best for which treatment setting, behavior, or patient profile (Rabins et al. 2014). However, despite the need for additional efficacy data, expert consensus indicates that nonpharmacological interventions should be used as first-line approaches, in part because the potential for adverse events with these interventions is extremely small (Lyketsos et al. 2006; Rabins et al. 2014; Salzman et al. 2008).

For the purposes of this chapter, we focus on nonpharmacological treatments that may be considered for use across treatment settings, even if the initial studies were performed outside of the hospital. These interventions will be discussed regarding 1) management of acute agitation; 2) consideration of specific precipitating factors; and 3) staff education, unit procedures, and facilities modification (Figure 16–1).

Management of Acute Agitation

First and foremost, during an episode of acute agitation, the primary goal is to safely de-escalate the situation. Several communication strategies may be helpful in accomplishing this, either alone or in combination with medication if nonpharmacological treatment alone does not sufficiently defuse the situation (Lyketsos et al. 2006). Many informational resources are available online from organizations such as the Alzheimer's Association. Table 16–3 lists commonly used communication techniques for de-escalation of acute agitation (Alzheimer's Association 2016; Gitlin et al. 2012).

It may also be helpful to provide distraction, such as a favorite snack, activity, or topic of conversation. In our case, when Mr. R resisted care, it was helpful to give him time and space and to provide a relaxing, soothing alternative. While flexibility in scheduling may be difficult in a hospital or other care environment, if at all possible, it is preferable to delay care until the patient is ready to receive it rather than forcing it at that time; this may avoid escalating the agitation or aggression.

Consideration of Specific Precipitating Factors

After the acute episode is de-escalated, additional attention should be paid to precipitating factors and how these might be avoided in the future. Behavioral problems often represent an expression of an unmet need. As conceptualized by Cohen-Mansfield (2000), this mind-set can help providers approach behaviors through a series of steps:

1. *Try to identify the unmet need that is driving the agitation.* Is the person scared? Hungry? In pain? Hot or cold? Overstimulated or understimulated?
2. *Consider how the behavior results from the need.* Is the patient using agitation to communicate that he or she has an unmet need? For instance, someone who is hungry may become more intrusive or loud if unable to state the need directly. Or is the person trying to meet the need himself or herself? For instance, a patient who wanders or tries to elope may be trying to "solve" the problem of being in an unfamiliar environment. In our case, the patient uses agitation to

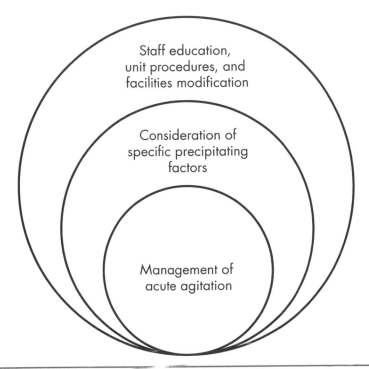

FIGURE 16–1. Nonpharmacological management of agitation.

TABLE 16–3. Communication techniques for de-escalation of acute agitation

Provide a quiet space with minimal distractions.

Be patient, supportive, and reassuring.

Speak slowly and clearly.

Ask yes/no questions, or offer no more than two choices.

Ask only one question at a time.

Give instructions one step at a time to avoid overwhelming detail.

Use positive phrasing ("Let's go over here") instead of negative ("Don't go over there").

Allow the person time to respond.

Avoid arguing with the patient. Go along with the patient's view and do not try to convince him or her otherwise.

Look for nonverbal cues, especially in a patient with limited verbal abilities.

express the unmet need (physical discomfort) and to attempt to address the need (physically preventing others from touching him in a way that would exacerbate the pain).

3. *Provide an appropriate intervention.* If the behavior is communicating a need, and that need can be identified, then that need may be provided for. If the patient is using behavior to try to alleviate the need, then providers can try to accommodate the behavior in a way that is less dangerous or disruptive. In our case, the agitation was a signal that the patient needed medical intervention for a painful and potentially dangerous condition. This allowed detection and treatment of the condition. Other expressions of discomfort, such as pacing, may need to be accommodated by providing a safe space to walk where the patient will not intrude on other patients' privacy or risk elopement.

In all of these considerations, the process should be specific both to the patient and to the unique situation. Regarding the patient, interventions should be tailored to the patient's cognitive status and personal preferences. Regarding the situation, this involves not only the patient's unmet needs but also the needs of the inpatient unit (including the needs of other patients) at that time. For instance, if other high-acuity patients are present, the staff will need to consider how the patient with behavioral disturbances may have an impact on their care. The staff also will need to consider if other patients who may have intrusive or otherwise disruptive behavior may pose a threat to a vulnerable patient with dementia.

Many studies provide examples of ways that specific patient needs may be accommodated. For instance, Gitlin et al. (2008) found that behaviors improved when patients were given activities appropriate to their level of functioning. Every inpatient unit will not have resources to provide detailed occupational therapy intervention as described in this study; however, any unit may be able to try simple interventions such as allowing patients to look at a newspaper, fold washcloths, or perform other activities that can be done repetitively. Distraction techniques that provide an activity for the individual's hands, such as rummage boxes, may also be useful in decreasing agitation (Crook et al. 2016).

For patients who have difficulty with hygiene tasks, bed baths may be a more acceptable alternative to conventional tub baths (Dunn et al. 2002). In a meta-analysis of psychosocial treatments of behavioral symptoms in dementia, O'Connor et al. (2009) found a moderate or large effect size with aromatherapy (lavender or lemon balm), playing the patients' preferred music, and muscle relaxation training (Ballard et al. 2002; Holmes et al. 2002). While this is not an exhaustive list, thoughtful use of such strategies could be effective in preventing escalation or providing redirection after an episode of acute agitation.

Staff Education, Unit Procedures, and Facilities Modification

While specific interventions should be targeted to individual patients, ongoing attention to unit policies and larger systems can help address these issues more effectively in the future. Not surprisingly, evidence supports education for nursing home staff as an effective method of decreasing agitation in nursing home residents (Burgio et al. 2002; Deudon et al. 2009), although the type of education provided varies from study to study (O'Connor et al. 2009; Richter et al. 2012). Although these studies have not been repeated on acute inpatient units, caregiver education often focuses on problem solving (Lyketsos et al. 2006), and this type of exercise may be a helpful group activity for unit staff who encounter similar challenges.

Similarly, ongoing consideration and clear communication of unit policies will help providers (especially those working after hours) implement appropriate interventions. For instance, it is helpful if the on-call provider can easily access information about what items patients are allowed on the unit. In the case of Mr. R, items such as a truss may be restricted or require additional supervision if they are to be used in areas with acutely suicidal patients. In other cases, a patient with dementia may want to hold on to a "security object" such as a wallet, and expedient and consistent communication of policies will allow the staff to work together to provide a more stable environment for the patient.

Lastly, even though not every hospital unit will be designed as a specialized dementia care unit, there may be simple fixes to help patients adjust to the hospitalization. As one example, we mentioned earlier having a safe place for this patient to walk, with clear stop points to prevent the patient from walking into other patients' rooms or toward the exit (or at least to help staff redirect him or her). A complete review would be beyond the scope of this chapter, but other considerations may be the removal of unnecessary objects, use of clear signage or visual cues (e.g., directing to the bathroom or patient rooms), or other attention to sound or temperature control (Gitlin et al. 2012).

Pharmacological Management

Pharmacological management is recommended for treatment of agitation in severe cases in which the agitated patient may be a harm to himself or herself or to others, or the patient's behaviors interfere with needed medical care (American Geriatrics Society Expert Panel on Postoperative Delirium in Older Adults 2015; Nassisi et al. 2006). In regard to management of agitation, most published evidence and guidelines address either acute agitation in the younger adult or long-term management of agitation in dementia patients. Data are still very limited in regard to acute treatment for older hospitalized patients.

Drug Classes

Antipsychotics and benzodiazepines are the most studied and used drug classes for acute agitation. Although effective, these drug classes are associated with many adverse effects that can occur even with short-term use, such as extrapyramidal symptoms (EPS), orthostasis, oversedation, respiratory depression, and falls. When pharmacological therapy is necessary, short-term use is recommended. Compared with younger adult patients, dosing should be conservative due to age-related changes in renal and hepatic function and drug distribution (American Geriatrics Society Expert Panel on Postoperative Delirium in Older Adults 2015; Nassisi et al. 2006). Parenteral formulations of benzodiazepines and antipsychotics are usually preferred in the hospital setting. The oral route is only recommended if the agitation symptoms are not severe or the oral medication is being given before a precipitating event (e.g., the patient has to be moved to radiology for a magnetic resonance imaging scan) (American Geriatrics Society Expert Panel on Postoperative Delirium in Older Adults 2015; Nassisi et al. 2006).

Antipsychotics

Haloperidol is the most studied antipsychotic for treatment of agitation in older adults. It is often preferred because of its lower risk of orthostatic hypotension and anticholinergic adverse effects compared with many other antipsychotics. However, patients should be monitored closely for EPS with haloperidol use (American Geriatrics Society Expert Panel on Postoperative Delirium in Older Adults 2015; Nassisi et al. 2006). In addition, prolonged QTc interval and risk of torsades de pointes are also associated with parenteral use of haloperidol; therefore, electrocardiogram monitoring is recommended (CredibleMeds 2019; Sharma et al. 1998; Wilt et al. 1993).

The second-generation antipsychotics olanzapine and ziprasidone have some efficacy data to support their use for acute agitation in older adults (Meehan et al. 2002; Oechsner and Korchounov 2005), which is discussed later in the subsection "General Medicine Setting." Antipsychotics are generally preferred over benzodiazepines when agitation is related to delirium (American Geriatrics Society Expert Panel on Postoperative Delirium in Older Adults 2015). However, antipsychotics should be used cautiously (or not at all) in patients with Parkinson's disease and Lewy body dementia because of the risk of worsening EPS (Nassisi et al. 2006). In addition, all antipsychotics carry a black box warning reporting an increased risk of mortality in elderly patients with dementia (Gill et al. 2005; Schneider et al. 2005; Wang et al. 2005).

Benzodiazepines

Lorazepam and diazepam are usually preferred for agitation because they come in parenteral dosing forms. Diazepam is not usually recommended for older adults because of its long half-life, active metabolite, and risk of accumulation in the body. Lorazepam is preferred over diazepam because it has a much shorter half-life and the risk of accumulation is low, even with subsequent dosing. Adverse effects associated with benzodiazepine use include orthostasis, falls, oversedation, and respiratory depression (Nassisi et al. 2006). Paradoxical agitation has also been noted with benzodiazepine administration, but evidence of this is limited to a few case reports (Robin and Trieger 2002).

Benzodiazepines are preferred over antipsychotics for agitation in patients at risk for alcohol withdrawal and those with contraindications to antipsychotics, such as Parkinson's patients and those at risk for torsades de pointes. Combination of an antipsychotic and benzodiazepine is a common treatment strategy for severely agitated younger adult patients. However, this treatment has not been well studied in older adults. Therefore, the use of one agent at a time is recommended in most cases (Nassisi et al. 2006).

Settings

General Medicine Setting

Intramuscular antipsychotics and lorazepam are often the treatments of choice for acutely agitated adults within the hospital setting (Table 16–4), but there is a paucity of data with regard to treating older adults. A study by Meehan et al. (2002) compared the use of intramuscular olanzapine 2.5 mg and 5 mg with intramuscular lorazepam 1 mg and placebo in 272 hospitalized or nursing home patients with dementia (mean age=77.6 years). Both olanzapine and lorazepam provided significant improvement in agitation and excitation symptoms 2 hours postinjection compared with placebo. There were no differences in efficacy between olanzapine and lorazepam. Treatment-emergent adverse effects were not significantly different between the active treatments compared with placebo. However, somnolence was observed more with the use of lorazepam than with olanzapine or placebo.

In a case series, Oechsner and Korchounov (2005) reported that intramuscular ziprasidone was useful for acute psychosis with agitation in five Parkinson's patients (mean age=71 years). All five patients experienced improvement in agitation symptoms by 2 hours postinjection, and a decline in motor function was not observed with the short use of ziprasidone.

Intensive Care Unit Setting

In the ICU, patients are given medications intravenously to induce sedation and prevent the onset of agitation. Treatment guidelines generally recommend the same sedating medications for both younger and older adults. Light sedation, rather than heavy sedation, is associated with better outcomes such as shorter duration of mechanical ventilation and shorter ICU length of stay. Dexmedetomidine (usual dose 0.15–1.5 µg/kg/hour) is recommended over benzodiazepines for light sedation. When compared with dexmedetomidine, benzodiazepines have been shown to increase the risk of ICU delirium, dependence on mechanical ventilation, and ICU length of stay (Barr et al. 2013). In addition, older adults are more sensitive to the sedative effects of benzodiazepines and more likely to accumulate the drugs due to reduced hepatic and renal function (Swart et al. 2006).

Patients who are administered dexmedetomidine can usually be aroused easily when it is necessary to do so, and the medication causes minimal respiratory depression. It is the only intravenous sedative approved by the U.S. Food and Drug Administration for use in nonintubated patients because of its low effect on respiratory drive. Adverse effects of dexmedetomidine include hypotension and bradycardia. A loss of oropharyngeal muscle tone has also been noted in case reports; therefore, patients who are not intubated should be monitored closely for this side effect (Barr et al. 2013).

To help minimize agitation, staff should ensure that ICU patients receive consistent pain treatment with around-the-clock analgesia. As a patient's condition improves, opioids and sedatives should be gradually

TABLE 16–4. Parenteral medications used for acute agitation in any setting

Drug	Intramuscular (IM) dosing	Possible adverse effects by drug class
Benzodiazepines		
Lorazepam	1–3 mg every 4–6 hours as needed	Central nervous system depression
Diazepam	2–5 mg every 4–6 hours as needed	Decreased concentration
		Psychomotor incoordination
		Abuse potential
		Anterograde amnesia
		Memory impairment
		Withdrawal symptoms
		Respiratory depression
		Orthostasis
		Paradoxical disinhibition
Antipsychotics		
Haloperidol	0.5–2 mg every 8–12 hours as needed	Central nervous system depression
Chlorpromazine	12.5–25 mg every 4–12 hours as needed	Dystonia
		Akathisia
		Parkinsonism
Olanzapine	2.5–5 mg every 4 hours as needed (no more than three doses in a 24-hour period)	Neuroleptic malignant syndrome
		Orthostasis
		Prolonged QTc interval
Ziprasidone	10–20 mg every 2–4 hours as needed (no more than 40 mg in a 24-hour period)	Anticholinergic effects (chlorpromazine and olanzapine)

reduced and discontinued. Clinicians should keep in mind that abrupt discontinuation of these agents can exacerbate agitation and delirium (Barr et al. 2013).

Palliative Care Setting

Antipsychotics are often preferred over benzodiazepines in the palliative care setting because agitation is commonly associated with delirium. Haloperidol has the most published data to support its use in this setting. Doses of 2 mg or less are usually effective and well tolerated. Occasionally, chlorpromazine may be a preferred antipsychotic, especially when sedation is needed (Dayer and Hutchinson 2015).

Adding benzodiazepines to antipsychotics may be beneficial when more sedation is needed to help calm the patient. A recent study that included 58 palliative care patients (mean age = 65 years) found that intravenous lorazepam 3 mg in combination with haloperidol 2 mg was more effective at reducing agitation symptoms 8 hours postinjection compared with haloperidol 2 mg monotherapy. In addition, caregivers and nurses reported better patient comfort for those who received combination therapy, and patients were not as likely to receive rescue doses of antipsychotics. Adverse effects were not statistically significantly different between the two treatment groups (Hui et al. 2017).

Notes for Nursing Staff

The nursing literature also shows benefit to implementing behavioral approaches for this patient population. McConnell and Karel (2016) have described an approach implemented in Veterans Health Administration community living centers (CLCs) or nursing homes. This approach, entitled STAR (Staff Training in Assisted living Residences), is an interprofessional behavioral intervention designed to reduce behavioral and psychological symptoms of dementia in various CLCs. It includes systematic assessment and individualized approaches to manage and prevent these symptoms. The training includes using behavioral assessment skills, developing a behavior plan in collaboration with the team, teaching other staff members knowledge and skills needed to implement the behavioral care plan, and translating the behavior plan into daily practice. The authors reported a 50%–60% decrease in ratings of severity and a 40%–45% decrease in ratings of frequency on average, with effect sizes of 1.0 or greater in addressing target symptoms of verbal or physical aggression, resistance to care, disruptive vocalization, and wandering. Moreover, there were improvements in staff outcomes such as sustained increases in staff self-efficacy in implementing behavioral approaches. Emphasis was placed on the interprofessional approach, leveraging complementary expertise of behavioral and nursing care experts. Behavioral health practitioners provide advanced expertise in behavioral assessment and coaching for behavior change, while nursing staff provide expertise in offering intimate personal care in a supportive, nonthreatening manner and are able to observe patients' response to treatment. When all members of the health care team work in conjunction, patient care can be optimized.

KEY POINTS

- Agitation is a common presenting complaint for geriatric patients transferred from home or a long-term care facility to an inpatient unit.
- It is optimal to use a stepwise approach when evaluating patients to determine the etiology of behavioral changes.
- An acute or subacute presentation warrants workup for urgent medical conditions such as delirium.
- Although the patient may have difficulty verbalizing his or her complaint, nonverbal cues and astute observations from staff can reveal the offending cause.
- Nonpharmacological interventions should be first-line options for reducing the likelihood of adverse events that can occur with pharmacological agents.
- Nonpharmacological strategies should focus on 1) de-escalating episodes of acute agitation, 2) problem solving to prevent future episodes, and 3) addressing larger system-wide needs such as unit policies, staff education, or facilities modification.
- Pharmacological management is indicated in severe cases in which the agitated patient may be a harm to self or others or in which behaviors interfere with needed medical care.

Resources

Alzheimer's Association: Behaviors: How to Respond when Dementia Causes Unpredictable Behaviors. Chicago, IL, Alzheimer's Association, 2017. Available at: www.alz.org/national/documents/brochure_behaviors.pdf

Alzheimer's Association: Downloadable Resources (website). Chicago, IL, Alzheimer's Association, 2018. Available at: www.alz.org/professionals/healthcare-professionals/for-patients-caregivers/downloadable-resources (Includes patient and caregiver educational packets [English and Spanish], topic sheets, resources in Spanish, Chinese, Japanese, Korean, Vietnamese.)

Hategan A, Bourgeois JA, Hirsch C: On-Call Geriatric Psychiatry: Handbook of Principles and Practice. Switzerland, Springer International Publishing, 2016

National Institute on Aging: Alzheimer's Caregiving: Coping With Agitation and Aggression in Alzheimer's Disease (website). Bethesda, MD, National Institute on Aging, 2017. Available at: www.nia.nih.gov/health/coping-agitation-and-aggression-alzheimers-disease

References

Alzheimer's Association: Communication: Tips for Successful Communication at All Stages of Alzheimer's Disease. Chicago, IL, Alzheimer's Association, 2016. Available at: https://www.alz.org/national/documents/brochure_communication.pdf. Accessed July 24, 2018.

American College of Emergency Physicians: Clinical policy for the initial approach to patients presenting with altered mental status. Ann Emerg Med 33(2):251–281, 1999 14765552

American Geriatrics Society Expert Panel on Postoperative Delirium in Older Adults: American Geriatrics Society abstracted clinical practice guideline for postoperative delirium in older adults. J Am Geriatr Soc 63(1):142–150, 2015 25495432

Ballard CG, O'Brien JT, Reichelt K, et al: Aromatherapy as a safe and effective treatment for the management of agitation in severe dementia: the results of a double-blind, placebo-controlled trial with Melissa. J Clin Psychiatry 63(7):553–558, 2002 12143909

Barr J, Fraser GL, Puntillo K, et al: Clinical practice guidelines for the management of pain, agitation, and delirium in adult patients in the intensive care unit. Crit Care Med 41(1):263–306, 2013 23269131

Borson S, Scanlan JM, Chen P, et al: The Mini-Cog as a screen for dementia: validation in a population-based sample. J Am Geriatr Soc 51(10):1451–1454, 2003 14511167

Burgio LD, Stevens A, Burgio KL, et al: Teaching and maintaining behavior management skills in the nursing home. Gerontologist 42(4):487–496, 2002 12145376

Cohen-Mansfield J: Nonpharmacological management of behavioral problems in persons with dementia: the TREA model. Alzheimers Care Q 1(4):22–34, 2000

Cohen-Mansfield J, Libin A: Assessment of agitation in elderly patients with dementia: correlations between informant rating and direct observation. Int J Geriatr Psychiatry 19(9):881–891, 2004 15352147

Cohen-Mansfield J, Dakheel-Ali M, Marx MS, et al: Which unmet needs contribute to behavior problems in persons with advanced dementia? Psychiatry Res 228(1):59–64, 2015 25933478

CredibleMeds: Risk Categories for Drugs that Prolong QT & induce Torsades de Pointes (TdP). Updated March 29, 2019. Available at: https://crediblemeds.org/index.php/?cID=328. Accessed April 14, 2019.

Crook N, Adams M, Shorten N, et al: Does the well-being of individuals with Down syndrome and dementia improve when using life story books and rummage boxes? A randomized single case series experiment. J Appl Res Intellect Disabil 29(1):1–10, 2016 25826476

Dayer L, Hutchinson LC: Palliative and hospice care, in Fundamentals of Geriatric Pharmacotherapy, 2nd Edition. Edited by Hutchinson LC, Sleeper RB. Bethesda, MD, ASHP, 2015, pp 124–154

Deudon A, Maubourguet N, Gervais X, et al: Non-pharmacological management of behavioural symptoms in nursing homes. Int J Geriatr Psychiatry 24(12):1386–1395, 2009 19370714

Dunn JC, Thiru-Chelvam B, Beck CH: Bathing. Pleasure or pain? J Gerontol Nurs 28(11):6-13, 2002 12465197

Fick DM, Cooper JW, Wade WE, et al: Updating the Beers criteria for potentially inappropriate medication use in older adults: results of a US consensus panel of experts. Arch Intern Med 163(22):2716–2724, 2003 14662625

Folstein MF, Folstein SE, McHugh PR: "Mini-mental state." A practical method for grading the cognitive state of patients for the clinician. J Psychiatr Res 12(3):189–198, 1975 1202204

Gill SS, Rochon PA, Herrmann N, et al: Atypical antipsychotic drugs and risk of ischaemic stroke: population based retrospective cohort study. BMJ 330(7489):445, 2005 15668211

Gitlin LN, Winter L, Burke J, et al: Tailored activities to manage neuropsychiatric behaviors in persons with dementia and reduce caregiver burden: a randomized pilot study. Am J Geriatr Psychiatry 16(3):229–239, 2008 18310553

Gitlin LN, Kales HC, Lyketsos CG: Nonpharmacologic management of behavioral symptoms in dementia. JAMA 308(19):2020–2029, 2012 23168825

Hategan A, Bourgeois JA, Hirsch C: On-Call Geriatric Psychiatry. Handbook of Principles and Practice. New York, Springer International, 2016, pp 231–249

Holmes C, Hopkins V, Hensford C, et al: Lavender oil as a treatment for agitated behaviour in severe dementia: a placebo controlled study. Int J Geriatr Psychiatry 17(4):305–308, 2002 11994882

Hui D, Frisbee-Hume S, Wilson A, et al: Effect of lorazepam with haloperidol vs haloperidol alone on agitated delirium in patients with advanced cancer receiving palliative care: a randomized clinical trial. JAMA 318(11):1047–1056, 2017 28975307

Husebo BS, Ballard C, Sandvik R, et al: Efficacy of treating pain to reduce behavioural disturbances in residents of nursing homes with dementia: cluster randomized clinical trial. BMJ 343:d4065, 2011 21765198

Inouye SK, van Dyck CH, Alessi CA, et al: Clarifying confusion: the confusion assessment method. A new method for detection of delirium. Ann Intern Med 113(12):941–948, 1990 2240918

Kales HC, Gitlin LN, Lyketsos CG: Management of neuropsychiatric symptoms of dementia in clinical settings: recommendations from a multidisciplinary expert panel. J Am Geriatr Soc 62(4):762–769, 2014 24635665

Kalish VB, Gillham JE, Unwin BK: Delirium in older persons: evaluation and management. Am Fam Physician 90(3):150–158, 2014 25077720

Lyketsos CG, Colenda CC, Beck C, et al: Position statement of the American Association for Geriatric Psychiatry regarding principles of care for patients with dementia resulting from Alzheimer disease. Am J Geriatr Psychiatry 14(7):561–572, 2006 16816009

McConnell ES, Karel MJ: Improving management of behavioral and psychological symptoms of dementia in acute care: evidence and lessons learned from across the care spectrum. Nurs Adm Q 40(3):244–254, 2016 27259128

Meehan KM, Wang H, David SR, et al: Comparison of rapidly acting intramuscular olanzapine, lorazepam, and placebo: a double-blind, randomized study in acutely agitated patients with dementia. Neuropsychopharmacology 26(4):494–504, 2002 11927174

Nasreddine ZS, Phillips NA, Bédirian V, et al: The Montreal Cognitive Assessment, MoCA: a brief screening tool for mild cognitive impairment. J Am Geriatr Soc 53(4):695–699, 2005 15817019

Nassisi D, Korc B, Hahn S, et al: The evaluation and management of the acutely agitated elderly patient. Mt Sinai J Med 73(7):976–984, 2006 17195883

National Institute for Health and Clinical Excellence: Delirium: Prevention, Diagnosis and Management (Clinical Guideline [CG103]). London, National Institute for Health and Clinical Excellence, 2010. Available at: https://www.nice.org.uk/guidance/cg103. Accessed July 24, 2018.

O'Connor DW, Ames D, Gardner B, et al: Psychosocial treatments of behavior symptoms in dementia: a systematic review of reports meeting quality standards. Int Psychogeriatr 21(2):225–240, 2009 18814806

Oechsner M, Korchounov A: Parenteral ziprasidone: a new atypical neuroleptic for emergency treatment of psychosis in Parkinson's disease? Hum Psychopharmacol 20(3):203–205, 2005 15799011

Rabins PV, Rovner BW, Rummans T, et al: Guideline Watch (October 2014): Practice Guideline for the Treatment of Patients With Alzheimer's Disease and Other Dementias. Arlington, VA, American Psychiatric Association, 2014. Available at: https://psychiatryonline.org/pb/assets/raw/sitewide/practice_guidelines/guidelines/alzheimerwatch.pdf. Accessed July 24, 2018.

Richter T, Meyer G, Möhler R, et al: Psychosocial interventions for reducing antipsychotic medication in care home residents. Cochrane Database Syst Rev 12:CD008634, 2012 23235663

Robin C, Trieger N: Paradoxical reactions to benzodiazepines in intravenous sedation: a report of 2 cases and review of the literature. Anesth Prog 49(4):128–132, 2002 12779114

Salzman C, Jeste DV, Meyer RE, et al: Elderly patients with dementia-related symptoms of severe agitation and aggression: consensus statement on treatment options, clinical trials methodology, and policy. J Clin Psychiatry 69(6):889–898, 2008 18494535

Schneider LS, Dagerman KS, Insel P: Risk of death with atypical antipsychotic drug treatment for dementia: meta-analysis of randomized placebo-controlled trials. JAMA 294(15):1934–1943, 2005 16234500

Sharma ND, Rosman HS, Padhi ID, et al: Torsades de pointes associated with intravenous haloperidol in critically ill patients. Am J Cardiol 81(2):238–240, 1998 9591913

Steffens DC, Blazer DG, Thakur ME (eds): The American Psychiatric Publishing Textbook of Geriatric Psychiatry, Fifth Edition. Arlington, VA, American Psychiatric Publishing, 2015

Swart EL, Zuideveld KP, de Jongh J, et al: Population pharmacodynamic modelling of lorazepam- and midazolam-induced sedation upon long-term continuous infusion in critically ill patients. Eur J Clin Pharmacol 62(3):185–194, 2006 16425056

Thakur ME, Gwyther LP: Agitation in older adults, in The American Psychiatric Publishing Textbook of Geriatric Psychiatry, 5th Edition. Edited by Steffens DC, Blazer DG, Thakur ME. Arlington, VA, American Psychiatric Association, 2015, pp 507–523

Wang PS, Schneeweiss S, Avorn J, et al: Risk of death in elderly users of conventional vs. atypical antipsychotic medications. N Engl J Med 353(22):2335–2341, 2005 16319382

Wilt JL, Minnema AM, Johnson RF, et al: Torsade de pointes associated with the use of intravenous haloperidol. Ann Intern Med 119(5):391–394, 1993 8338292

Witlox J, Eurelings LS, de Jonghe JF, et al: Delirium in elderly patients and the risk of postdischarge mortality, institutionalization, and dementia: a meta-analysis. JAMA 304(4):443–451, 2010 20664045

Yohanna D, Cifu AS: Antipsychotics to treat agitation or psychosis in patients with dementia. JAMA 318(11):1057–1058, 2017 28975291

Post–Intensive Care Syndrome

"He's Just Not Himself"

Duane Allen, M.D.
Babar Khan, M.D., M.S.
Sophia Wang, M.D.

Clinical Presentation

Chief Complaint

"He's just not himself."

Vignette 1

A 77-year-old African American man presents to his primary care doctor at the insistence of his wife, who states, "He's just not himself." The patient was recently hospitalized in the intensive care unit (ICU) for an episode of necrotizing pancreatitis that was complicated by severe alcohol withdrawal and acute respiratory distress syndrome, which required intubation and mechanical ventilation. He required restraints and medications for agitation during his ICU stay. After 9 days in the ICU, he was transferred to the ward and then to a subacute rehabilitation center for 8 weeks. He comes in today shortly after returning home. His wife reports that he has difficulty managing his finances, forgets recent conversations, and is now getting lost driving to areas he was familiar with. He tends to have "mood swings" and will yell at his wife whenever he is frustrated. He requires a walker to ambulate but frequently leaves it behind despite his wife's insistence that he use it. His wife reports that prior to his hospitalization, he had mild

CHAPTER 17

memory difficulties that occurred on a daily basis but was able to manage his finances independently and drive without any difficulty. He has a past medical history of alcohol abuse, hypertension, coronary artery disease, and pancreatitis. His medications include aspirin, amlodipine, atorvastatin, clonazepam, metoprolol, lisinopril, quetiapine, and trazodone.

Vignette 2

A 62-year-old white woman presents to her primary care doctor complaining of worsening anxiety since her recent ICU stay. She was recently hospitalized in the ICU with pneumonia and an exacerbation of chronic obstructive pulmonary disease (COPD). During her ICU stay, she required intubation and mechanical ventilation for 6 days and was administered multiple doses of intravenous lorazepam to help manage her anxiety. Her sister confides that the patient has a history of being sexually assaulted and now has frequent nightmares about both this past trauma and her recent ICU stay. She was eventually discharged to a subacute rehabilitation facility and has recently returned home. She has a history of COPD, extensive tobacco use, congestive heart failure (CHF), coronary artery disease, hypertension, and osteoarthritis. Her medications include lorazepam, albuterol inhaler, aspirin, budesonide-formoterol, amlodipine, metoprolol, tiotropium, naproxen, acetaminophen, and atorvastatin.

Discussion

Post–intensive care syndrome (PICS) refers to the long-term cognitive, physical, and psychological impairments observed in ICU survivors, including family members (Table 17–1). As ICU survivorship has increased over the past few decades, managing these impairments has becoming the defining challenge of critical care medicine (Desai et al. 2011; Iwashyna 2010). About 50%–70% of ICU survivors will experience at least one PICS impairment. Although many of these impairments improve over the first year, these effects can persist for as long as 5–15 years after discharge (Desai et al. 2011).

Differential Diagnosis, Workup, and Questions to Ask When Determining Treatment Strategies

Vignette 1 Patient

This patient has new-onset cognitive changes that started after his episode of delirium during his ICU hospitalization. The most important

TABLE 17–1. Key clinical characteristics of post–intensive care syndrome (PICS)

Domain	Prevalence in all ICU survivors	Risk factors	Diagnostics	Treatment
Cognitive	30%–80% have cognitive impairment 15% of ICU patients are newly diagnosed with dementia (major neurocognitive disorder)	Prior cognitive impairment Delirium Severe sepsis Acute dialysis	Screening with MoCA Referral for neuropsychological testing	Cognitive rehabilitation
Physical	50% have functional recovery Two-thirds require new services on discharge More than 50% require inpatient rehabilitation or long-term care	Low body mass Mechanical ventilation Vision and hearing impairment	Neurological examination Get up and go test Physical therapy evaluation	Physical and occupational therapy Support devices as needed
Mental health	Depression: 19%–37% Anxiety: 32%–40% PTSD: 12%–22% More likely to have premorbid psychiatric illness	Premorbid mental health disorder Older age for depression Younger age for PTSD	Depression: PHQ-9 or GDS-15 Anxiety: GAD-7 PTSD: PC-PTSD-5	Referral to mental health professional SSRI
Family	Depression: 4.7%–36% Anxiety: 15%–24% PTSD: 35%–57%	Spouse Female gender Prior mental health disorder Younger patient	Depression: PHQ-9 or GDS-15 Anxiety: GAD-7 PTSD: PC-PTSD-5	ICU: diaries, educational materials Limited evidence for post-ICU interventions

Note. GAD-7 = Generalized Anxiety Disorder, 7-item scale; GDS-15 = Geriatric Depression Scale 15-item version; ICU = intensive care unit; MoCA = Montreal Cognitive Assessment; PHQ-9 = Patient Health Questionnaire, 9-item instrument; PC-PTSD-5 = Primary Care PTSD Screen for DSM-5; PTSD = posttraumatic stress disorder; SSRI = selective serotonin reuptake inhibitor.

part of the clinical assessment of post-ICU cognitive changes is a thorough history from a reliable informant. Assessment of the cognitive complaints should focus on specific examples of the nature of the problems; their frequency, severity, and progression; and their impact, if any, on daily functioning. Clinicians should also clarify the patient's premorbid cognitive and functional status. Understanding the progression or changes in the nature of cognitive issues since the patient's critical illness will guide the future workup. The most important disorder to consider on the differential diagnosis when a patient or informant complains of post-ICU cognitive changes is persistent ICU delirium or subsyndromal delirium. Older adults are more likely to have hypoactive delirium. The key to distinguishing delirium from long-term cognitive impairment requires determining whether the cognitive changes are fluctuating (suggestive of delirium) or persistent (suggestive of long-term cognitive impairment). The likelihood of delirium decreases as the length of time since the ICU hospitalization increases. Cognitive symptoms that persist more than a month later should be examined more carefully, and although cognition can improve as much as a year later, studies suggest that many older adults who have a sudden cognitive decline during hospitalization do not return to their cognitive baseline (Desai et al. 2011; Hopkins et al. 2005).

The physical examination should include a thorough neurological examination to determine whether the patient has focal or asymmetric neurological findings. Asymmetric findings would raise concern for neurological disorders such as a stroke or severe traumatic brain injury. Parkinsonism (cogwheel rigidity, resting tremor, shuffling gait) can also be due to primary neurological disorders (e.g., Parkinson's disease, stroke, traumatic brain injury) or be medication induced (e.g., antipsychotics). Basic laboratory workup should also be performed to rule out a metabolic contribution to his symptoms. This workup should include a complete blood count, chemistry panel including liver function, thyroid testing, and folate and B_{12} levels. While the patient denies current substance abuse, urine toxicology and ethyl glucuronide should be collected to confirm this. Neuroimaging may also be helpful, especially if a stroke is suspected. Brain magnetic resonance imaging is more sensitive than head computed tomography for structural changes. White matter changes have also been observed in ICU delirium, but this is a nonspecific finding.

Medication reconciliation should focus on identifying unnecessary medications, especially those that may impact cognition. When this patient was discharged, he was taking quetiapine and clonazepam, a regimen that is not uncommon to see following an ICU hospitalization. Both of these medications may be decreasing his attention and processing speed. Tapering these medications should be considered.

This patient should be screened for cognitive impairment using a standardized screen. This standardized screen would ideally be widely available and sensitive to the impairments the clinician might expect following critical illness. Executive function, the cognitive domain required for planning, insight, and judgment, is the most affected domain in ICU-related cognitive impairment. While the Mini Mental State Examination (MMSE; Folstein et al. 1975) is widely used, it is not sensitive to executive dysfunction. The Montreal Cognitive Assessment (MoCA; Nasreddine et al. 2005) has a higher sensitivity to executive dysfunction and is widely and freely available. If his cognitive deficits continue to persist 3–6 months after hospitalization, a referral for detailed neuropsychological testing may also be appropriate to characterize the nature of his cognitive deficits and serve as a baseline for future testing if he should continue to decline.

The differential diagnosis suggests that the most likely disorder is long-term cognitive impairment from ICU delirium (part of PICS). Other possibilities include mild cognitive impairment, early-stage Alzheimer's disease (AD), early-stage vascular dementia (major neurocognitive disorder), alcohol-related dementia (major neurocognitive disorder), and cognitive impairment secondary to medications. These disorders may also be comorbid (e.g., long-term cognitive impairment from ICU delirium and cognitive impairment secondary to medications). The first step is to make sure that all potentially reversible causes of cognitive impairment, such as depression or mood disorders, alcohol use, or cognitively impairing drugs, have been addressed. Afterward, a cognitive reassessment is appropriate. Patients who have premorbid normal cognition, mild cognitive impairment, or early-stage dementia (major neurocognitive disorder) usually see improvement in their cognition within the first year, although they may not return to their pre-ICU level of cognitive performance. Patients who have premorbid moderate or severe dementia (major neurocognitive disorder) may or may not see a period of recovery but frequently decline to a new baseline. On the other hand, patients with AD, vascular dementia (major neurocognitive disorder), and mixed dementia (major neurocognitive disorder; AD and vascular etiologies) have progressive cognitive decline.

Vignette 2 Patient

Although the initial referral was for anxiety, the patient's and sister's histories indicate that there are concerns for other comorbid psychiatric disorders, most notably posttraumatic stress disorder (PTSD). The most concerning details of the history for PTSD include a previous traumatic event, benzodiazepine exposure while in the ICU, and nightmares about the patient's ICU trauma. Diagnostic questions should clarify the nature and timeline of the patient's mental health symptoms before and after her ICU stay. The effects of the current symptoms on her life should also be evaluated. It will be important to also clarify whether she had any mental health treatments prior to her time in the ICU, especially whether she had a prior diagnosis of depression, anxiety, or PTSD for her sexual assault. If she received mental health treatment in the past, the clinician should ask both about the type of treatment (e.g., dosage and duration of medications, type of psychotherapy, electroconvulsive therapy) and effectiveness of the treatments.

Medical disorders should also be considered in the differential diagnosis (e.g., poorly controlled COPD and CHF). Her current medication use should be examined for new medications and medications that may be contributing to her symptoms, such as excessive use of albuterol. The differential diagnosis for a psychiatric disorder in this patient would include generalized anxiety disorder, panic disorder, major depressive disorder, and PTSD.

This patient should be screened for depression, anxiety, and PTSD. Widely available and sensitive screens for depression include the Geriatric Depression Scale–15 item (Sheikh and Yesavage 1986) and the Patient Health Questionnaire–9 (Kroenke et al. 2001; Sheikh and Yesavage 1986). Anxiety screening can be completed with the Generalized Anxiety Disorder–7 (Spitzer et al. 2006). The Primary Care PTSD Screen for DSM-5 (Prins et al. 2003) would be useful for PTSD.

If this patient screens positive on these scales, treatment options should be discussed. Medications used to treat this patient's symptoms would include antidepressants, either a selective serotonin reuptake inhibitor (SSRI) or a serotonin-norepinephrine reuptake inhibitor (SNRI). Generally, patients require a low starting dosage (usually half of the usual starting dosage) and slow titration to avoid paradoxical anxiety; longer periods to response (8–12 weeks); and high dosages to see benefit. Benzodiazepines should ideally be minimized and tapered off in older adults once anxiety symptoms have improved. Possible nonpharmacological approaches for anxiety include cognitive-behavioral therapy for anxiety, deep breathing exercises, and progressive muscle relaxation. Evidence-based treatments for PTSD include exposure-based therapies and cognitive processing psychotherapy.

The differential diagnosis, workup, and questions to ask when determining treatment strategies for both patients described in the preceding vignettes are summarized in Table 17–2.

TABLE 17–2. **Quick review of assessment after ICU hospitalization**

Vignette 1: Cognitive impairment	Vignette 2: Anxiety

History and physical

Establish the timeline of symptoms:
  How was his cognition before his critical illness?
  What domains seem to be affected now? Memory? Executive function? Attention?
  How have symptoms progressed since the illness? Are they worsening? Are they improving?
 	
Assess for contributing factors:
  Is there any history or suspicion of substance abuse?
  What medications have been added since his critical illness?
 	
Evaluate for alternative diagnoses:
  What does the neurological examination show?
  Is there asymmetry suggesting cerebrovascular accident?
  Are there signs of parkinsonism (e.g., cogwheel rigidity)?
	Evaluate previous mental health history:
	  What type of mental health symptoms did the patient have before the ICU?
	  What type of mental health treatment, if any, did she receive before she went to the ICU?
	  If she received mental health treatment or psychiatric medications before, what worked and what did not work?
	
	Define current symptoms:
	  What is the frequency and severity of current symptoms?
	  How do these symptoms affect her everyday life?
	
	Consider alternative diagnoses:
	  Are there any other undiagnosed psychiatric disorders, such as depression or PTSD, that could be complicating her mental health symptoms?
	  Are there medical disorders, such as COPD, that could be complicating her mental health symptoms?

Testing

Complete blood count, metabolic panel including liver function testing
Thyroid panel, folate levels, B_{12} levels
Urine drug screen, ethyl gluconuride
Screening with MoCA
Can consider brain MRI
	Screening
	  Depression screening: GDS-15 or PHQ-9
	  Anxiety screening: GAD-7
	  PTSD screening: PC-PTSD-5

TABLE 17–2. Quick review of assessment after ICU hospitalization _(continued)_

Vignette 1: Cognitive impairment	Vignette 2: Anxiety
Treatment and referral	
Should the patient be referred for neuropsychological testing so that a comprehensive cognitive examination can be carried out?	What treatment should be offered? Does the patient prefer medication and/or therapy?
Should this patient be referred to a dedicated ICU survivor clinic, if one is available?	If the patient has required treatment in the past, why did she stop going?
Would this patient benefit from cognitive rehabilitation?	Treatments to consider:
	Psychotropics such as antidepressants (SSRI or SNRI)
	Evidence-based depression- and anxiety-focused psychotherapies such as CBT and IPT
	Evidence-based PTSD-focused psychotherapies such as exposure-based therapies and cognitive processing psychotherapy
	Benzodiazepines ideally minimized or tapered off in older adults once their symptoms are improved

Note.   CBT=cognitive-behavioral therapy; COPD=chronic obstructive pulmonary disease; GAD-7=Generalized Anxiety Disorder, 7-item scale; GDS-15=Geriatric Depression Scale 15-item version; ICU=intensive care unit; IPT=interpersonal therapy; MoCA = Montreal Cognitive Assessment; MRI=magnetic resonance imaging; PHQ-9=Patient Health Questionnaire, 9-item instrument; PC-PTSD-5=Primary Care PTSD Screen for DSM-5; PTSD=posttraumatic stress disorder; SNRI=serotonin-norepinephrine reuptake inhibitor; SSRI=selective serotonin reuptake inhibitor.

Clinical Pearl

When patients and their family members describe multiple cognitive, behavioral, and mental health symptoms, it is important to clarify in what order the symptoms first appeared (cognitive, behavioral, or psychological) and which one is bothering the patient and family the most. Clinicians should not settle for patients or families' self-diagnoses and instead focus on examples and descriptions. For example, families may come in stating patients are depressed, but they are actually apathetic from cognitive impairment. To be able to capture this information, clinicians should elicit detailed descriptions, usually of patients' daily activities. Possible questions include "Describe for me the *very first* thing you noticed was different about your loved one. Give me a specific example." Family members often have difficulty describing changes, although they know patients are now different. "I know it's hard to tell me what differences you've seen in your loved one. Think back a few years ago when you said she was normal. What activities does she have trouble doing now? How is her behavior now?" "Describe to me her daily activities. What time does she get up? When does she get out of the house?"

Sequelae of Critical Illness

Cognitive Impairment

Patients who survive ICU hospitalization are at high risk of developing new cognitive impairment. Between 30% and 80% will have PICS-related cognitive deficits that can persist for years (Girard et al. 2010; Myers et al. 2016). Fifteen percent of survivors will have a new diagnosis of dementia (major neurocognitive disorder) after their illness, with 40% of those diagnoses being made in the first year (Guerra et al. 2015).

Risk factors for ICU-acquired long-term cognitive impairment (LTCI) include neurological dysfunction, severe sepsis, and acute dialysis (Guerra et al. 2012) (Figure 17–1). The mechanism of how delirium contributes to LTCI is incompletely understood, but hypoxia and proinflammatory cytokines are thought to be involved (Jutte et al. 2015). LTCI is distinct from other causes of dementia (major neurocognitive disorder) in several ways. It appears to affect multiple cognitive domains, including executive function, memory, and attention, whereas AD primarily affects memory (Pandharipande et al. 2013). Although LTCI can persist for several years, it generally improves within the first year, unlike AD, in which there is a progressive decline (Pandharipande et al. 2013).

Physical Impairment

Critical illness represents a significant risk for future physical impairment. Only one half of older adult ICU survivors have functional recovery after their critical illness, and for those that do, the median recovery time is 3 months (Ferrante et al. 2016). They are more likely to need additional assistance with instrumental activities of daily living and/or activities of daily living, compared to their prehospital baseline, and more than two-thirds of patients require new support services on discharge (Ferrante et al. 2015; Iwashyna et al. 2012). More than half of these patients require inpatient rehabilitation or long-term care (Ferrante et al. 2015). These new impairments are a major source of stress for these pa-

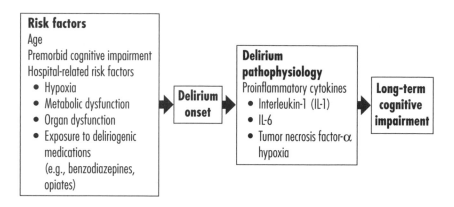

FIGURE 17–1. **Relationship between age and long-term cognitive impairment secondary to delirium.**

Source. Reprinted from Wang S, Allen D, Kheir YN, et al.: "Aging and Post-Intensive Care Syndrome: A Critical Need for Geriatric Psychiatry." *American Journal of Geriatric Psychiatry* 26(2):212–221, 2018. Copyright © 2018 with permission from Elsevier.

tients and contribute significantly to depression at 3 and 12 months after ICU hospitalization (Jackson et al. 2014).

Mental Health Impairments

ICU survivors experience increased mental health impairments. The most commonly described are depression, anxiety, and PTSD, with prevalence rates of 19%–37%, 32%–40%, and 12%–22%, respectively (Wang et al. 2017). These rates may be artificially high, because psychiatric comorbidity is four to six times more common in ICU survivors than in the general population and many of these patients have premorbid psychiatric disorders (Bienvenu et al. 2015; Davydow et al. 2008a, 2008b, 2009; Kessler et al. 2005; Nikayin et al. 2016; Rabiee et al. 2016; Wang et al. 2017; Wolters et al. 2016). It may be that patients who develop critical illness are more likely to have premorbid psychiatric illness compared with patients on the general wards and the general population.

Caregiver Stress: PICS-Family

Patients who survive critical illness are known to have the physical, cognitive, and psychological impairments mentioned, but their caregivers undergo a significant life change as well. The term PICS-Family (PICS-F) is used to describe the psychological impact of ICU hospitalization and recovery on family members and caregivers of survivors (Needham et al.

2012). They experience anxiety, depression, and PTSD, with prevalence rates of 15%–24%, 4.7%–36%, and 35%–57%, respectively, at 6 months after the ICU stay (van Beusekom et al. 2016). The symptoms often start in the ICU and persist throughout recovery. Female gender, younger patient age, being the spouse of the patient, previous mental health disorder, and family history of mental health disorder are all risk factors for the development of PICS-F (van Beusekom et al. 2016). There are interventions aimed at minimizing this risk, including ICU diaries, in which the family members record ICU events and the recovery process, as well as educational materials about PICS (Locke et al. 2016). Condolence letters written to family members have shown to worsen depression and PTSD-related symptoms (Kentish-Barnes et al. 2017).

Treatment and the Critical Care Recovery Center

There are no widely accepted treatment guidelines for patients with PICS. They should be assessed for cognitive, physical, and psychological impairment and ideally be referred to specialized care depending on their impairments. An important opportunity to minimize harm to these patients is a careful examination of their medication list. ICU survivors are often discharged on inappropriate medications, which can impact PICS symptoms. Benzodiazepines, antipsychotics, anticholinergics, and opioids represent potential contributors to PICS. These medications should be weaned and stopped if possible, especially in the geriatric population.

Since 2011, there has been a growth in dedicated ICU survivor clinics in the United States. These clinics have been seen in the United Kingdom since the 1980s, but the first U.S. clinic was not opened until 2011. This clinic, the Critical Care Recovery Center, is affiliated with Indiana University (Wang et al. 2018). Patients of this clinic undergo an initial assessment that includes a comprehensive neuropsychological examination, a physical function battery, pharmacist-directed medication reconciliation, and additional laboratory and imaging workup as indicated. A team consisting of a critical care physician, a registered nurse, a social worker, and a pharmacist meets with the patient and the family after this initial battery to discuss the findings and develop a personalized treatment plan. There are care coordinators who function as recovery coaches to assist the patient and family throughout this process and also assist with coordinating care with other providers, as part of a collaborative care model (Figure 17–2). The Society of Critical Care Medi-

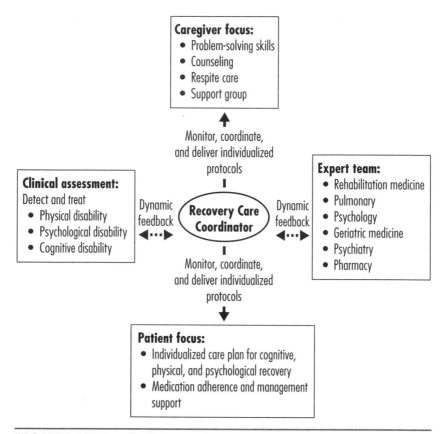

Caregiver focus:
- Problem-solving skills
- Counseling
- Respite care
- Support group

Monitor, coordinate,
and deliver individualized
protocols

Clinical assessment:
Detect and treat
- Physical disability
- Psychological disability
- Cognitive disability

Dynamic
feedback

**Recovery Care
Coordinator**

Dynamic
feedback

Expert team:
- Rehabilitation medicine
- Pulmonary
- Psychology
- Geriatric medicine
- Psychiatry
- Pharmacy

Monitor, coordinate,
and deliver individualized
protocols

Patient focus:
- Individualized care plan for cognitive, physical, and psychological recovery
- Medication adherence and management support

FIGURE 17–2. Collaborative care model of the Critical Care Recovery Center.

Source. Reprinted from Wang S, Allen D, Kheir YN, et al.: "Aging and Post-Intensive Care Syndrome: A Critical Need for Geriatric Psychiatry." *American Journal of Geriatric Psychiatry* 26(2):212–221, 2018. Copyright © 2018 with permission from Elsevier.

cine has developed a network of these ICU survivor clinics, promoting their expansion throughout the United States. If such clinics are available, ICU survivors should be referred to them.

KEY POINTS

- The long-term effects of critical illness are known as post-intensive care syndrome (PICS) and include impairments in cognition, mental health, and physical functioning.

- Delirium is a major risk factor for cognitive impairment after critical illness.
- PICS-Family is used to describe the psychological impact of intensive care unit (ICU) hospitalization and recovery on family members and caregivers of survivors.
- ICU survivors are often discharged on inappropriate medications, such as benzodiazepines, antipsychotics, and opioids. These medications should be weaned and stopped if possible, especially in the geriatric population.

Resources

Organization

Society of Critical Care Medicine: www.myicucare.org/thrive

Measures

Generalized Anxiety Disorder–7: www.phqscreeners.com/sites/g/files/g10016261/f/201412/GAD-7_English.pdf
Geriatric Depression Scale–15: www.aafp.org/dam/AAFP/documents/patient_care/cognitive_care_kit/gds.pdf
Patient Health Questionnaire–9: www.cqaimh.org/pdf/tool_phq9.pdf
Primary Care PTSD Screen for DSM-5: www.integration.samhsa.gov/clinical-practice/PC-PTSD.pdf

References

Bienvenu OJ, Colantuoni E, Mendez-Tellez PA, et al: Cooccurrence of and remission from general anxiety, depression, and posttraumatic stress disorder symptoms after acute lung injury: a 2-year longitudinal study. Crit Care Med 43(3):642–653, 2015 25513784

Davydow DS, Desai SV, Needham DM, et al: Psychiatric morbidity in survivors of the acute respiratory distress syndrome: a systematic review. Psychosom Med 70(4):512–519, 2008a 18434495

Davydow DS, Gifford JM, Desai SV, et al: Posttraumatic stress disorder in general intensive care unit survivors: a systematic review. Gen Hosp Psychiatry 30(5):421–434, 2008b 18774425

Davydow DS, Gifford JM, Desai SV, et al: Depression in general intensive care unit survivors: a systematic review. Intensive Care Med 35(5):796–809, 2009 19165464

Desai SV, Law TJ, Needham DM: Long-term complications of critical care. Crit Care Med 39(2):371–379, 2011 20959786

Ferrante LE, Pisani MA, Murphy TE, et al: Functional trajectories among older persons before and after critical illness. JAMA Intern Med 175(4):523–529, 2015 25665067

Ferrante LE, Pisani MA, Murphy TE, et al: Factors associated with functional recovery among older intensive care unit survivors. Am J Respir Crit Care Med 194(3):299–307, 2016 26840348

Folstein MF, Folstein SE, McHugh PR: "Mini-mental state." A practical method for grading the cognitive state of patients for the clinician. J Psychiatr Res 12(3):189–198, 1975 1202204

Girard TD, Jackson JC, Pandharipande PP, et al: Delirium as a predictor of long-term cognitive impairment in survivors of critical illness. Crit Care Med 38(7):1513–1520, 2010 20473145

Guerra C, Linde-Zwirble WT, Wunsch H: Risk factors for dementia after critical illness in elderly Medicare beneficiaries. Crit Care 16(6):R233, 2012 23245397

Guerra C, Hua M, Wunsch H: Risk of a diagnosis of dementia for elderly Medicare beneficiaries after intensive care. Anesthesiology 123(5):1105–1112, 2015 26270938

Hopkins RO, Weaver LK, Collingridge D, et al: Two-year cognitive, emotional, and quality-of-life outcomes in acute respiratory distress syndrome. Am J Respir Crit Care Med 171(4):340–347, 2005 15542793

Iwashyna TJ: Survivorship will be the defining challenge of critical care in the 21st century. Ann Intern Med 153(3):204–205, 2010 20679565

Iwashyna TJ, Cooke CR, Wunsch H, et al: Population burden of long-term survivorship after severe sepsis in older Americans. J Am Geriatr Soc 60(6):1070–1077, 2012 22642542

Jackson JC, Pandharipande PP, Girard TD, et al: Depression, post-traumatic stress disorder, and functional disability in survivors of critical illness in the BRAIN-ICU study: a longitudinal cohort study. Lancet Respir Med 2(5):369–379, 2014 24815803

Jutte JE, Erb CT, Jackson JC: Physical, cognitive, and psychological disability following critical illness: what is the risk? Semin Respir Crit Care Med 36(6):943–958, 2015 26595053

Kentish-Barnes N, Chevret S, Champigneulle B, et al: Effect of a condolence letter on grief symptoms among relatives of patients who died in the ICU: a randomized clinical trial. Intensive Care Med 43(4):473–484, 2017 28197680

Kessler RC, Chiu WT, Demler O, et al: Prevalence, severity, and comorbidity of 12-month DSM-IV disorders in the National Comorbidity Survey Replication. Arch Gen Psychiatry 62(6):617–627, 2005 15939839

Kroenke K, Spitzer RL, Williams JB: The PHQ-9: validity of a brief depression severity measure. J Gen Intern Med 16(9):606–613, 2001 11556941

Locke M, Eccleston S, Ryan CN, et al: Developing a diary program to minimize patient and family post–intensive care syndrome. AACN Adv Crit Care 27(2):212–220, 2016 27153310

Myers EA, Smith DA, Allen SR, et al: Post-ICU syndrome: rescuing the undiagnosed. JAAPA 29(4):34–37, 2016 27023654

Nasreddine ZS, Phillips NA, Bédirian V, et al: The Montreal Cognitive Assessment, MoCA: a brief screening tool for mild cognitive impairment. J Am Geriatr Soc 53(4):695–699, 2005 15817019

Needham DM, Davidson J, Cohen H, et al: Improving long-term outcomes after discharge from intensive care unit: report from a stakeholders' conference. Crit Care Med 40(2):502–509, 2012 21946660

Nikayin S, Rabiee A, Hashem MD, et al: Anxiety symptoms in survivors of critical illness: a systematic review and meta-analysis. Gen Hosp Psychiatry 43:23–29, 2016 27796253

Pandharipande PP, Girard TD, Jackson JC, et al: Long-term cognitive impairment after critical illness. N Engl J Med 369(14):1306–1316, 2013 24088092

Prins A, Bovin M, Kimerling R, et al: The Primary Care PTSD Screen for DSM-5 (PC-PTSD-5): development and operating characteristics. Prim Care Psychiatry 9(1):9–14, 2003

Rabiee A, Nikayin S, Hashem MD, et al: Depressive symptoms after critical illness: a systematic review and meta-analysis. Crit Care Med 44(9):1744–1753, 2016 27153046

Sheikh JI, Yesavage JA: Geriatric Depression Scale (GDS): recent evidence and development of a shorter version. Clin Gerontol 5(1–2):165–173, 1986

Spitzer RL, Kroenke K, Williams JB, et al: A brief measure for assessing generalized anxiety disorder: the GAD-7. Arch Intern Med 166(10):1092–1097, 2006 16717171

van Deusekom I, Bakhshi-Raiez F, de Keizer NF, et al: Reported burden on informal caregivers of ICU survivors: a literature review. Crit Care 20:16, 2016 26792081

Wang S, Mosher C, Perkins AJ, et al: Post-intensive care unit psychiatric comorbidity and quality of life. J Hosp Med 12(10):831–835, 2017 28991949

Wang S, Allen D, Kheir YN, et al: Aging and post-intensive care syndrome: a critical need for geriatric psychiatry. Am J Geriatr Psychiatry 26(2):212–221, 2018 28716375

Wolters AE, Peelen LM, Welling MC, et al: Long-term mental health problems after delirium in the ICU. Crit Care Med 44(10):1808–1813, 2016 27513540

Physical Activity

"I Can Only Go About a Block Before Running Out of Breath"

J. Kaci Fairchild, Ph.D., ABPP
Kathryn Phillipps, M.S.
Peter Louras, M.S.

CHAPTER 18

Clinical Presentation

Chief Complaint

"I can only go about a block before running out of breath."

Vignette

Mr. Q is a 75-year-old retired, widowed man who presents to a new primary care provider to establish care. He recently moved to the area to be closer to his children and grandchildren after the death of his wife. He currently lives alone in a large senior living community that is approximately 5 miles from his son's house. He regularly sees his son and grandchildren and has made some friends in his new community.

Mr. Q denies any significant health problems, although his family history is positive for cardiovascular disease. Mr. Q is adjusting well to his new home and has kept busy exploring the area with his family. He has, however, noticed that he grows tired more easily and at times becomes winded when he exerts himself. The results of his examination reveal that he has high blood pressure (132/85) and elevated blood glucose levels. Mr. Q also reports that he has gained 15 pounds over the past 4 years. During that time, Mr. Q was the primary caregiver for his wife, who had dementia (major neurocognitive disorder). He reports that he struggled to manage all of the responsibilities in his caregiving role and that he frequently did not have the time be physically active or exercise. Prior to his wife's illness, Mr. Q routinely played tennis and golf with a group of friends. Mr. Q estimates that it has been at least 3 years since he engaged in any regular physical activity. He states that he knows exercise is important and that he feels better when he is more active. He reports that his senior living community has a nice gym that he has visited. However, his most recent visit to the gym resulted in sore, painful muscles that restricted his mobility and kept him in his apartment for 2 days.

Discussion

The Problem of Physical Inactivity

Physical inactivity among older adults is a problem of epidemic proportions. The Centers for Disease Control and Prevention (CDC) estimates that one in four older adults is physically inactive. Physical activity is integral in the prevention and management of many age-related illnesses and health conditions. The concept of "use it or lose it" is not a new one, because older adults have long been encouraged to be physically active as a means of maintaining functional independence. Yet the role of physical activity and exercise in a healthy lifestyle has taken on greater importance because of its widespread benefits, which include the primary and secondary prevention of multiple chronic diseases, such as cardiovascular disease, diabetes, cancer, hypertension, obesity, depression, cognitive impairment, and osteoporosis (Petersen et al. 2018; Warburton et al. 2006). Moreover, in light of the growing evidence of benefits of exercise to late-life cognitive function, the American Academy of Neurology now advises that providers should recommend regular exercise to older adults at risk for dementia (Petersen et al. 2018). In addition to these widespread health benefits, exercise and physical activity are not as costly as traditional treatments for these chronic diseases, nor do they have significant side effects associated with them. Because both cost and side effects can lead to reduced treatment adherence and compliance in older patients, exercise and physical activity may be more acceptable than traditional pharmacological options.

Factors Associated With Physical Inactivity

There is little disagreement as to the wide-ranging benefits of physical activity, yet physical inactivity is prevalent in older adults. Rates of physical activity are highest in children and youth; however, the onset of young adulthood heralds a sharp decline in physical activity that continues through midlife and accelerates into old age (Clarke et al. 2017). Physical inactivity in older adults is due to a complex set of demographic, physiological, emotional, and environmental factors. Effective recommendations for increasing physical activity and exercise should include consideration of these underlying factors.

Demographic Factors

Physical activity behavior is influenced by a number of demographic factors, including age, gender, race/ethnicity, level of education, and marital status. People grow more physically inactive as they age, with prevalence rates of inactivity rising from roughly 25% in people ages 65–74 years to over 35% in people age 75 years or older. Physical inactivity tends to be higher in older women compared with older men and higher among Hispanics and non-Hispanic blacks compared with non-Hispanic whites and those of other ethnicities (Watson et al. 2016). Older adults with less education are more likely to be physically inactive compared with those with at least some secondary education, and those older adults who are not married are more likely to be physically inactive than those who are married (Park et al. 2014). Many of these demographic risk factors are not modifiable; however, providers should be sensitive to the presence of these risk factors in their older patients and screen for inactivity accordingly.

Physiological Factors

As people age, widespread changes in the physiology of the musculoskeletal system occur that impact a person's ability to engage in physical activity. Older adults have bones that are weaker and more brittle and thus are more susceptible to fracture. Muscle tissue is fundamentally altered by the aging process because people lose muscle tissue and muscle strength declines. This loss of muscle mass and strength increases stress on joints, and the increased stress heightens the risk for arthritis and falls. Joints also experience some ill effects of the aging process as structural changes compromise their integrity, reducing the joints' resiliency and increasing their vulnerability to damage. Stiff joints result in reduced range of motion and consequently limited mobility. Changes in the bones, muscles, and joints contribute to the loss of height that can occur with age. When this height loss is coupled with age-associated increases in body fat and loss of muscle mass, a person's overall body mass index increases, even in weight-stable persons (Fairchild et al. 2017).

Certain chronic medical conditions that impact physical activity are also more prevalent in older adults. These chronic conditions include arthritis, cancer, diabetes, coronary heart disease, chronic obstructive pulmonary disease (COPD), and stroke. Importantly, an analysis of 2014 Behavioral Risk Factor Surveillance System data found that rates of physical inactivity in older adults with at least one of these medical conditions were 40% higher than in older adults with no chronic medical condition (Watson et al. 2016).

Physiological risk factors must be considered when treatment recommendations are being made for older patients. Importantly, some of these risk factors are modifiable and will improve with exercise. For example, sedentary older adults may have reduced muscle mass, muscle strength, and mobility. These conditions make weight-bearing exercises difficult; thus, providers can recommend non-weight-bearing exercises such as water aerobics or swimming for more deconditioned or physically inactive patients. Regular participation in these activities will increase muscle mass, strength, and mobility, and this in turn will increase the ability to more fully participate in weight-bearing activities such as walking or bike riding. Furthermore, exercise recommendations must also include consideration of chronic medical conditions such as atrial fibrillation or COPD. Specifically, the severity of these conditions will have direct implications for the type, duration, and intensity of exercises and activities that a person is able to do in a safe manner.

Emotional Factors

Emotional factors, such as depression, social isolation, and loneliness, affect physical activity behavior throughout the lifespan. However, in older adults, these emotional factors often interact with physiological changes to result in pronounced changes in physical activity. Depression is one of the most commonly occurring mental health concerns in older adults. Older adults with symptoms of depression are often less physically active. As physical inactivity increases, older adults participate in fewer enjoyable activities, which in turn intensifies depressive symptoms, further reducing physical activity (Chang et al. 2016). Social isolation and loneliness are also associated with physical inactivity in older adults (Hawkley et al. 2009). Social support is a strong determinant of physical activity. People are more likely to engage in regular physical activity and exercise if they have social support; thus, those older adults who are socially isolated or lack quality relationships with others may be missing a key reinforcement for physically active behavior.

Among older adults, factors such as self-efficacy and self-regulation skills are also important determinants of physical activity (Park et al.

2014). Older adults who are more confident in their ability to exercise or engage in physical activity (i.e., have higher self-efficacy) are more likely to be physically active, as are those older adults who are better able to set goals and track progress toward meeting those goals. Many things can impact older adults' confidence in their ability to exercise. One important factor to consider is *fall-related concerns*, which is a term that encompasses fear of falling, falls self-efficacy or lack of balance confidence, and consequence concerns (Pauelsen et al. 2018). Fall-related concerns are prevalent, as they occur in up to 55% of community-dwelling older adults. This prevalence increases with age and occurs more frequently in women. Importantly, fall-related concerns are associated with activity avoidance, which in turn results in a higher fall risk. Furthermore, fall-related concerns are associated with morbidity and mortality (Auais et al. 2018; Wetherell et al. 2018). Fall-related concerns are not limited to those older adults who have experienced a fall; thus, providers who work with older adults should consider screening their patients for fall-related concerns regardless of fall history.

Several screening instruments exist to screen for emotional factors that are associated with physical inactivity. For instance, the Geriatric Depression Scale (Yesavage et al. 1982–1983) is a brief self-report measure of depression that exists in multiple formats, although the 15-item (short form) and 30-item (long form) scales are the most frequently used. Three commonly used scales to assess for social isolation and loneliness are the Campaign to End Loneliness Measurement Tool (Campaign to End Loneliness 2019), the De Jong Gierveld Loneliness Scale (De Jong and Van Tilburg 2006), and the UCLA Loneliness Scale (Hughes et al. 2004). Fall-related concerns can be easily assessed with the Short Falls Efficacy Scale–International (Kempen et al. 2008). Providers should be cognizant of these factors and the role that they play in the success or failure of an exercise prescription. Although many of these factors may be successfully addressed through exercise (e.g., improved mood, reduced loneliness), they may also prove to be obstacles to beginning the exercise program and thus necessitate focused intervention (e.g., pharmacological intervention or psychotherapy) before beginning the exercise program.

Environmental Factors

Older adults face multiple environmental factors that can serve as barriers to engaging in physical activity and exercise. The costs associated with gym memberships, exercise classes, and exercise equipment can be prohibitive for many older adults. Some health insurance programs, such as Medicare, include basic fitness services as a benefit for older adults, and many senior centers offer no- or low-cost exercise classes at their facilities. Accessibility may be an issue for those older adults without regular transportation to the gym or senior center. For those older adults who do venture to the gym, they may find that gyms lack exercise classes for seniors or complementary introductory training sessions to teach the proper use of gym equipment.

Exercise and increased physical activity can easily be accomplished outside of the gym. Walking is one of the most popular physical activities in older adults, yet many lack access to safe, well-lit, and evenly graded walking paths with available benches or other resting spots. Several federally funded programs have been developed to teach older adults how to safely exercise in their homes. Older adults report that health care providers influence their physical activity behavior by discussing the importance of exercise and providing concrete instruction about exercise programs (Bethancourt et al. 2014). Consequently, older adults may not learn about these programs if their health care providers do not discuss these programs with them.

Many resources are available to assist providers in helping older patients problem-solve environmental obstacles to exercise. The reader is directed to the "Resources" section at the end of the chapter for suggested materials for providers and patients.

Assessment of Physical Activity

Particularly important in older adults is the recommendation to check with their physician before beginning an exercise regimen. The American College of Cardiology and American Heart Association (AHA) recognize the increased cardiovascular risk for older adults engaging in exercise and recommend comprehensive testing before beginning any exercise regimen (Fletcher et al. 2013). Screening tools can range from simple checklists and logs to lengthy tests requiring professional administration and interpretation. Because of the number of diagnostic tests available, selecting a proper approach should consider clinical judgment, evidence-based models, and cost-effectiveness.

The American College of Sports Medicine (2014) offers guidelines for selecting appropriate assessment tools and narrows interventions based on the patient's current level of exercise, underlying health concerns, and short- and long-term exercise goals. The intent of testing before beginning any exercise regimen is to reduce the amount of unnecessary medical interventions while addressing major risk factors to ensure safe exercise participation (Riebe et al. 2015). There may also be limitations to the use of certain testing instruments with older adults due to changing sensory and cognitive abilities, physical limitations, and ease of use. Thus, it is important for providers to recognize how these factors may influence a patient as well as the results of testing.

Activity assessment is just one tool in evaluating older adults' overall health and should be considered in collaboration with medical histories, physical problems, disabilities, and sensory impairments. With this in mind, it is important for a patient to receive medical clearance from a primary care provider or undergo a physical examination and diagnostic laboratory testing to rule out any barriers to exercise. Initial screening tools such as the Physical Activity Readiness Questionnaire and the American Heart Association/American College of Sports Medicine Health/Fitness Facility Preparticipation Screening Questionnaire offer quick and easy-to-complete checklists that can identify cardiovascular conditions, pain, and balance issues that may impair further exercise and physical assessments (Balady et al. 1998). Practitioners should use clinical judgment when obtaining results from these measures regarding treatment recommendations, appropriate alternative assessments, or referral for further diagnostic workup.

Self-Assessment

Self-report measures are simple methods for patients and clinicians to establish baseline health and fitness levels as well as track daily and weekly habits over time. Physical activity questionnaires typically ask patients to account for activities over the past week or month and consider a range of physical efforts from vigorous walking, running, and swimming to less vigorous activities such as shopping, housework, and gardening.

The Physical Activity Scale for the Elderly (Washburn et al. 1993) and the Yale Physical Activity Survey (Dipietro et al. 1993) demonstrate consistent objectivity, validity, and reliability for indirect self-assessment with older adults recalling regular exercise and leisure routines (Krol-Zielinska and Ciekot 2015). Older adults may also be encouraged to track their activities via daily logs to capture subjective data, duration of activity, and intensity of activity. Keeping daily logs may help patients be more aware of daily activities and reflect slightly more complete representations of daily activity. Although these methods are inexpensive and easy to administer, self-reports may have limitations, especially with older adult populations, who may have difficulties with memory, cognition, and recall bias of past activities, especially over longer time frames (Helmerhorst et al. 2012). When compared with objectively measured physical activity, self-reported measures tend to demonstrate over-estimation of moderate and vigorous activity with older adults (Tucker et al. 2011) and underestimation of light activities and daily tasks that may go unreported (Schrack et al. 2016). Therefore, self-assessment alone may not be comprehensive, and all materials should be reviewed with the patient for accuracy and completeness.

Physical Tests

Physical tests can add prognostic information to assessments of older adults through direct observations of body regions, strength, balance, and endurance. Physical tests increase the objectivity of functionality and physical ability in older adults, with many tests requiring minimal equipment. At the same time, formal tests should always be performed and interpreted by licensed or certified clinicians who are familiar with the assessments and equipment. This creates an obligation for training observers and administrators so that tests are conducted with consistent and accurate readings; such training is imperative with advanced tests requiring specialized equipment, calibration, and upkeep (Fletcher et al. 2013). Before performing physical tests, clinicians should review physical screening tools to assess patients for gait or balance issues and consider medical history for falls and cardiac or other medical difficulties.

An easy first step can be performance-oriented assessments of gross motor and fine motor skills, particularly through observing tasks that replicate everyday functions such as sitting, standing, balance, turning, and gait. One example is the Timed Up and Go (TUG) test that asks patients to stand up from a chair, walk 3 meters forward, turn, walk back to the chair, and sit down. The TUG test serves the dual purpose of observing and measuring the balance of an individual (based on a scale of 1 to 5) as well as allowing comparisons with confidence intervals of timed performance (Bohannon 2006). Walk tests additionally observe cardiac abilities by measuring the maximum distance a person can cover in a set amount of time. In the 6-Minute Walk Test, a participant walks back and forth between two cones 30 meters (100 feet) apart to complete as many laps as possible in 6 minutes. Blood pressure and heart rate are taken before and after testing, as well as estimations on the modified Borg Scale, and Borg Rating of Perceived Exertion (RPE) Scale, for breathlessness and perceived levels of exertion. Walk tests require minimal equipment such as a stopwatch and blood pressure cuff, as well as space for participants to ambulate. These studies integrate aerobic capacity and endurance and have been demonstrated to be a submaximal test of aerobic capacity (Steffen et al. 2002).

A stress test, or cardiopulmonary exercise test, is considered the standard for assessing maximal oxygen uptake and aerobic capacity with older adults (Peritz et al. 2017). Exercise stress testing typically uses a treadmill or stationary bicycle ergometer to gradually increase exercise resistance while monitoring patients' cardiopulmonary system through electrocardiography. Many variations of protocols and interpretive algorithms exist that vary in intensity and duration, although those with gradual inclines and increases in speed appear most appropriate for testing older adults (Huggett et al. 2005). Stress testing provides the most technical results of physical assessment because of its reliance on detailed equipment and trained technicians. As such, fees, equipment malfunction, and scheduling may create barriers for testing older adults, and exercise stress testing may be contraindicated for individuals with abnormal baseline cardiac health or those demonstrating signs of poor perfusion (Riebe et al. 2015). In the event of a suspected cardiac or health issue (e.g., shortness of breath, chest pain, dizziness, increased heart rate), a stress test should be immediately stopped.

Wearable Devices

Wearable technology can help providers directly track patients' physical activity as well as help patients self-monitor their current activity levels and personal health via immediate feedback. Devices can range from simple pedometers to watches and smartphone technology with built-in accelerometer or gyroscope, global positioning system (GPS) tracking, and skin sensors. Wearable devices can be one of the easiest forms of daily tracking and can monitor everything from steps to sleep patterns and heart rate levels and have proven feasible for older adults depending on size, ease of use, and price (Dobkin and Dorsch 2011).

Pedometers are one of the simplest forms of wearable devices on the market and come in inexpensive and compact designs. Pedometers provide the luxury of tracking a person's steps while being lightweight, easy to wear, and simple in operational use. Wearing a pedometer has been shown to help increase older adults' awareness of physical activity as well as cause increases in daily steps when paired with goal setting and intervention programs (Bravata et al. 2007). At the same time, pedometers are limited to measuring only steps and may be difficult for older adults to remember or keep track of.

Recent advances in smart technology have opened the door to a range of wearable devices for consumers. New technology utilizes accelerometer, gyroscope, and GPS sensors that tend to be more precise in tracking daily activity and provide useful information for older adult populations who monitor their health. Commercial watches have advanced in style, size, and functionality over the years depending on brand and price (Schrack et al. 2016). At the same time, corresponding software has advanced to become more user friendly, with features able to explore personal attributes in greater detail.

Older adult populations may experience difficulties with wearable devices, especially with those who demonstrate sensory declines or gait disorders or who walk at slower speeds (de Bruin et al. 2008). When a device is being chosen, it is important to consider variable changes in older adults, including loss of fine motor skills, sensitivity to touch, and hearing and visual acuity. For example, when working with patients with hearing impairment, providers should recommend a smartwatch that includes an alternative alarm system that vibrates or flashes.

Physical Activity Guidelines

Federal guidelines, based on recommendations from the CDC, advise that older adults engage in a minimum of 150 minutes (or 2.5 hours) of moderate-intensity aerobic activity each week. Alternatively, older adults can achieve adequate aerobic activity in 75 minutes of vigorous-intensity aerobic activity, or an equivalent mixture of moderate-intensity and vigorous-intensity aerobic activity. For even greater health benefits, the CDC recommends that older adults engage in 300 minutes (or 5 hours) of moderate-intensity aerobic activity each week. Alternatively, older adults can engage in 150 minutes (or 2.5 hours) of vigorous-intensity aerobic activity, or an equivalent mixture of moderate-intensity and vigorous-intensity aerobic activity. Aerobic activity (also known as "cardio") is that in which breath rate and heart rate increase. CDC guidelines call for any kind of activity in which an individual is breathing faster, and their heart is beating harder, to occur for a minimum of 10 minutes at a time in order to qualify as exercise. In addition to this aerobic activity, the CDC recommends that older adults engage in 2 or more days a week of muscle-strengthening activities that stimulate all major muscle groups. Muscle-strengthening activities can include strength training, resistance training, and endurance exercises—essentially, any activities that increase strength, power, and endurance of skeletal muscles (U.S. Department of Health and Human Services 2008).

Exercise intensity, a key component of the recommended dosage of exercise and physical activity, can be defined as the amount of work a body uses when exercising. Put another way, exercise intensity describes how difficult exercise feels while the individual is engaged in it. Three common ways of measuring exercise intensity include target heart rate, Borg RPE Scale, and the "talk test" (Table 18–1). Most physical activity guidelines, including current federal guidelines for physical activity, present exercise intensity in terms of low, moderate, and vigorous levels of exercise. These levels represent percentages of a person's age-related maximum heart rate. The maximum heart rate represents the maximum number of times a person's heart should beat per minute of exercise or physical activity. A person's maximum heart rate is most commonly calculated using the formula: 220−your age. For example, a 75-year-old person's maximum heart rate would be 145 bpm (beats per minute). The maximum heart rate is then used to calculate a person's target heart rate zones. This calculation is only a rough estimate of a person's maximum heart rate, because the formula does not consider important variables such as level of physical fitness, medical conditions, or medication usage, all of which can raise or lower a person's maximum heart rate. Heart rate can be measured through use of wrist-based heart rate monitors as well as those that employ a chest strap. For those who do not have access to a heart rate monitor, a patient's heart rate can be calculated by taking his or her pulse. When taking the pulse, the pulse taker should count the beats for 10 seconds, then multiply that number by six to calculate the beats per minute.

A second approach to identifying exercise intensity is through the use of self-report scales. These scales often use physical indicators experienced during exercise, such as increased perspiration, shortness of breath or change in breathing rate, and muscle fatigue, to identify level of exercise intensity. One such scale, the Borg RPE Scale, allows patients to rate how hard it feels like their body is working while engaged in physical activity or exercise. Ratings on the Borg RPE can range from 0 to 10 or 6 to 20. Using the latter scale as an example, a rating of 6 represents "no exertion at all," an 11 represents "light exertion," a 15 represents "heavy exertion or hard work," and a 20 represents "maximal exertion." The Borg RPE Scale correlates well with target heart rate zones, so a person's rating can be a fairly good estimate of actual heart rate during exercise (Borg 1998). Scales such as the Borg RPE Scale may be preferable when the clinician is working with patients who have health conditions or take medications that affect heart rate.

A third method of quantifying exercise intensity is the "talk test." In this method, levels of exercise intensity are correlated with the ease with which a person can talk while engaged in exercise. Using this method, a person is able to sing while engaged in low-intensity exercise, to talk but not sing while engaged in moderate-intensity exercise, and to only say a few words at a time during vigorous intensity exercise. The talk test requires no specialized equipment or familiarity with RPEs and thus may

TABLE 18–1. Assessment of physical activity intensity

Intensity category	Objective measures[a]	Subjective measures[b]	Descriptive measures	Talk test
Maximum	90%–100% of HR_{max}	17–20	Out of breath, fatigue, heavy sweating; activity cannot be maintained for more than 10 minutes	Cannot speak or converse
Vigorous	70%<90% of HR_{max}	14–16	Difficulty breathing, moderate sweating; activity can be maintained for up to 30 minutes	Speaks in syllables, broken sentences
Moderate	55%<70% of HR_{max}	11–13	Heavy breathing, light sweating; activity can be maintained for 30–60 minutes	Can converse, one or two sentences at a time
Low	40%<55% of HR_{max}	8–10	Easy breathing; activity can be maintained can maintained for at least 60 minutes	Can engage in normal conversation
Warm-up	<40% of HR_{max}	<8	Very mild exertion; activity involves sitting or lying down with little to no energy exertion	Can engage in normal conversation

[a] HR_{max} = maximum heart rate.
[b] Ratings correspond to the Borg Rating of Perceived Exertion Scale (Borg 1998).

be preferable for those patients who do not have access to heart rate monitors or who struggle to calculate their own pulse.

Tips for Talking With Patients

Health care providers should talk to their patients about physical activity and exercise not only because of the importance of exercise and physical activity to patients' health but also because older adults want to discuss exercise and physical activity with their providers (Bethancourt et al. 2014). Providers may feel unsure as to how to begin this conversation or uncomfortable in making concrete recommendations for exercise or physical activity programs. Health care providers can begin with a discussion of the benefits of physical exercise, because patients who understand the benefits of exercise as it relates to their own health may be more motivated to begin an exercise program. Patients may or may not have past experience with exercise; thus, it is important for providers to inquire about both past and current physical activity.

Exercise plans are tailored to each patient as they take into account that patient's specific fitness goals, preferences, level of physical fitness, and any health conditions that require accommodations. For example, older adults who have an increased risk of falls can engage in balance exercises and other activities that may improve or maintain balance. Patients who are sedentary may struggle to meet the recommended guidelines of 150 minutes of moderate-intensity exercise each week. For these patients, providers should encourage the patients to exercise in 10-minute increments until such time that they have increased their stamina and are able to exercise for longer periods of time. This highlights the fact that exercise plans are not static programs but are best designed to evolve based on changes in the patient's goals and physical fitness.

Table 18–2 provides an overview of how to introduce the topic of physical activity and exercise as well as tips to help guide the discussion.

Most people understand and accept the importance of exercise, yet many struggle to begin or maintain an exercise program. A common scenario might be one in which a patient with chronic medical conditions (e.g., hypertension and hyperlipidemia) presents for an annual checkup with reports of increased shortness of breath and headaches. The provider and patient have discussed the importance of exercise in past clinic visits, and the patient even agreed to become more active. Yet despite the patient's awareness of the importance of exercise and commitment to exercising, the patient remained sedentary.

TABLE 18–2. Talking to patients about physical activity and exercise

Discuss both the benefits of physical activity and exercise and how those benefits pertain to the patient. Highlighting the personal relevance of the benefits can increase motivation to begin exercising.

Ask patients about their daily activities and if they participate in any regular physical activity or exercise. People may engage in incidental physical activity without recognizing it as such (e.g., taking the stairs). Patients should be encouraged to continue with this incidental physical activity and empowered to incorporate new exercises or activities into their daily routine.

Work with patients to develop fitness goals for both the short term (i.e., next week or two) and the long term (i.e., 6 months, 1 year, 2 years). Fitness goals should be both specific and reasonable to increase the likelihood that patients can successfully achieve them. Goal setting is an important element of any exercise plan.

Write an exercise plan or prescription that includes specific information about the type of exercise or activity (e.g., walking); the intensity (e.g., walking speed); and frequency and duration of exercise or activity (e.g., 4 days a week for 60 minutes).

Identify any health conditions that may require accommodations. Although some severe health conditions may preclude participation in physical activity and exercise, most can be accommodated, and those accommodations should be included in the exercise plan.

Ask patients to identify any potential barriers to completing the exercise plan. Actively problem-solve these barriers with patients and include potential solutions in the exercise plan.

Refer patients to community resources as well as federally funded exercise programs specifically for older adults.

Situations such as this are common and can lead to both provider frustration and patient discouragement. In these instances, providers may try to "fix" the problem by telling the patient what to do using language that includes "must," "should," or "have to" statements. These statements are rarely effective and in fact can put the patient on the defensive, effectively shutting down communication. Providers may also use scare tactics to try to initiate behavior change; however, fear is only effective in the short term and rarely leads to lasting behavioral changes.

In frustrating situations such as this, providers may choose to employ motivational interviewing (MI) techniques to facilitate lasting behavior change (Miller and Rollnick 2012). Briefly, the principles of MI include the following:

1. **Resist the righting reflex** (put another way, resist the urge to immediately help the patient or "fix" the problem). In the scenario just described, the provider would begin by listening to the patient discuss the struggle with starting an exercise program while also trying not to advise the patient. In this first step, providers should also reflect back what they have heard the patient say. For instance, in this scenario, the provider might reflect back that "It's hard to find the time to exercise."
2. **Understand the patient's motivation.** In the scenario, the provider should work to spend more time learning about the patient's obstacles to and concerns about exercise than in planning how the patient will become more active.
3. **Listen to the patient** (seek the patient's ideas and insights about the problem). In the scenario, the provider might ask, "What are your ideas about how you can become more active?" This question opens up communication between the patient and the provider, thus allowing change-oriented talk to enter their conversation.
4. **Empower the patient** (use respectful collaboration—that is, collaboration that empowers the patient to take the lead in conversation). The patient in this scenario may have endorsed bike riding as an enjoyable activity. The provider could then ask, "So you like bike riding?" and then listen to the patient share any thoughts or feelings about the matter. The provider can then build on this suggestion by discussing with the patient how bike riding might fit into the patient's life.

The use of MI is at times in stark contrast to how providers traditionally communicate with patients, and thus providers are encouraged to review Miller and Rollnick's (2012) book for a thorough discussion of the use of MI in health care settings.

Vignette *(continued)*

In light of his familial history of cardiovascular disease, Mr. Q is concerned about his blood pressure and elevated glucose levels. He prefers to manage these symptoms through increased exercise and identified this as his fitness goal. Mr. Q has played golf and tennis in the past; however, he has not had anyone to do these activities with since he moved to the area. He identified using the gym at his facility as an alternative to tennis and golf. Mr. Q reported that he is most familiar with the treadmill, so he identified walking as his preferred activity. Because he has been more inactive over the past 4 years, Mr. Q's exercise prescription included walking on the treadmill for 20 minutes 4 days a week at a low to moderate intensity, followed by muscle-strengthening exercises targeting each major muscle group. His exercise prescription also included a plan for ramping up the duration and intensity of his walking as his physical fitness improved. Finally, Mr. Q's exercise plan also included information about the Go4Life program as well as community resources for older adults who want to become more active.

Two weeks after Mr. Q's appointment, clinic staff checked in with him by phone to assess how he was progressing with his exercise prescription. Mr. Q noted that he had not been to the gym since his clinic appointment. He expressed his embarrassment over not starting his exercise prescription and said he "felt bad" for "letting us down." Clinic staff reassured Mr. Q that many people struggle to begin exercise programs. They then worked with him to identify his obstacles to going to the gym. Mr. Q revealed that he was unfamiliar with the equipment in the facility, and thus he lacked the confidence to independently begin his exercise program. Clinic staff and Mr. Q brainstormed potential ways to become more familiar with the equipment and gain more confidence in his ability to use the gym. Mr. Q noted that the gym was staffed by trainers who were available to residents for exercise consultations. He agreed to set up a meeting with a trainer at the gym so that he could be formally oriented to the equipment in the facility. Clinic staff also encouraged Mr. Q to invite a fellow resident to work out with him once a week, as peer support increases both motivation and accountability.

Mr. Q acknowledged that he would be more likely to use the gym if he met a friend there, so he agreed to invite his neighbor to the gym for one of his workouts each week. Finally, clinic staff worked with Mr. Q to adjust the initial frequency of his workouts to twice a week. It is important for patients to have a sense of achievement and accomplishment in achieving their fitness goals. By decreasing the initial number of daily workouts, Mr. Q is more likely to hit his weekly goal of working out twice a week. Once Mr. Q is able to consistently workout twice a week, clinic staff will work with Mr. Q to adjust his exercise prescription to meet his evolving fitness needs.

KEY POINTS

- Physical inactivity in older adults is due to a complex set of demographic, physiological, emotional, and environmental factors.
- Effective recommendations for increasing physical activity and exercise should include consideration of these underlying factors.
- Activity assessment is just one tool in evaluating older adults' overall health and should be considered in collaboration with medical histories, physical problems, disabilities, and sensory impairments.
- Health care providers should talk to their patients about physical activity and exercise not only because of the importance of exercise and physical activity to patients' health but also because older adults want to discuss exercise and physical activity with their providers.

Resources for Clinicians

Screening Tools: Readiness to Engage in Physical Activity

American Heart Association/American College of Sports Medicine Health/Fitness Facility Preparticipation Screening Questionnaire (Balady et al. 1998)

Self-Report Measures of Physical Activity

Centers for Disease Control and Prevention: Physical Activity Diary. Available at: www.cdc.gov/healthyweight/pdf/physical_activity_ diary_cdc.pdf

Dipietro L, Caspersen CJ, Ostfeld AM, et al: A survey for assessing physical activity among older adults. Med Sci Sports Exerc 25(5):628–642, 1993

National Heart Lung and Blood Institute: Weekly Physical Activity Log: Aerobic and Strengthening Activities. Bethesda, MD, National Institutes of Health, 2013. Available at: www.nhlbi.nih.gov/health/ educational/healthdisp/pdf/tipsheets/Weekly-Physical-Activity-Log.pdf

U.S. Department of Health and Human Services: Keeping Track of What You Do Each Week (2008 Physical Activity Guidelines for Americans; ODPHP Publ No U0050). Rockville, MD, Office of Disease Prevention and Health Promotion, U.S. Department of Health and Human Services, 2008. Available at: https://health.gov/paguidelines/ guidelines/keepingtrack.pdf

Washburn RA, Smith KW, Jette AM, et al: The Physical Activity Scale for the Elderly (PASE): development and evaluation. J Clin Epidemiol 46(2):153–162, 1993

Emotional Factors Associated With Physical Inactivity

Depression

Yesavage JA, Brink TL, Rose TL, et al: Development and validation of a geriatric depression screening scale: a preliminary report. J Psychiatr Res 17(1):37–49, 1982–1983

Social Isolation and Loneliness

Campaign to End Loneliness: Measuring Your Impact on Loneliness in Later Life. Available at: www.campaigntoendloneliness.org/measuring-loneliness

De Jong Gierveld J, Van Tilburg T: A 6-item scale for overall, emotional, and social loneliness. Confirmatory Tests on Survey Data 28(5):582–598, 2006

Hughes ME, Waite LJ, Hawkley LC, et al: A short scale for measuring loneliness in large surveys: results from two population-based studies. Res Aging 26(6):655–672, 2004

Fall-Related Concerns

Kempen GI, Yardley L, van Haastregt JC, et al: The Short FES-I: a shortened version of the Falls Efficacy Scale–International to assess fear of falling. Age Ageing 37(1):45–50, 2008

Website

National Institute on Aging: Encouraging Wellness in Older Patients. Available at: www.nia.nih.gov/health/encouraging-wellness-older-patients

Books

Chodzko-Zajko W: ACSM's Exercise for Older Adults. Philadelphia, PA, Lippincott Williams & Wilkins, 2013

Miller WR, Rollnick S: Motivational Interviewing, Helping People Change, 3rd Edition. New York, Guilford, 2012

Resources for Patients

Websites

American Heart Association: Healthy Living and Fitness: www.heart.org/en/healthy-living/fitness

Centers for Disease Control and Prevention: Physical Activity Needs for Older Adults: www.cdc.gov/physicalactivity/basics/older_adults/index.htm

National Heart, Lung, and Blood Institute: Physical Activity and Your Heart: www.nhlbi.nih.gov/health/health-topics/topics/phys/recommend

Office of Disease Prevention and Health Promotion: 2008 Physical Activity Guidelines for Older Adults: https://health.gov/paguidelines/guidelines/older-adults.aspx

Book

National Institute on Aging: Exercise and Physical Activity: Your Everyday Guide from the National Institute on Aging at NIH. Bethesda, MD, National Institute on Aging, 2018. Available at: https://order.nia.nih.gov/sites/default/files/2018-04/nia-exercise-guide.pdf

References

American College of Sports Medicine: ACSM's Guidelines for Exercise Testing and Prescription, 9th Edition. Edited by Pescatello LS, Arena R, Riebe D, et al. Philadelphia, PA, Wolters Kluwer/Lippincott Williams and Wilkins Health, 2014

Auais M, French S, Alvarado B, et al: Fear of falling predicts incidence of functional disability 2 years later: a perspective from an international cohort study. J Gerontol A Biol Sci Med Sci 73(9):1212–1215, 2018 29220420

Balady GJ, Chaitman B, Driscoll D, et al: Recommendations for cardiovascular screening, staffing, and emergency policies at health/fitness facilities. Circulation 97(22):2283–2293, 1998 9631884

Bethancourt HJ, Rosenberg DE, Beatty T, Arterburn DE: Barriers to and facilitators of physical activity program use among older adults. Clin Med Res 12(1–2):10–20, 2014 24415748

Bohannon RW: Reference values for the timed up and go test: a descriptive meta-analysis. J Geriatr Phys Ther 29(2):64–68, 2006 16914068

Borg G: Borg's Perceived Exertion and Pain Scales. Champaign, IL, Human Kinetics, 1998

Bravata DM, Smith-Spangler C, Sundaram V, et al: Using pedometers to increase physical activity and improve health: a systematic review. JAMA 298(19):2296–2304, 2007 18029834

Campaign to End Loneliness: Measuring Your Impact on Loneliness in Later Life. Available at: https://www.campaigntoendloneliness.org/wp-content/uploads/Loneliness-Measurement-Guidance1.pdf. Accessed March 21, 2019.

Chang S-C, Pan A, Kawachi I, Okereke OI: Risk factors for late-life depression: a prospective cohort study among older women. Prev Med 91:144–151, 2016 27514249

Clarke TC, Norris T, Sachiller JS: Early Release of Selected Estimates Based on Data From 2016 National Health Interview Survey. Hyattsville, MD, National Center for Health Statistics, May 2017. Available at: https://www.cdc.gov/nchs/data/nhis/earlyrelease/earlyrelease201705.pdf. Accessed March 21, 2019.

de Bruin ED, Hartmann A, Uebelhart D, et al: Wearable systems for monitoring mobility-related activities in older people: a systematic review. Clin Rehabil 22(10–11):878–895, 2008 18955420

De Jong Gierveld J, Van Tilburg T: A 6-item scale for overall, emotional, and social loneliness. Confirmatory Tests on Survey Data 28(5):582–598, 2006

Dipietro L, Caspersen CJ, Ostfeld AM, et al: A survey for assessing physical activity among older adults. Med Sci Sports Exerc 25(5):628–642, 1993 8492692

Dobkin BH, Dorsch A: The promise of mHealth: daily activity monitoring and outcome assessments by wearable sensors. Neurorehabil Neural Repair 25(9):788–798, 2011 21989632

Fairchild JK, Haws K, Mead C: The aging body and age-related health conditions, in Psychology of Aging: A Biopsychosocial Perspective. Edited by Yochim B, Woodhead E. New York, Springer, 2017, pp 49–86

Fletcher GF, Ades PA, Kligfield P, et al: Exercise standards for testing and training: a scientific statement from the American Heart Association. Circulation 128(8):873–934, 2013 23877260

Hawkley LC, Thisted RA, Cacioppo JT: Loneliness predicts reduced physical activity: cross-sectional and longitudinal analyses. Health Psychol 28(3):354–363, 2009 19450042

Helmerhorst HJ, Brage S, Warren J, et al: A systematic review of reliability and objective criterion-related validity of physical activity questionnaires. Int J Behav Nutr Phys Act 9(103):103, 2012 22938557

Huggett DL, Connelly DM, Overend TJ: Maximal aerobic capacity testing of older adults: a critical review. J Gerontol A Biol Sci Med Sci 60(1):57–66, 2005 15741284

Hughes ME, Waite LJ, Hawkley LC, et al: A short scale for measuring loneliness in large surveys: results from two population-based studies. Res Aging 26(6):655–672, 2004 18504506

Kempen GI, Yardley L, van Haastregt JC, et al: The Short FES-I: a shortened version of the Falls Efficacy Scale–International to assess fear of falling. Age Ageing 37(1):45–50, 2008 18032400

Krol-Zielinska M, Ciekot M: Assessing physical activity in the elderly: a comparative study of most popular questionnaires. Trends in Sports Sciences 22(3):133–144, 2015

Miller WR, Rollnick S: Motivational Interviewing, Helping People Change. New York, Guilford, 2012

Park C-H, Elavsky S, Koo K-M: Factors influencing physical activity in older adults. J Exerc Rehabil 10(1):45–52, 2014 24678504

Pauelsen M, Nyberg L, Röijezon U, et al: Both psychological factors and physical performance are associated with fall-related concerns. Aging Clin Exp Res 30(9):1079–1085, 2018 29264814

Peritz DC, Chung EH, Ryan JJ: The Role of Stress Testing in the Older Athlete. Expert Analysis. Washington, DC, American College of Cardiology, 2017. Available at: https://www.acc.org/latest-in-cardiology/articles/2017/11/06/10/32/the-role-of-stress-testing-in-the-older-athlete. Accessed March 21, 2019.

Petersen RC, Lopez O, Armstrong MJ, et al: Practice guideline update summary: Mild cognitive impairment: Report of the Guideline Development, Dissemination, and Implementation Subcommittee of the American Academy of Neurology. Neurology 90(3):126–135, 2018

Riebe D, Franklin BA, Thompson PD, et al: Updating ACSM's recommendations for exercise preparticipation health screening. Med Sci Sports Exerc 47(11):2473–2479, 2015 26473759

Schrack JA, Cooper R, Koster A, et al: Assessing daily physical activity in older adults: unraveling the complexity of monitors, measures, and methods. J Gerontol A Biol Sci Med Sci 71(8):1039–1048, 2016 26957472

Steffen TM, Hacker TA, Mollinger L: Age- and gender-related test performance in community-dwelling elderly people: six-minute walk test, Berg Balance Scale, Timed Up and Go test, and gait speeds. Phys Ther 82(2):128–137, 2002 11856064

Tucker JM, Welk GJ, Beyler NK: Physical activity in U.S.: adults compliance with the Physical Activity Guidelines for Americans. Am J Prev Med 40(4):454–461, 2011 21406280

U.S. Department of Health and Human Services: 2008 Physical Activity Guidelines for Americans. Washington, DC, U.S. Department of Health and Human Services, 2008. Available at: https://health.gov/paguidelines/2008/pdf/paguide.pdf. Accessed March 21, 2019.

Warburton DER, Nicol CW, Bredin SSD: Health benefits of physical activity: the evidence. CMAJ 174(6):801–809, 2006 16534088

Washburn RA, Smith KW, Jette AM, et al: The Physical Activity Scale for the Elderly (PASE): development and evaluation. J Clin Epidemiol 46(2):153–162, 1993 8437031

Watson KB, Carlson SA, Gunn JP, et al: Physical inactivity among adults aged 50 years and older—United States, 2014. MMWR Morb Mortal Wkly Rep 65(36):954–958, 2016 27632143

Wetherell JL, Bower ES, Johnson K, et al: Integrated exposure therapy and exercise reduces fear of falling and avoidance in older adults. a randomized pilot study. Am J Geriatr Psychiatry 26(8):849–859, 2018 29754811

Yesavage JA, Brink TL, Rose TL, et al: Development and validation of a geriatric depression screening scale: a preliminary report. J Psychiatr Res 17(1):37–49, 1982–1983 7183759

The Social Worker in Geriatric Outpatient Care

"Can You Help Me With This Patient?"

Laura Clayton, LCSW

CHAPTER 19

Clinical Presentation

Chief Concern of Referring Provider

"I have a patient with a complicated clinical picture who is also struggling to navigate daily needs due to isolation, limited mobility, and lack of support. Can you help me with this patient?"

Vignette

The social worker received a consult for Ms. S, age 85 years, because her providers were concerned that Ms. S was experiencing stress in multiple areas of functioning. Ms. S was living at home with her husband and was reliant on him for much of her day-to-day care, although they no longer had a loving or nurturing relationship. She had multiple debilitating medical conditions in addition to a long history of mental health issues. These challenges were compounded by worsening cognitive impairment. Upon first speaking with the social worker, Ms. S loudly pronounced, "My life is shit!"

During the assessment, Ms. S described no meaningful relationships. She was estranged from her living family members and had no close friendships. She described her husband as irritating and said that she felt stuck being in a relationship with him. She was involved with no social groups. Her closest relationships were with paid helpers who helped with household chores once or twice a week. She identified her sole reason for living was to care for her beloved pets.

Discussion

What Can Social Workers Bring to the Table?

Social workers can be very helpful in supporting patients in a primary care or geriatric mental health setting and within a multidisciplinary team approach. Social workers provide crucial psychosocial support to patients in navigating complex systems of care. In addition, social workers provide individual, family, and group therapy. Social workers are invaluable advocates for patients and critical members of multidisciplinary teams.

According to the National Association of Social Workers Code of Ethics,

> The primary mission of the social work profession is to enhance human well-being and help meet the basic human needs of all people, with particular attention to the needs and empowerment of people who are vulnerable, oppressed, and living in poverty. A historic and defining feature of social work is the profession's focus on individual well-being in a social context and the well-being of society. Fundamental to social work is attention to the environmental forces that create, contribute to, and address problems in living. (National Association of Social Workers 2017)

Social workers practice from a variety of theoretical frameworks. One framework that is extremely helpful in working with geriatric patients is systems theory. This framework emphasizes the connection between person and environment, specifically looking at the interactional dynamics between the person and the systems he or she interacts with on a regular basis. Systems involved in a particular patient's life could include family, friends, work, health care, and community. Systems theory recognizes the fact that small changes can have exponentially large effects on the individuals' life.

The social worker on a multidisciplinary team will utilize a person-centered and strengths-based approach. Social workers place high emphasis on building on the strengths of patients and will attempt to meet patients "where they are" currently when developing initial treatment recommendations. In other words, social workers will aim to vary their interventions for each patient based on the system and current set of resources available to them. Above all else, they emphasize patient self-determination and will serve as the patient's advocate within a multidisciplinary team to set goals that align with the patient's wishes.

Psychosocial Assessment

Prior to commencement of social work interventions, a psychosocial assessment is necessary. The depth and scope of the assessment will vary for each practice setting. A psychosocial assessment often includes cognitive, social, psychological, spiritual, financial, and legal dimensions of the client system (Swerdlow et al. 2017). As a social worker gathers information, genograms and eco-maps can be helpful tools in the assessment process and provide additional information to all members of the treatment team regarding the patient's current living situation, family history, and currently available psychosocial support. A *genogram* is a visual depiction of a patient's family system, including family members who are deceased, and the social relationships between members. A genogram is similar to a family tree, but information on relationships between family members is also included (Figure 19–1). An *eco-map* can be similar to a genogram, in that it may include information on family members; however, an eco-map is a more flexible way to include information on the systems a patient is involved with (Figure 19–2). Eco-maps often include nonfamily entities such as friends and organizations that are sources of support, stress, or conflict. Common psychosocial stressors include changes in social relationships, social isolation, financial problems, housing issues, and ageism. Perceived stress can also negatively impact an individual's mental health. Within a multidisciplinary team, social workers are in a prime position to help patients address psychosocial stressors and reduce overall levels of stress.

Vignette *(continued)*

In a psychosocial assessment with Ms. S from a systems perspective, the social worker was struck by Ms. S's interactions with her family, health care providers, and social systems. Of great concern was that Ms. S had very few systems involved in her life, and this became a goal for work. Increasing the number of connections and level of support Ms. S received from community agencies could provide an opportunity to change the overall functioning of her support system. When the treatment team considered the concept of

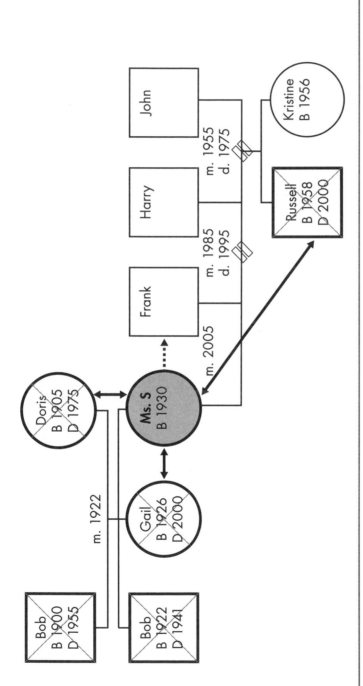

FIGURE 19–1. Genogram.

This genogram highlights Ms. S in the middle as the patient. Notice that she has very few connections. The *thicker lines* depict "good" relationships from Ms. S's perspective. The *dotted line* depicts conflict. Birth (B) and death (D) dates are included when known. The X through individuals is another way to depict that the specific person is deceased. The *diagonal equals sign* is another way to depict divorce (d). As much or as little detail can be included to make a genogram helpful, such as marriages (m), estrangements, domestic violence, mental health issues, or substance abuse issues.

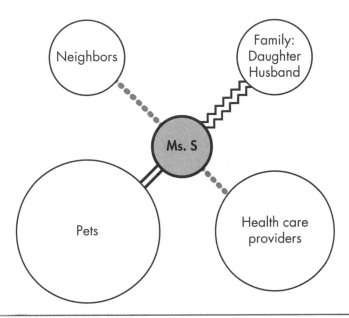

FIGURE 19-2. Eco-map.

In this eco-map, Ms. S is depicted by the *shaded circle* in the middle of the diagram. Similar to the genogram in Figure 19–1, notice how few systems are involved with Ms. S. In this map, the social worker adjusted the size of the circles based on importance to Ms. S. The connecting lines also vary depending on Ms. S's relationship with the system. Notice the *zigzagged* lines that connect Ms. S to her family. This conveys that Ms. S often has conflictual relationships with her family but is reliant on them on a daily basis.

"goodness of fit" between Ms. S and her environment, it was clear that Ms. S was experiencing severe disruptions. Ms. S's goals were not supported by the systems she interacted with, yet she was unable or unwilling without external support to add systems into her environment that would potentially improve the fit and support her goals.

In the case of Ms. S, transportation was also a major stressor, because she was unable to drive, which increased her isolation. Ms. S described this worsening isolation as directly contributing to worsening symptoms of depression. The team provided local resources to assist Ms. S in exploring transportation programs in her community. Two community programs that offered free or low-cost services to seniors in her community were identified.

Social Determinants of Health

Social determinants of health also fall within the psychosocial picture of geriatric mental health from a broader social work perspective. Social determinants of health are conditions in the environments in which people are born, live, learn, work, play, worship, and age that affect a wide range of health, functioning, and quality-of-life outcomes and risks (Office of Disease Prevention and Health Promotion 2018). These social and economic conditions impact the health and wellness of individuals and communities (Centers for Disease Control and Prevention 2018). Social work interventions with individual, families, and communities that help address these conditions can reduce health inequities and improve patient care outcomes.

According to the Office of Disease Prevention and Health Promotion (2018; see website, www.HealthyPeople.gov) and the Centers for Disease Control and Prevention (2018), examples of social determinants of health can include the following:

- Availability of resources to meet daily needs (e.g., safe housing and local food markets)
- Access to educational, economic, and job opportunities
- Access to health care services
- Quality of education and job training
- Availability of community-based resources in support of community living and opportunities for recreational and leisure-time activities
- Transportation options
- Public safety
- Social support
- Social norms and attitudes (e.g., discrimination, racism, distrust of government)
- Exposure to crime, violence, and social disorder (e.g., presence of trash, lack of cooperation in a community)
- Socioeconomic conditions (e.g., concentrated poverty and the stressful conditions that accompany it)
- Residential segregation
- Language/literacy
- Access to mass media and emerging technologies (e.g., cell phones, the internet, social media)
- Culture
- How a person develops during the first few years of life (early childhood development)
- Amount of education a person obtains
- Ability to get and keep a job
- Kind of work a person does
- Food security (having food or being able to get food)
- Access to health services and the quality of those services

- Housing status
- Amount of money a person earns
- Discrimination and social support

Vignette *(continued)*

When the treatment team considered the social determinants of health in Ms. S's situation, they noted that her social supports were extremely lacking and that improvements were likely to yield overall gains in her health. She also had difficulty accessing health care services because of transportation gaps and worsening cognitive impairment. This led to greater health inequity and warranted social work advocacy and assistance. Targeted referrals to transportation assistance were given in order to address this unmet need; however, Ms. S struggled to engage these resources on her own. In session, efforts were made to place calls with Ms. S to help start the process and engage outside agencies. The team also discussed linkage to memory support programs or an adult day program that could provide socialization and structure to Ms. S's day, which could reduce her social isolation and improve social support. Engaging a geriatric care manager might also be helpful, because this would provide Ms. S with direct, personalized support in navigating the complex health care system and improve her overall access to health care.

Social Work Interventions

Common social work interventions include community linkage and referral, psychoeducation, advocacy, individual therapy, and family therapy. Interventions will vary based on the social worker's assessment of the patient's unique situation and needs. Interventions will also vary depending on the social worker's training and scope of practice.

Social work interventions often include finding ways to empower the patient to initiate change. This concept is vital to social work practice because it decreases patient reliance on others and can strengthen the patient's sense of self-efficacy in creating sustainable improvements in his or her quality of life and health.

Vignette *(continued)*

In working with Ms. S, the team social worker attempted all the interventions identified thus far. Unfortunately, Ms. S did not follow up on the recommendations and referrals. As part of the social worker's continued efforts to help Ms. S, further assessment and rapport building were done and goals were pursued more aggressively. It became clearer that Ms. S's overall goal was to move into a senior living community. By narrowing in on this desire as the ultimate goal, the social worker was able to honor Ms. S's self-determination, and work was done to empower Ms. S in pursuit of this goal. This concept—start where the patient is—is a key point in empowering patients and achieving progress in treatment. Efforts to link Ms. S with transportation, social support, and a geriatric care manager were unsuccessful, in part due to Ms. S's desire to work on a different goal. Although transportation, social support, and a geriatric care manager would have all likely been helpful to Ms. S's well-being, those were not her goals. She was, however, ultimately able to identify an assisted-living environment in her community and moved in with her husband. At this point, her care was transferred to local providers.

Ethical Considerations

Although self-determination is crucial in successful interventions with patients, social workers must pay special attention to geriatric patients to ensure they are safe from abuse and neglect. Abuse and neglect laws vary in each state, so it is very important for clinicians to be familiar with the nuances where they practice.

Vignette *(continued)*

In the case of Ms. S, the team monitored her closely for self-neglect. Some of the interventions attempted with Ms. S, such as linkage to transportation assistance and a geriatric care manager, may have mitigated some of her risk factors, but she did not follow up on these referrals. This increased the team's concern for Ms. S and prompted increased monitoring until her situation was more stable.

During work with Ms. S before her move to assisted living, the social worker did end up reaching out to Adult Protective Services (APS) on more than one occasion. Involving APS can challenge the relationship and rapport between providers and patients. To preserve rapport with Ms. S, the social worker informed Ms. S directly when her situation rose to a level where the team needed to function as a mandated reporter and notify APS. Although Ms. S was frustrated by the decision, she did not disagree with her need for increased support, and Ms. S and the team were able to continue their work together. The social worker emphasized to Ms. S that her greatest concern was Ms. S's safety, and Ms. S appreciated the social worker's directness in informing her of the need to report before doing so, so that she wasn't blindsided.

KEY POINTS

- Social workers can be extremely valuable members of a multidisciplinary team.

- Social workers focus on patient-centered, strengths-based care.
- Social workers value patient self-determination and attempt to help patients develop greater self-efficacy.
- Social workers often practice from a systems perspective, assessing the patient as a person-in-environment and the goodness of fit between the patient and his or her environment.

Resources

Alzheimer's Association: www.alz.org (Has numerous and broad resources for patients with dementia and their caregivers, such as basic information on dementia, web training, and resource finding. Caregivers may find helpful the Northern California Chapter training "Savvy Caregivers," which is a multisession offering to build knowledge and skills of the caregiver.)

Family Caregiver Alliance: www.caregiver.org (Focuses on caregivers of adults with a variety of diagnoses. This website provides a wide array of resources for family caregivers, including caregiver education, online support groups, and links to state-specific caregiving information, as well as other useful resources through the "Family Care Navigator" feature.)

John A. Hartford Foundation: www.johnahartford.org (This website and the National Institute on Aging site [below] offer extensive information on a variety of topics related to health and aging. Their newsletters include helpful information on working with older adults.)

National Institute on Aging: www.nia.nih.gov

University of Michigan School of Social Work's Web-Based Certificate in Advanced Clinical Dementia Practice: https://ssw.umich.edu/offices/continuing-education/certificate-courses/clinical-dementia (This web-based training program is a 34-hour, self-paced certificate course on dementia assessment, care planning, and intervention.)

References

Centers for Disease Control and Prevention: Social Determinants of Health: Know What Affects Health. Atlanta, GA, Centers for Disease Control and Prevention, 2018. Available at: https://www.cdc.gov/socialdeterminants. Accessed June 9, 2018.

National Association of Social Workers: Code of Ethics. Washington, DC, National Association of Social Workers, 2017. Available at: https://www.socialworkers.org/About/Ethics/Code-of-Ethics/Code-of-Ethics-English. Accessed March 22, 2019.

Office of Disease Prevention and Health Promotion: Social Determinants of Health. Rockville, MD, Department of Health and Human Services, 2018. Available at: https://www.healthypeople.gov/2020/topics-objectives/topic/social-determinants-of-health. Accessed June 9, 2018.
Swerdlow S, Morano C, Morano B: Psychosocial assessment in care management, in Handbook of Geriatric Care Management. Edited by Cress CJ. Burlington, MA, Jones and Bartlett Learning, 2017, pp 35–62

Initial Evaluation and Management of Frontotemporal Dementia

"My Wife Seems Different"

Eveleigh Wagner, M.D.
Warren Taylor, M.D., MHSc
R. Ryan Darby, M.D.

CHAPTER 20

> We hold the opinion that Pick's disease does not belong to the extreme rarities, but that it remains often unrecognized by the clinician as well as the anatomist because not enough attention is directed to it.
>
> K. Onari and H. Spatz (1926)
> (quoted in Galimberti et al. 2015)

Clinical Presentation

Chief Complaint

"My wife seems different."

Vignette

Ms. T is a 65-year-old woman who was referred by her primary care physician for psychiatric consultation regarding changes in behavior, including notable social withdrawal. Ms. T has no significant past psychiatric history and a medical history relevant only for mild hypertension. She denies a family history of psychiatric illnesses aside from a family history of Alzheimer's disease (AD) in her mother and an alcohol use disorder in her son. She previously worked as a teacher but retired approximately 4 years ago. In recent years, she has spent her time volunteering with local women's groups.

In May 2017, she arrived with her husband for an initial psychiatric appointment. She was quiet and minimally interactive in the office. Her husband provided most of the history. He reported that 6 months ago his wife began "acting differently." She became more withdrawn, declined lunch invitations, and stopped volunteering. This was around the same time that her only son relapsed on alcohol and was readmitted for rehabilitation. At the time, her husband presumed she was overwhelmed by the stress. A few months later, Ms. T exhibited word-finding difficulties, where she would pause midsentence and occasionally appear frustrated with her speech. Her primary care physician recommended she see a psychiatrist for an evaluation out of concern that depression was the driving cause of these changes. The psychiatrist agreed with the diagnosis, started her on sertraline, and referred her to therapy.

Three months later, in August, she had increased difficulty with speech to the point that she could not speak to anyone but her husband. Despite titration and augmentation with bupropion, the antidepressant had not provided benefit. Given her worsening symptoms, she was referred to a neurologist, who ordered a magnetic resonance imaging (MRI) scan and "written tests," but the results were inconclusive. She continued taking her antidepressants and attended therapy weekly with her husband. A few months later, in a follow-up visit with the psychiatrist, her husband reported worsening social avoidance; she now refused to go to the grocery store. She was also exhibiting new episodes of odd behavior, including feeding expensive steaks to her dogs and serving soup with her hands, which resulted in a mild burn. Ms. T rarely spoke more than 5–10 words a day.

Ms. T was largely indifferent to these changes, which frustrated her husband. The psychiatrist again suspected a neurological cause for these changes, given that Ms. T had not improved with psychiatric treatment and was experiencing progressive behavior and speech changes. She was referred to a new neurologist with expertise in dementia for a second opinion on her condition.

By the time of Ms. T's second neurology appointment in December, she was no longer bathing or grooming and had developed incontinence. Her husband described her as staring at the wall for hours and at times inappropriately disrobing. She was seen by the neurologist, who discussed the likely diagnosis of dementia based on the progressive behavioral changes, apathy, and reduction of speech. The positron emission tomography (PET) scan ordered 14 months after symptom onset demonstrated the characteristic pattern for frontotemporal degeneration.

Discussion

Frontotemporal dementia (FTD) was initially described in 1892 by the Czech neurologist Arnold Pick in a patient with progressive deterioration of speech and evidence of left temporal lobe atrophy (Olney et al. 2017). In the early 1900s, the anatomy of Pick's cases was studied by Alois Alzheimer, who identified characteristic cell inclusions within the frontal and temporal lobes (Olney et al. 2017). Today, FTD describes clinical disorders whose symptoms include alterations in behavior, language, executive dysfunction, and motor symptoms (Olney et al. 2017). Although previously diseases of the frontotemporal lobes were collectively known as Pick's disease, currently there are three main variants of FTD: behavioral variant FTD (bvFTD), semantic variant primary progressive aphasia, and nonfluent/agrammatic variant primary progressive aphasia (Olney et al. 2017). The hallmark feature of these disorders is progressive atrophy of the frontal and temporal lobes (Karageorgiou and Miller 2014).

The incidence of FTD is estimated to be between 1.61 and 4.1 cases per 100,000 people annually, with approximately 20,000–30,000 people in the country having FTD at any one time (Coyle-Gilchrist et al. 2016; Knopman and Roberts 2011). The peak prevalence of the disorder is between 65 and 69 years of age, and FTD is the second most common dementing illness in persons under the age of 65 (Coyle-Gilchrist et al. 2016; Knopman and Roberts 2011). Within FTD, the behavioral variant is the most common, comprising approximately 60% of cases (Onyike and Diehl-Schmid 2013). BvFTD is defined by disinhibition, apathy, lack of empathy, compulsive behaviors, alterations in dietary habits, and reduced executive function (Olney et al. 2017). A summary of these criteria can be found in Table 20–1. The remainder of cases include the primary progressive aphasias (Olney et al. 2017). The semantic variant is identified by impaired object naming and word comprehension, while the nonfluent variant is defined by effortful speech and agrammatic language production (Laforce 2013). Upward of 15% of FTD patients have a concurrent motor neuron disease, such as amyotrophic lateral sclerosis (Olney et al. 2017). As the disorder progresses, patients can experience overlapping behavioral, language, and motor symptoms (Mann and Snowden 2017). From diagnosis, the average survival time is typi-

TABLE 20–1. Making the diagnosis of behavioral variant frontotemporal dementia (bvFTD)

Summary of criteria for bvFTD

1. Patient must show evidence of progressive deterioration in cognition, behavior, or both.

2. Patient must exhibit three of the following six symptoms:
    a. Early behavioral disinhibition
        i.   Inappropriate social behavior
        ii. Impulsive or reckless actions
    b. Early apathy
    c. Early loss of sympathy or empathy
        i.   Reduced response to others' needs
        ii. Reduced interpersonal attachment
    d. Early repetitive or compulsive behavior
        i.   Repetitive movements or speech
        ii. Ritualistic behavior or obsessions
    e. Changes in diet
        i.   Excess consumption of food (esp. sweets)
        ii. Ingesting inedible objects
    f. Executive dysfunction
        i.   Poor decision making
        ii. Impaired moral judgment

Note. Episodic memory and visuospatial skills are typically spared.
Source. Summarized from International Behavioral Variant FTD Criteria Consortium: Criteria for Behavioral Variant FTD, 2011. Available at https://www.theaftd.org/wp-content/uploads/2018/03/Table-3-International-consensus-criteria-for-behavioural-variant-FTD.pdf. Accessed August 22, 2018.

cally between 3 and 14 years, although isolated longer cases are reported (Lanata and Miller 2016).

While the majority of FTD cases occur sporadically, between 30% and 50% of cases appear to be familial. Approximately 10% of cases exhibit a clear autosomal dominant inheritance pattern, with three major genes identified: *C9orf72, MAPT,* and *GRN* (Mann and Snowden 2017). Almost all FTD cases are linked to one of four proteins, with tau and TDP-43 being the most common (Lanata and Miller 2016). In FTD these proteins misfold and form insoluble inclusions, resulting in cell death and brain dysfunction (Hock and Polymenidou 2016). One hypothesis proposes that the progressive nature of FTD is similar to that of the prion disease Creutzfeldt-Jakob disease (Hock and Polymenidou 2016). The misfolded proteins propagate throughout the brain much like a virus, which could account for the spread of atrophy across connected regions, and result in the variety of clinical syndromes.

Clinical Evaluation and Differential Diagnosis

In the early stages, bvFTD appears strikingly similar to primary psychiatric disorders, particularly as changes in behavior often precede cognitive decline (Lanata and Miller 2016). Persons eventually diagnosed with bvFTD frequently are first evaluated by mental health professionals. Given the overlap of psychiatric symptoms, it can be challenging to correctly diagnose FTD in its early stages. For example, symptoms of psychosis and apathy are common in patients with FTD, but these are also hallmarks of schizophrenia. Disinhibition, another key feature of FTD, can present as impulsivity, substance abuse, or excessive spending, behaviors often seen in bipolar disorder. More commonly, patients with bvFTD are diagnosed with depression due to social withdrawal and apathy. A significant delay can occur between initial presentation of symptoms and accurate diagnosis, which increases stress and burden on patients and families (Cardarelli et al. 2010; Lanata and Miller 2016). Overall, FTD is probably underdiagnosed because of the lack of awareness about the disease among nonneurologists, particularly in providers with limited experience working with geriatric populations (Olney et al. 2017). It is important to include FTD in the differential diagnosis of any older adult with first-episode onset of an apparent psychiatric disorder, particularly if there is a family history of dementia (Lanata and Miller 2016).

The evaluation of an adult patient with new behavioral change should include medical and psychiatric history, physical examination, lab testing, imaging, and referrals (Cardarelli et al. 2010). To begin, a provider should elicit a thorough history from both the patient and family members. Particular attention should be paid to the onset and progression of symptoms, including changes in behavior, mood, and speech as well as the development of functional impairment. A detailed family history of any psychiatric or neurological illnesses should include the age at onset when possible. Importantly, FTD can have different clinical presentations arising from a common genetic mutation, accounting for different presentations within families (Karageorgiou and Miller 2014).

Standardized assessment practices are important. Brief cognitive screening with tools such as the Montreal Cognitive Assessment can identify gross cognitive abnormalities, but can often be normal in early stages (Cardarelli et al. 2010). The patient-completed Frontal Assessment Battery and the caregiver-completed Frontal Behavioral Inventory can be useful in assessing frontal lobe dysfunction (Cardarelli et al. 2010; Slachevsky et al. 2004). The physical examination should focus on any new motor symptoms, including parkinsonism, seen on initial evaluation in approximately 20% of patients with bvFTD (Cardarelli et al. 2010; Karageorgiou and Miller 2014). Patients with clinical FTD symptoms accompanied by muscle twitching, weakness, or spasticity on examination may warrant electromyography testing for motor neuron disease (Laforce 2013; Olney et al. 2017). Completing the initial clinical evaluation, laboratory testing for reversible causes of dementia such as hypothyroidism and B_{12} deficiency is recommended (Sanford 2017).

Late-onset psychiatric illnesses and early FTD can be difficult to distinguish. Particular cases—such as late-onset depression or bipolar disorder, especially those with a progressive course, poor treatment response, or unusual medication reactions—should raise concern for a neurocognitive disorder (Galimberti et al. 2015). A similar concern is present for late-onset psychosis with cognitive features and poor response to antipsychotics. When differentiating FTD from psychiatric disorders such as late-onset schizophrenia, the clinician should assess symptoms that are not typically present in the psychiatric illness, such as hyperorality and predilection for sweets (Karageorgiou and Miller 2014). Red flags for further workup or referral, highlighted in Table 20–2, would include family history of dementia, deteriorating course, poor treatment response, or presence of cognitive impairment (Galimberti et al. 2015).

Should a diagnosis of FTD be suspected, the next steps include neuropsychological testing and imaging studies, recognizing that at any point in the timeline a patient can be referred to a neurologist for a second evaluation or completion of the workup. Because memory deficits may not be observable early in the disease course, neuropsychological testing can be tailored to evaluate for subtle language changes and can be essential for identifying primary progressive aphasia. A structural brain MRI is a key test that can evaluate for other causes of mental status change including tumors or vascular disease, while also assessing the pattern of cerebral atrophy (Gordon et al. 2016; Karageorgiou and Miller 2014). In comparisons of FTD with AD, patients with FTD typically exhibit volume loss primarily in the frontal and temporal lobes, whereas AD would exhibit more global atrophy, including parietal and

TABLE 20–2. Could it be frontotemporal dementia? Important clues and red flags from the initial evaluation

History
New psychiatric symptoms in an adult over age 45 years
New symptoms of functional impairment
Family history of dementia (especially early-onset)
Family history of psychiatric problems (especially late-onset)
Noted changes in personality
New bizarre, inappropriate behavior in an adult over age 45 years

Physical examination
Motor symptoms such as tremor, weakness
Difficulties with speech production

Cognitive testing
Impairments in language or executive planning on Montreal Cognitive Assessment
Difficulty following complex directions on Frontal Assessment Battery

temporal volume loss (Olney et al. 2017). Figures 20–1 and 20–2 illustrate findings of frontal and temporal atrophy associated with a diagnosis of FTD. Should specific atrophy patterns not be observed on a structural MRI when FTD is suspected, a fluorodeoxyglucose-PET scan—which measures metabolism within the brain—can provide better diagnostic accuracy (Karageorgiou and Miller 2014). Should a strong family history of cognitive disorders be present, it may be useful to conduct genetic testing for the known *C9orf72, MAPT,* and *GRN* mutations linked to FTD (Cardarelli et al. 2010).

Diagnostic certainty is captured as possible, probable, or definite FTD. *Possible* is based only on clinical evaluation of symptoms, whereas *probable* and *definite* are based on imaging and biopsy, respectively (Lanata and Miller 2016). Timely and accurate diagnosis of FTD allows for appropriately educating caregivers and connecting patients with resources while also helping to avoid unnecessary interventions that may be detrimental. With future scientific developments, early diagnosis could increase the effectiveness of disease-modifying therapies early in the disease course. Figure 20–3 illustrates a practical flow for workup and referral of suspected FTD. At any time along the diagnostic journey a patient can be referred to neurology for specialized evaluation.

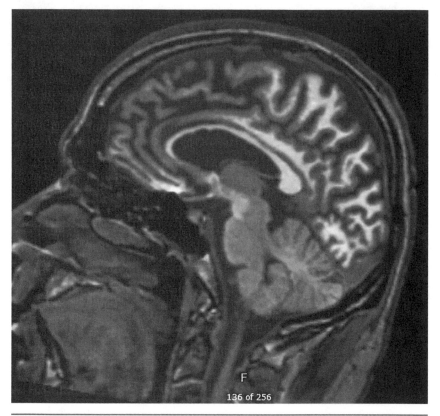

FIGURE 20–1. Sagittal magnetic resonance imaging (MRI) scan of a patient with frontotemporal dementia.

This MRI scan shows evidence of frontal atrophy in a patient with symptoms of behavioral variant frontotemporal dementia.

See Plate 1 to view this image in color.

Treatment

There are currently no U.S. Food and Drug Administration (FDA)–approved treatments for FTD. Because there are no disease-modifying treatments, medication treatment focuses on symptom management. Patients often lack insight about their limitations or are unable to communicate how they are feeling to others; therefore, the caregiver's observation of behavioral symptoms often guides both nonpharmacological and pharmacological treatment (Dinand et al. 2016). Nonpharmacological therapies focus on behavioral management and caregiver education. Medication management may be necessary when nonpharmacological efforts fail; however, medications have limited efficacy and a considerable side-effect burden in this population (Barton et al. 2016).

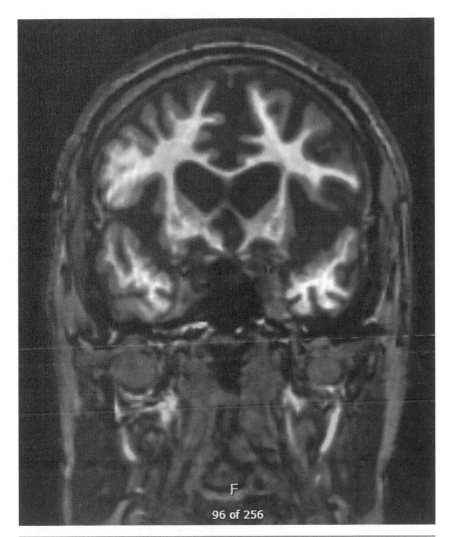

FIGURE 20–2. Coronal magnetic resonance imaging (MRI) scan of a patient with frontotemporal dementia.

This is a coronal slice of the same MRI scan from Figure 20–1, which shows additional evidence of frontal and temporal atrophy in a patient with symptoms of behavioral variant frontotemporal dementia.

See Plate 2 to view this image in color.

Nonpharmacological Interventions

One nonpharmacological model for the management of behavioral symptoms is the ABC model first described by Buckwalter, which focuses on identifying triggers and environmental responses that may contribute to the particular behavior (Barton et al. 2016). Some of the

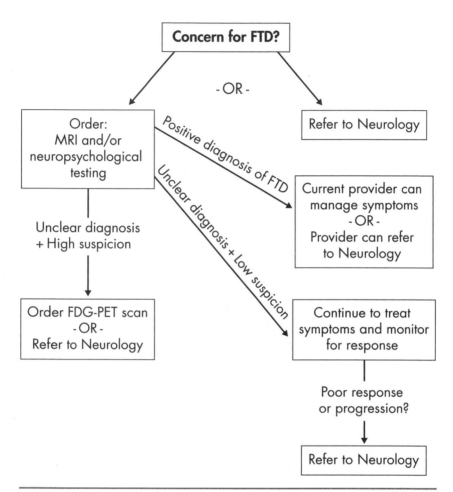

FIGURE 20–3. Steps to confirming a diagnosis of frontotemporal dementia (FTD).

FDG-PET = fluorodeoxyglucose-positron emission tomography; MRI = magnetic resonance imaging.

behaviors seen in FTD may be a result of overstimulation or misinterpretation of the environment, so reducing noise, clutter, and stimulation may be helpful. Problems with impulsivity can be mitigated by limiting access to credit cards, internet, or cars. As the disease progresses, it is important to be mindful of the patient's needs, because he or she may have difficulty communicating hunger, pain, fatigue, or warmth. When appropriate, modest exercise may be helpful for behavioral symptoms, while calming techniques such as distraction with music can reduce agitation (Barton et al. 2016). Caregivers should be cautioned against confronting or challenging the patient's inappropriate behavior or delusions, which could increase agitation. If wandering is a concern, it may be necessary to use identification bracelets, phone locators, or home monitoring devices for safety (Morhardt et al. 2015).

One particularly troubling behavioral symptom is sexual disinhibition. This can range from "sex talk," or provocative, inappropriate conversations, to "sexual acts" of disrobing or touching self or others. This type of behavior is frequently related to broader problems with impaired judgment and lesions in the frontal lobe (Cipriani et al. 2016). However, such behavior is not always sexual in nature and instead may be related to unverbalized discomfort, such as temperature in the case of disrobing or pain in the case of self-touching (Cipriani et al. 2016). The first step in managing these behaviors is to evaluate the frequency and context in which they occur and identify any triggers. Treatment can begin with the reduction of triggers, distraction with other activities, or modified clothing that opens in the back.

The CARE Pathway Model for Dementia emphasizes the importance of connecting patients and families with resources to enhance the network of care (Morhardt et al. 2015). This process involves broad input from multidisciplinary referrals. For example, providers can, when indicated, refer a patient to physical therapy for motor symptoms or speech therapy for aphasia symptoms (Morhardt et al. 2015). Home safety evaluations and driving evaluations are two other vital resources for caregivers and families to maintain a safe environment. Social work referrals can be useful to assess the family's individual needs and the impact of the disease on the family structure. Day programs may provide respite for caregivers or a safe space for patients when they can no longer be left at home alone, while referrals to occupational therapy can create structured activities attuned to the person's functional level (Barton et al. 2016). Such programs can also provide structure and mental stimulation for patients, who might otherwise remain sedentary (Shnall et al. 2013). While many providers routinely discuss medicolegal issues such as power of attorney and code status, some families may benefit from the input of an elder law attorney.

Pharmacological Interventions

Because there are no FDA-approved medications for FTD and no disease-modifying agents, medications are used off-label to reduce the severity of distressing symptoms. Notably, treatments used commonly for AD have not shown equal benefit for patients with FTD, and acetylcholinesterase inhibitors may worsen behavioral symptoms (Olney et al.

2017). Selective serotonin reuptake inhibitors (SSRIs) are largely used as first-line agents to assist with behavioral symptoms and underlying anxiety or depression, which could exacerbate symptoms of agitation or apathy (Olney et al. 2017). SSRIs can also be used to treat compulsive and repetitive behaviors. Atypical antipsychotics should be considered as second-line agents and used with caution because of the side-effect burden and black box warning in the elderly, but at times these may be necessary in the case of extreme agitation (Olney et al. 2017). When atypical antipsychotics are used, dosages should start out low and be increased at a slow rate. Additionally, if successful, atypical antipsychotic use should be reviewed regularly to ensure the medications are still required, and patients may benefit from attempts to taper and discontinue them. Other agents, such as benzodiazepines, should be avoided because of the risks of further disinhibition and falls, and substantial benefit has not been found for mood stabilizers in FTD (Olney et al. 2017). In cases of inappropriate sexual behavior, should nonpharmacological efforts fail, medications such as SSRIs can be used to reduce sexual urges (Cipriani et al. 2016). Future treatment approaches may include use of antibodies targeted at the proteins, such as tau, as a form of immunotherapy to eliminate the aggregates within cell bodies and reduce disease progression (Hock and Polymenidou 2016).

Patients with FTD can be treated by neurologists, psychiatrists, or even general practitioners depending on the complexity of the individual patient and comfort level of the provider with the patient's active symptoms. Reasons to refer a patient to a neurologist would be an unclear diagnosis, presence of motor symptoms, identified family history of the disease, or difficulty obtaining the proper workup. Neurologists within academic centers are often connected to clinical trials, which may be of interest to some families. Once the diagnosis is made, patients may benefit from longer-term treatment by a geriatric psychiatrist to manage behavioral symptoms.

Considerations for Caregivers

Given the limited therapeutic options, family members and caregivers are at the front line for nonpharmacological treatment. Caregivers of patients with dementia experience higher stress levels than those caring for loved ones without dementia (Cheng 2017). The reaction of family members toward a new diagnosis of FTD can be a mixture of both relief in finally having an answer for the change in their loved one and fear of a difficult future. Typical responses for caregivers can include anger, anxiety, embarrassment, and helplessness. It is important to normalize these feelings as natural responses to the diagnosis of a devastating illness (Caceres et al. 2016). Recent studies have shown that the presence of neuropsychiatric symptoms contributes to caregiver burnout, particularly for disruptive behaviors that strain the emotional connection between caregivers and their loved ones and increase the difficulty of assisting with activities of daily living (Cheng 2017). The burden of direct caretaking is high, but institutionalization can also impose an emotional toll, with feelings of guilt or inadequacy. Family members benefit from taking part in support groups early in the disease process, where they can receive education and emotional encouragement and share experiences (Cardarelli et al. 2010; Shnall et al. 2013).

Challenges for the caregiver extend beyond those related to direct patient care. Caregivers are also likely taking on previously shared responsibilities of household work, finances, or child care. There is also a significant sense of grief that their loved one will no longer be the same person he or she once was. Caregivers will need support as they adjust to the changed nature of the relationship with the patient (Caceres et al. 2016). Caring for a loved one with FTD is isolating, because patients are often unable to reciprocate social interaction or affection due to the apathetic symptoms (Shnall et al. 2013). As a coping mechanism, family members may find it helpful to view the behavioral symptoms as a part of the illness and not the individual (Caceres et al. 2016). Support for caregivers is vital, and they may benefit from disclosing the diagnosis to other family and close friends, which can increase awareness and foster understanding (Morhardt et al. 2015). It is important to encourage family members in self-care, because caring for a loved one with FTD is emotionally taxing over time.

KEY POINTS

- Frontotemporal dementia (FTD) is often misdiagnosed in its early stages due to the overlap in symptoms with common psychiatric disorders.
- It is important to keep FTD on the differential diagnosis for patients, in particular those presenting with late-life psychiatric symptoms.
- Atypical presentations of psychiatric symptoms, cognitive features, or nonresponse to traditional medications should heighten suspicion for the diagnosis of FTD.

- Additional testing, such as magnetic resonance imaging, positron emission tomography scan, or a neuropsychological battery, is essential to making the diagnosis. These can be either ordered by the initial provider or enveloped within a referral to neurology.
- Treatment at present is focused on symptom management; however, there is the potential for disease-modifying treatments in the future.
- Caregivers of those with FTD serve on the front lines for treatment. They should be encouraged to engage in support groups and other activities that bolster self-care.
- Referrals to other departments, such as physical therapy, occupational therapy, speech pathology, and social work, can help extend the network of care for the patient and family.

Resources

Resources for Clinicians

Consortium for Frontotemporal Dementia Research: www.bluefieldproject.org (Offers up-to-date information on clinical trials and treatment research.)

Frontal Assessment Battery: http://psychogeriatricsos.com.au/images/ pdf/frontal_fab_scale.pdf (Brief test for specific frontal symptoms found in FTD.)

Frontal Behavioral Inventory: www.virtualhospice.ca/Assets/ FBI_test_Nov0907_20151210172144.pdf (Questionnaire for caregivers regarding patient behavior.)

Montreal Cognitive Assessment (MoCA): www.parkinsons.va.gov/ resources/MOCA-Test-English.pdf (Brief test for cognitive function.)

Resources for Families

Organizations and Online Resources

Alzheimer's Association: 225 N. Michigan Ave., Floor 17, Chicago, IL 60601; (800) 272-3900; www.alz.org

Association for Frontotemporal Degeneration (AFTD): Radnor Station Building 2, Suite 320, 290 King of Prussia Road, Radnor, PA 19087; (866) 507-7222; www.theaftd.org

Family Caregiver Alliance, 101 Montgomery Street, Suite 2150, San Francisco, CA 94104; (800) 445-8106; www.caregiver.org

FTD Support Forum: http://ftdsupportforum.com (online group for caregivers to connect and share information)

National Institute of Neurological Disorders and Stroke: www.ninds.nih.gov (Provides information on FTD, treatment options, resources and active clinical trials; for information about FTD for caregivers, see Frontotmeporal Disorders: Hope Through Research: www.ninds.nih.gov/Disorders/Patient-Caregiver-Education/Hope-Through-Research/Frontotemporal-Disorders)

National Institute on Aging: Building 31, Room 5C27, 31 Center Drive, MSC 2292, Bethesda, MD 20892; (800) 438-4380 (Alzheimer's Disease and Related Dementias Education and Referral Center; www.nia.nih.gov; www.nia.nih.gov/alzheimers/clinical-trials)

Books

Lipton AM, Marshall CD: The Common Sense Guide to Dementia for Clinicians and Caregivers. New York, Springer, 2013

Mace NL, Rabins PV: The 36 Hour Day: A Family Guide to Caring for People Who Have Alzheimer's Disease, Other Dementias, and Memory Loss, 6th Edition. Baltimore, MD, Johns Hopkins University Press, 2017

Radin G, Radin L (eds): What If It's Not Alzheimer's? A Caregiver's Guide to Dementia, 3rd Edition. Amherst, NY, Prometheus Books, 2014

References

Barton C, Ketelle R, Merrilees J, et al: Non-pharmacological management of behavioral symptoms in frontotemporal and other dementias. Curr Neurol Neurosci Rep 16(2):14, 2016 26750129

Caceres BA, Frank MO, Jun J, et al: Family caregivers of patients with frontotemporal dementia: an integrative review. Int J Nurs Stud 55:71–84, 2016 26612696

Cardarelli R, Kertesz A, Knebl JA: Frontotemporal dementia: a review for primary care physicians. Am Fam Physician 82(11):1372–1377, 2010 21121521

Cheng ST: Dementia caregiver burden: a research update and critical analysis. Curr Psychiatry Rep 19(9):64, 2017 28795386

Cipriani G, Ulivi M, Danti S, et al: Sexual disinhibition and dementia. Psychogeriatrics 16(2):145–153, 2016 26215977

Coyle-Gilchrist IT, Dick KM, Patterson K, et al: Prevalence, characteristics, and survival of frontotemporal lobar degeneration syndromes. Neurology 86(18):1736–1743, 2016 27037234

Dinand C, Nover SU, Holle D, et al: What is known about the subjective needs of people with behavioural variant frontotemporal dementia? A scoping review. Health Soc Care Community 24(4):375–385, 2016 25827780

Galimberti D, Dell'Osso B, Altamura AC, et al: Psychiatric symptoms in frontotemporal dementia: epidemiology, phenotypes, and differential diagnosis. Biol Psychiatry 78(10):684–692, 2015 25958088

Gordon E, Rohrer JD, Fox NC: Advances in neuroimaging in frontotemporal dementia. J Neurochem 138 (suppl 1):193–210, 2016 27502125

Hock EM, Polymenidou M: Prion-like propagation as a pathogenic principle in frontotemporal dementia. J Neurochem 138 (suppl 1):163–183, 2016 27502124

Karageorgiou E, Miller BL: Frontotemporal lobar degeneration: a clinical approach. Semin Neurol 34(2):189–201, 2014 24963678

Knopman DS, Roberts RO: Estimating the number of persons with frontotemporal lobar degeneration in the US population. J Mol Neurosci 45(3):330–335, 2011 21584654

Laforce R Jr: Behavioral and language variants of frontotemporal dementia: a review of key symptoms. Clin Neurol Neurosurg 115(12):2405–2410, 2013 24446563

Lanata SC, Miller BL: The behavioural variant frontotemporal dementia (bvFTD) syndrome in psychiatry. J Neurol Neurosurg Psychiatry 87(5):501–511, 2016 26216940

Mann DMA, Snowden JS: Frontotemporal lobar degeneration: pathogenesis, pathology and pathways to phenotype. Brain Pathol 27(6):723–736, 2017 28100023

Morhardt D, Weintraub S, Khayum B, et al: The CARE pathway model for dementia: psychosocial and rehabilitative strategies for care in young-onset dementias. Psychiatr Clin North Am 38(2):333–352, 2015 25998120

Olney NT, Spina S, Miller BL: Frontotemporal dementia. Neurol Clin 35(2):339–374, 2017 28410663

Onyike CU, Diehl-Schmid J: The epidemiology of frontotemporal dementia. Int Rev Psychiatry 25(2):130–137, 2013 23611343

Sanford AM: Mild cognitive impairment. Clin Geriatr Med 33(3):325–337, 2017 28689566

Shnall A, Agate A, Grinberg A, et al: Development of supportive services for frontotemporal dementias through community engagement. Int Rev Psychiatry 25(2):246–252, 2013 23611354

Slachevsky A, Villalpando JM, Sarazin M, et al: Frontal assessment battery and differential diagnosis of frontotemporal dementia and Alzheimer disease. Arch Neurol 61(7):1104–1107, 2004 15262742

Legal Issues in Cognitive Disorders

"Mom Changed Her Will"

Leah McGowan, J.D.
Michael Kelly, M.D.

CHAPTER 21

Clinical Presentation

Chief Complaint

"We're worried about Mom. Her home health aide won't let us talk to her, and Aunt Genie said that Mom changed her will."

Vignette

Ms. U is an 89-year-old woman who was diagnosed with Alzheimer's disease (AD) 2.5 years ago. A full-time home health aide has been living with her for the past year. Ms. U's three adult children live several hours away in a metropolitan area and visit their mother every 2–3 months. Ms. U's adult children have become increasingly concerned in recent months due to their mother's refusal to see them or speak with them over the phone. Ms. U's sister, Genie, recently called the children to tell them that their mother had changed her will and listed the home health aide as the sole recipient of her estate. Ms. U's children subsequently called an attorney, who recommended a forensic psychiatrist to evaluate their mother's testamentary capacity.

Discussion

Cognitive Disorders and the Law

At its best, the law functions to protect individuals with vulnerabilities while preserving, to the maximum extent practical, individual autonomy. Instances of government involvement with the life choices of the sick, disabled, or elderly date back to the thousands-years-old doctrines of *parens patriae* ("parent of the nation"—a doctrine with roots in English Common Law that allows the state to serve as a guardian for children, the mentally ill, the elderly, or disabled persons who are unable to care for themselves) and *De Praerogativa Regis* ("The Prerogative of the King"—a 1324 statute in the English legal system that gave jurisdiction over the persons and property of "idiots" and those who "happen to fail their wit" to the monarch). The spectrum for the court's allocation of a person's life choices ranges from ordering the implementation of an individual's own advance directive to appointing a guardian or conservator to make all significant decisions for the individual.

The law can also validate or invalidate an individual's actions or choices through the concepts and doctrines of *capacity* and *competency*. Such decisions by a court may lead, for example, to declaring a will invalid, granting a judgment of nullity on a marriage, reducing the sentence for a charged crime, or finding an accused innocent in criminal court.

The individual, his or her family, the government (a court or government agency such as the Department of Human Services, Social Security, prosecutor's office, or public defender's office), or an unrelated but financially interested individual may ask for a capacity assessment to inform his or her decision or support his or her position on any of these issues. Assessing capacity is also relevant for providers who need to determine whether their patient has the capacity to consent to treatment.

In this chapter, we introduce some of the legal concepts and issues relevant to the care of geriatric individuals who have cognitive disorders.

Legal Concepts in Geriatric Decision Making: Competency, Capacity, and Consent

In the medicolegal context, the terms *competency, capacity,* and *consent* are distinct but related terms. An understanding of these terms is useful to navigate issues in geriatric decision making. *Capacity* is a time- and situation-specific determination made by health care providers. Decisions regarding "capacity" or "decisional capacity" are based on the clinical appraisal of an individual's ability to function in regard to a specific demand or situation (Mishkin 1989). *Competence* is a legal determination. It can be specific to an issue (e.g., a judge can find an individual competent to stand trial) or a global determination. Bringing the terms together, a court will make a finding regarding an individual's *competence* based on a physician or other health care worker's opinion of that individual's *capacity*. Competence is a legal term that refers to the capacity to perform or make decisions in a specific context.

The terms *competence* and *capacity* are often used interchangeably, however, in both the psychiatric and the legal literature (Appelbaum 2007). For example, the Uniform Probate Code (UPC 2010; an act that sets standards for how inheritance and estates are allocated) now uses the term "incapacitated" rather than "incompetent," and the Uniform Adult Guardianship and Protective Proceedings Jurisdiction Act (UAGPPJA) (2007); an act aimed at clarifying jurisdiction and providing a procedural roadmap for handling dilemmas that arise when more than one state is involved in a guardianship) also reflects this trend. Both the UPC and the UAGPPJA offer standard rules, but individual states must adopt these acts, or particular provisions of the acts, before they become enforceable in an individual state. At the time of this writing, all states except for Kansas, Florida, Michigan, and Texas have adopted the UAGPPJA in its entirety, and 18 states have adopted the UPC in its entirety.

As to *consent,* an individual must have the capacity to consent in order for the consent to be valid. To provide consent to treatment, a patient must possess the capacity, or decisional capacity, to do so. Paul Appelbaum (2007) summarized the four key factors of decisional capacity as follows: "Legal standards for decision-making capacity for consent to treatment vary somewhat across jurisdictions, but generally they embody the abilities to communicate a choice, to understand the relevant information, to appreciate the medical consequences of the situation, and to reason about treatment choices" (p. 1835).

Forensic Assessment of Competencies and Capacities

It is beyond the scope of this chapter to describe methods that mental health professionals use to help assess the decision-making abilities of persons with cognitive decline. In general, however, a number of tools are available to assist practitioners in making such determinations, including formal neuropsychological testing and functional assessment scales. The MacArthur Competence Assessment Tool for Treatment (Grisso and Appelbaum 1995) and the Aid to Capacity Evaluation (ACE; Etchells et al. 1999) are two instruments that can help assess a patient's capacity to make medical decisions. The ACE is free and available online at http://jcb.utoronto.ca/tools/ace_download.shtml. Forensic evaluators may also rely on forensic assessment instruments designed to determine whether the evaluee is able to meet a specific legal requirement (Sousa et al. 2014). Such evaluations are typically carried out by mental health professionals who have training and expertise in performing forensic evaluations on geriatric populations.

Legal Instruments to Convey or Allocate Decision Making

Recent trends in geriatric care and decision making focus on honoring the individual's own choices whenever possible. Legal mechanisms that facilitate this goal include advance directives and the newer legal trend of supported decision making (SDM).

Advance Directives

Under the Patient Self-Determination Act (1990), providers must inform patients about the right to refuse or accept treatment and to create advance directives. *Advance directives* are legal documents that allow patients to make future health care decisions for themselves that are to be implemented if the patient lacks decision-making capacity at some future time. The subjects covered by an advance directive differ by state and may or may not include psychiatric care.

A *psychiatric advance directive* (PAD) allows a patient with chronic or severe mental disabilities to outline treatment desires for periods when the patient may become incapacitated due to mental illness (Swanson et al. 2006). Clinicians may override a PAD, however, if a choice in the PAD 1) conflicts with the doctor's view of the standard of care or 2) conflicts with civil commitment law. According to the National Resource Center on Psychiatric Advance Directives (2017), 25 U.S. states have PAD statutes. The National Resource Center on Psychiatric Advance Directives provides state-by-state information on PADs (see "Resources").

A court order is not required to make and execute advance directives. A patient's advance directive takes effect once a physician determines the patient lacks capacity to make medical decisions. A patient can change the advance directive at any time while the patient is capable of making the decision to change and then refuse the treatment he or she had previously chosen to accept. Advance directives are facile when the advance directive permits the treatment recommended by the care provider and the patient who lacks capacity assents to that recommended treatment. If a patient who lacks capacity refuses treatment or tries to change an advance directive, however, a guardian or court order may be needed.

Advance directives can express personal treatment preferences (e.g., decision directives or living wills), create proxy directives (e.g., durable power of attorney), or do both. Generally, if a patient has both a durable power of attorney and a living will, the living will overrides the former.

Proxy Directives (Durable Power of Attorney)

Proxy directives designate a particular individual to make financial and/or medical decisions for a person in the event that person ever lacks capacity. Most states in the United States have statutes authorizing proxy directives, or "durable powers of attorney for health care." (See the "Resources" section for the American Bar Association's state-by-state guide to power of attorney statutes.) The statute will specify when the power of attorney will take effect, typically when the patient's physician determines that he or she lacks decision-making capacity. At that point, the physician must obtain informed consent from the designated proxy. The health care proxy is the actual document the person signs to allow another individual to make health care decisions on his or her behalf in the event of incapacity.

Decision Directives (Living Wills)

Decision directives, or living wills, allow patients to outline preferences for health care treatment. Like proxy directives, they typically become effective when a patient lacks decisional capacity. Patients can use living wills to declare their wishes regarding the use of life-sustaining treatment in the event they become terminally ill or permanently unconscious. Thus, the living will authorizes physicians to follow instructions regarding medical treatment that was previously designated by the patient.

Only a patient can revoke his or her own living will. A patient can change or revoke the living will at any time, as long as he or she is capable of making the decision to change the living will. Unfortunately, a patient's living will may not envision all potential scenarios or take into account advances in medical science that might change prognoses.

Vignette *(continued)*

Upon inquiry, the forensic psychiatrist learned that Ms. U had a proxy directive that designated her oldest daughter to make financial decisions for her in the event Ms. U ever lost the capacity to manage her own money. Pending conclusion of a capacity assessment, the oldest daughter may be able to override financial decisions Ms. U made when she lacked financial capacity.

Supported Decision Making

SDM has recently emerged as an alternative to guardianship (American Bar Association Commission on Law and Aging 2017a). It places the individual with a disability at the center of the decision-making process. SDM describes a process that utilizes input from friends, family, social services, community organizations, and other sources of support to weigh the pros and cons of a decision, review potential outcomes, and make a choice. SDM takes many forms, from recognition of informal, yet practical, decision-making networks to formal, written, supported decision-making agreements.

According to the American Bar Association Commission on Law and Aging (2017a), lawyers, courts, state legislatures, and the U.S. Department of Health and Human Services have started to endorse SDM. Readers interested in learning more about SDM and other alternatives to guardianship may explore the resources and research available at the American Bar Association's Commission on Law and Aging website, referred to in the "Resources" section.

Conservatorship/Guardianship

The law's most drastic allocation of a person's life choice is the appointment of a guardian or conservator. *Guardianships* and *conservatorships* are formal legal processes in which a court declares that a person lacks the capacity for making life decisions or managing his or her financial affairs. The court then appoints someone to act on behalf of the incapacitated person. The purpose of the appointment is to protect the incapacitated individual from exploitation and neglect, but the appointment comes at great cost to the individual's freedom, agency, and self-determination.

Standards and definitions vary across jurisdictions and are often vague, but the UPC defines "incapacitated person" as follows:

> An individual who, for reasons other than being a minor, is unable to receive and evaluate information or make or communicate decisions to

such an extent that the individual lacks the ability to meet essential requirements for physical health, safety, or self-care, even with appropriate and reasonably available technological assistance. (Uniform Probate Code 2010).

Some states have moved to a more functional definition requiring that the person lack the ability to provide for his or her basic personal needs for food, clothing, and shelter. The American Bar Association Commission on Law and Aging et al. (2006) offer a model "Clinical Evaluation Report" for guardianship proceedings, referred to in the "Resources" section, which gives insight into the factors analyzed by a court in these proceedings.

In most jurisdictions, conservatorships and guardianships *of the estate* are proceedings to appoint someone to manage financial affairs (Schouten and Brendel 2017). Guardianships *of the person* appoint someone to make one or more nonfinancial decisions, such as decisions about health care or housing (Schouten and Brendel 2017). Some states use the term "guardianship" for both protection of the person and protection of the estate; some states use the term "conservatorship" for both purposes (Schouten and Brendel 2017).

An appointment of a guardianship means that the subject individual may not enter contracts, manage funds, file lawsuits, vote, or consent to surgery. A "rebuttable presumption" applies to the individual's testamentary capacity, which means that unless proven otherwise, the law assumes the person lacks the capacity to make a will.

The guardians and conservators appointed by the court must make decisions on behalf of the incapacitated person according to one of two basic standards, or a combination of them. The traditional standard is the "best interest standard." By this standard, the guardian must act according to the "best interest" of the incapacitated person. The second standard is the "substituted judgment" standard, under which the guardian must choose as the incapacitated person would have chosen before becoming incapacitated. Under the substituted judgment standard, advance directives serve as good evidence of what the incapacitated person would have chosen. Because there is no uniform standard across the United States, it is important for clinicians to know the standard in their jurisdiction.

In guardianship/conservatorship proceedings, courts may seek the guidance of experts to evaluate whether a person is "incapacitated." The evaluation of capacity calls for an assessment of the functional abilities the individual lacks and retains. The court will then consider whether to authorize a guardianship or conservatorship, and if so, the appropriate terms. Moye et al. (2007) identified six factors to be assessed as part of the evaluation:

1. Underlying medical condition that is causing functional disability
2. Level of cognitive functioning
3. Person's ability to function on a daily basis, including self-care and medical decision making
4. Preferences of the individual in question
5. Risk of harm and need for supervision
6. Means to enhance capacity

Guardianship deprives an individual of virtually all legal rights to make decisions and choices. Before a guardian is appointed, the court generally must find that there is a need for a guardian and that no less restrictive alternative would be possible and effective (Uniform Guardianship, Conservatorship, and Other Protective Arrangements Act 2017). Less-restrictive alternatives include a limited guardianship, in which the guardian is granted only the powers that are required for the safety and protection of the incapacitated person, who retains as many abilities and powers as possible (i.e., guardian of estate only). Other alternatives include making advance directives, discussed earlier; appointing a representative payee for Social Security benefits; designating a custodian of Veterans Administration funds; or creating a trust.

The American Bar Association has advocated for less-restrictive alternatives to guardianship. It takes the position that courts, family members, and others tend to assume that the decision-making abilities of persons with disabilities (including older individuals with dementia) are compromised, resulting in guardians for people who could continue to make their own decisions with the right supports and services (American Bar Association Commission on Law and Aging 2017b). The American Bar Association Commission on Law and Aging, Commission on Disability Rights, Section on Civil Rights and Social Justice, and Section on Real Property, Trust and Estate Law created a tool for identifying and implementing decision-making options for persons with disabilities that are less restrictive than guardianship. Readers can find a link to the tool in the "Resources" section of this chapter.

Testamentary Capacity

Testamentary capacity is the legal and mental ability to create or alter a will (Sousa et al. 2014). Individuals need to have testamentary capacity if they want to make or change a will. If someone wants to enforce or challenge a will, that person may need to prove that the testator (person making the will) either did or did not have testamentary capacity when he or she made or changed the will.

Standards differ across jurisdictions, but generally speaking, to have testamentary capacity, an individual must 1) generally understand the nature and extent of his or her assets; 2) be aware of the people who would naturally be his or her heirs; 3) understand the nature of a will and that he or she is signing a will; and 4) be free of delusion (Schouten and Brendel 2017).

Testamentary capacity is determined based on capacity at the time of writing the will. This means that if someone loses his or her testamentary capacity hours after executing a will, the will is still valid. Similarly, if someone wants to invalidate a will executed by someone who may experience temporary lapses in testamentary capacity, he or she will have to prove that the person lacked capacity at the exact time the will was executed. To avoid the challenges of assessing capacity at a time in the past, patients should be advised to obtain an evaluation of testamentary capacity at the time they want to make or change their will (Schouten and Brendel 2017).

Even if a testator had testamentary capacity, undue influence can still void a will. *Undue influence* occurs when someone exerts enough influence over a testator to overcome the testator's free will and cause the testator to act in a way he or she otherwise would not have acted (The Restatement [Third] of Property 2003). Undue influence may occur in the caregiver/patient context, for example, if a caregiver threatens to withhold standard care unless the testator includes the caregiver in the testator's will. Undue influence impairs the testator's ability to decide freely about the distribution of his property. The law will not recognize a will that does not represent the wishes of the testator as a result of undue influence.

Susceptibility to undue influence may include advancing age, the mental and physical condition of the testator, and the relationship between the testator and the person who is being alleged to have unduly influenced the testator. It is reasonable, however, for certain parties, such as a spouse, to exert reasonable influence over a testator or to legitimately persuade a testator. This type of influence is not considered to be "undue." Thus, it is "undue influence," not mere "influence," that invalidates a will.

Delusional beliefs can also invalidate a will. A delusion is a "fixed false belief that is held despite evidence to the contrary" (Kennedy 2012, p. 193). (Some state statutes and case law still use the dated term "insane delusion.") In order to invalidate a will on the basis of a delusional belief, the individual would have to show that the testator was experiencing the delusion at the time he or she executed the will and that the delusion affected the substance of the will (Kennedy 2012). For example, the testator may have held the delusional belief that aliens had inhabited her son's body and were controlling her son's actions. If the testator removed her son from her will because she did not want to give aliens access to her inheritance, the removal would be invalidated if the son could prove the delusional belief caused the change to his mother's will. There are several guidelines for evaluating testamentary capacity but no specific instruments (Sousa et al. 2014).

Financial Capacity

Financial capacity is "the capacity to manage money and financial assets in ways that meet a person's needs and which are consistent with his/her values and self-interest" (Marson et al. 2011, p. 41). Financial capacity is considered an advanced activity of daily living (Moye and Marson 2007) that is highly sensitive and vulnerable to mild cognitive impairment and mild AD (Marson 2015). Financial capacities of the general elderly population, as well as individuals who have dementia, depression, anxiety, psychotic disorder, or hypomania, are often questioned, giving rise to the need for a financial capacity determination (Sousa et al. 2014). To find a person incompetent to manage his or her finances, the court must find that the person lacks the capacity to manage finances. If it makes this finding, the court may appoint a guardian of estate or a conservator (depending on the term used by the jurisdiction). Reasons for appointing a guardian of estate or conservator include squandering money, hoarding money, or being easily victimized.

As for assessments, the functional approach (as opposed to a diagnostic approach) is the widely accepted model in the determination of financial capacity (Sousa et al. 2014). The Financial Capacity Instrument (FCI; Marson et al. 2000) assesses domain-level financial activities and task-specific financial abilities. It directly tests performance on financial tasks, financial domains, and overall financial capacity (Marson et al. 2000). The Financial Capacity Instrument—Short Form (FCI-SF; Marson 2015) is a performance measure developed from the FCI. The FCI-SF was designed to detect financial skill declines in early phases of AD. It measures task completion time and directly tests performance on monetary calculation, financial conceptual knowledge, use of a checkbook/registry, and use of bank statements (Marson 2015). However, when an assessment of financial capacity is being made, Sousa and colleagues also recommend considering medical conditions or mental disorders, the values and preferences of the individual, cognition, emotional functioning, personality, and financial, social, and cultural factors (Sousa et al. 2014).

In sum, the functional assessment measures may be able to detect functional impairment in preclinical AD. For purposes of assessing financial capacity for legal and other functional determinations, however, an individual's functionality should be considered within the context of additional factors.

Abuse and Neglect

Abuse and neglect in the elderly population are fairly common yet highly underreported (Cooper et al. 2008). Types of elder abuse include physical abuse, psychological or verbal abuse, sexual abuse, financial exploitation, and neglect (Lachs and Pillemer 2015). A study conducted by Cooper et al. (2008) reviewed the prevalence of elder abuse and found that about a quarter of older people dependent on another for care reported significant psychological abuse. A fifth reported neglect. Interestingly, over a third of family members who provided the care for dependent elders reported perpetrating significant abuse. These findings suggest that vulnerable older people are at high risk of abuse and that they and their family members are often willing to report it. Cooper et al. (2008) concluded that routinely asking individuals and those who care for them about abuse will often lead to its detection.

Financial exploitation is a form of elder abuse. It includes taking, hiding, or using the money or property of an elder or dependent adult wrongfully or with intent to defraud (i.e., using undue influence to get a victim to sign documents such as a will, trust, property transfer, and so forth without a financial power of attorney or conservator). It also includes consumer fraud by businesses. The appointment of a conservator, discussed earlier, is one legal mechanism designed to protect against financial elder abuse.

Most states have elder and dependent adult abuse reporting laws. These statutes require helping professions, such as physicians and home health providers, to report suspected elder abuse or neglect. In some states, everyone is a mandated reporter. Mandatory reporting laws differ in regard to the language used to describe the standard for reporting; however, most include language akin to having a cause to reasonably suspect that an elderly individual (or other vulnerable person, such as a child or a developmentally disabled adult) has been abused or neglected.

Mandatory reporters can satisfy their reporting obligation by contacting an adult protective services agency. Most states have these agencies, which help elders and dependent adults when these adults are unable to meet their own needs or are victims of abuse, neglect, or exploitation. These agencies typically provide investigatory, protective, and social services and are usually administered by state or county human services. Readers interested in learning more about elder abuse or the reporting requirements in their jurisdiction are encouraged to visit the website run by the National Center on Elder Abuse (https://ncea.acl.gov).

In general, mandated reporters are not held criminally or civilly liable for reports of abuse made in good faith. On the other hand, liability may arise from knowingly submitting a false report. Failure to report, or impeding or inhibiting a report of elder abuse, is a misdemeanor in many jurisdictions.

Vignette *(continued)*

During the capacity evaluation, the psychiatrist addressed the potential for elder abuse. The psychiatrist asked indirect questions to make the interview less threatening (e.g., "Ms. U, do you feel safe at home?").

Family Disagreements

In the absence of an enforceable advance directive, some states (e.g., Utah, Louisiana, Georgia) have statutes that recognize family members as appropriate decision makers for health care choices in the event of decisional incapacity. Other states do not have statutes but have case law that authorizes allocating health care decisions to family according to a hierarchy. These statutes and case law typically set forth the following hierarchy: 1) spouses, 2) adult children, 3) parents, 4) siblings, and 5) more distant relations (e.g., see Louisiana 2005). The omission of long-term partners and significant others from this list can create complex issues for those who may not have legal standing to make decisions for their beloved ones. It can also create tension when family members disagree on the best health care decision for the sick individual. Ideally, an advance directive can avoid or minimize these issues.

Marriage and Divorce

What if, at age 82, your patient divorces her husband of 40 years and marries a 30-year-old suitor? Marriage is a type of contract. The capacity to marry and divorce incorporates elements of contractual and financial capacities. A contract is not valid if one of the parties did not have a true understanding of what he or she was doing at the time of entering the contract, due to mental illness. As with other competency evaluations, it must be shown that a mental disability (including cognitive disabilities) rendered the individual unable to appreciate the nature of the transaction or its ramifications. Simple ignorance or lack of sophistication is not enough to invalidate a contract. In most jurisdictions, to be competent to marry, the individual must be capable of understanding the nature of the marriage contract and the duties and financial responsibilities it creates (*Dunphy v. Dunphy* 1911).

Typically, courts will annul a marriage if either party was of "unsound mind" or unable to understand the nature of the marriage or domestic partnership, including the obligations that come with it (California Family Code 1992a). Unlike actions for a dissolution (divorce), which must be brought by one of the individuals in the marriage, suits to annul a marriage may be brought by a conservator of the person of unsound mind, or by a relative (California Family Code 1992b). Suits to annul a marriage must be brought before the death of either party, however. So, with the elderly population, the individual or the individual's family should act to annul a marriage as soon as it is recognized that the marriage did not result from a cogent choice.

Vignette *(continued)*

The forensic psychiatrist obtained collateral information from Ms. U's family, reviewed her medical records, collaborated with a psychologist who administered neuropsychological testing, and performed a thorough evaluation. The psychiatrist's evaluation included the use of several functional assessment scales and forensic assessment instruments to help investigate her testamentary capacity. The psychiatrist ultimately concluded that Ms. U lacked the capacity to make decisions regarding her will both presently and around the time she removed her children as beneficiaries. It was later determined that the home health aide had sold several family heirlooms that had been "gifted" to her by Ms. U, and some of Ms. U's savings had been depleted. The psychiatrist's report caused the home health aide to abandon plans to enforce the changed will, and she returned some of the money she received from the sale of the family heirlooms. The family did not file a lawsuit against the home health aide, but the forensic psychiatrist reported the home health aide to adult protective services. Because Ms. U did not have the testamentary capacity to change her will, the changes to the will were not valid, and Ms. U's original will remains enforceable. Ms. U's oldest daughter consulted with her siblings, and they all agreed to employ a new home health aide service and to interview jointly the next home health aide candidate.

KEY POINTS

- A range of legal documents can help patients make legally binding decisions regarding their future health care and the disposition of their financial resources.
- Patients with diagnoses of early dementia and other psychiatric illness should be encouraged to work with an attorney to make financial arrangements and end-of-life health care decisions.
- Courts examine capacity at the time a person makes or changes a legal instrument. To avoid future uncertainty, patients should be encouraged to obtain a capacity evaluation concurrent with the execution of these legal instruments.
- Elder abuse is fairly common and underreported; practitioners should routinely ask elders and those who provide care for elders about abuse. Physicians and other care providers are mandatory reporters of elder abuse.
- To assess capacity, forensic evaluators may employ formal neuropsychological testing, functional assessment scales, and forensic assessment instruments designed to determine whether an evaluee is able to meet a specific legal requirement.

Resources

American Bar Association Commission on Law and Aging: Resources and Research (website). Washington, DC, American Bar Association, 2018. Available at: www.americanbar.org/groups/law_aging/resources.html

American Bar Association Commission on Law and Aging: State Health Care Power of Attorney Statutes. Washington, DC, American Bar Association, January 2018. Available at: www.americanbar.org/content/dam/aba/administrative/law_aging/state-health-care-power-of-attorney-statutes.authcheckdam.pdf

American Bar Association Commission on Law and Aging, American Psychological Association, National College of Probate Judges: Judicial Determination of Capacity of Older Adults in Guardianship Proceedings: A Handbook for Judges. Washington, DC, American Bar Association and the American Psychological Association, 2006. Available at: www.americanbar.org/content/dam/aba/administrative/law_aging/2011_aging_bk_judges_capacity.authcheckdam.pdf (Includes a model clinical evaluation report)

American Bar Association Commission on Law and Aging, Commission
  on Disability Rights, Section on Civil Rights and Social Justice, et al:
  Practical Tool for Lawyers: Steps in Supporting Decision Making.
  Washington, DC, American Bar Association, 2016. Available at:
  www.americanbar.org/content/dam/aba/administrative/law_aging/
  PRACTICALTool.authcheckdam.pdf
Etchells E: Aid to Capacity Evaluation (ACE). Toronto, ON, Canada,
  University of Toronto Joint Centre for Bioethics, n.d. Available at:
  http://jcb.utoronto.ca/tools/ace_download.shtml (Instrument to
  aid assessment of a patient's capacity to make medical decisions)
National Center on Elder Abuse: https://ncea.acl.gov
National Resource Center on Psychiatric Advance Directives: State-by-
  State Information: www.nrc-pad.org/states

References

American Bar Association Commission on Law and Aging: ABA urges supported
  decision making as less-restrictive alternative to guardianship. Bifocal: A Journal of the ABA Commission on Law and Aging 38(6):95, 2017a. Available at:
  https://www.americanbar.org/content/dam/aba/publications/bifocal/
  2017_july_aug_bfcl.authcheckdam.pdf. Accessed July 8, 2018.
American Bar Association Commission on Law and Aging: Resources and Research: Guardianship and Supported Decision-Making (website). Washington,
  DC, American Bar Association, 2017b. Available at: https://www.americanbar.org/
  groups/law_aging/resources/guardianship_law_practice.html#sdm. Accessed July 08, 2018.
American Bar Association Commission on Law and Aging, American Psychological
  Association, National College of Probate Judges: Judicial Determination of Ca-
  pacity of Older Adults in Guardianship Proceedings: A Handbook for Judges.
  Washington, DC, American Bar Association and the American Psychological As-
  sociation, 2006. Available at: https://www.americanbar.org/content/dam/aba/
  administrative/law_aging/2011_aging_bk_judges_capacity.authcheckdam.pdf.
  Accessed November 19, 2017.
Appelbaum PS: Clinical practice: assessment of patients' competence to consent
  to treatment. N Engl J Med 357(18):1834–1840, 2007 17978292
California Family Code § 2210(c) (1992a)
California Family Code § 2211(c) (1992b)
Cooper C, Selwood A, Livingston G: The prevalence of elder abuse and neglect:
  a systematic review. Age Ageing 37(2):151–160, 2008 18349012
Dunphy v Dunphy 161 C 380, 383 (1911)
Etchells E, Darzins P, Silberfeld M, et al: Assessment of patient capacity to con-
  sent to treatment. J Gen Intern Med 14(1):27–34, 1999 9893088
Grisso T, Appelbaum PS: The MacArthur Treatment Competence Study, III:
  abilities of patients to consent to psychiatric and medical treatments. Law
  Hum Behav 19(2):149–174, 1995, 11660292
Kennedy KM: Testamentary capacity: a practical guide to assessment of ability
  to make a valid will. J Forensic Leg Med 19(4):191–195, 2012 22520369

Lachs MS, Pillemer KA: Elder abuse. N Engl J Med 373(20):1947–1956, 2015 26559573

Louisiana Rev Stat § 40:1299.53 (2005)

Marson D: Investigating functional impairment in preclinical Alzheimer's disease. J Prev Alzheimers Dis 2(1):4–6, 2015 26855935

Marson DC, Sawrie SM, Snyder S, et al: Assessing financial capacity in patients with Alzheimer disease: a conceptual model and prototype instrument. Arch Neurol 57(6):877–884, 2000 10867786

Marson DC, Triebel K, Knight A: Financial capacity, in Civil Capacities in Clinical Neuropsychology: Research Findings and Practical Applications (National Academy of Neuropsychology: Series on Evidence-Based Practices). Edited by Demakis G. New York, Oxford University Press, 2011, pp 39–68

Mishkin B: Determining the capacity for making health care decisions. Adv Psychosom Med 19:151–166, 1989 2686360

Moye J, Marson DC: Assessment of decision-making capacity in older adults: an emerging area of practice and research. J Gerontol B Psychol Sci Soc Sci 62(1):P3–P11, 2007 17284555

Moye J, Butz SW, Marson DC, et al: A conceptual model and assessment template for capacity evaluation in adult guardianship. Gerontologist 47(5):591–603, 2007 17989401

National Resource Center on Psychiatric Advance Directives: State by State Information (website), 2017. Available at: https://www.nrc-pad.org/states. Accessed July 8, 2018.

Patient Self-Determination Act of 1990 (H.R. 4449–101st Congress 1989–1990)

The Restatement (Third) of Property (Wills and Don, Trans) § 8.3 cmt. c (2003)

Schouten R, Brendel RW: Guardianships, conservatorships, and alternative forms of substitute decision making, in Primer on Mental Health Practice and the Law. Edited by Schouten R. New York, Oxford University Press, 2017, pp 118–119, 127

Sousa LB, Simões MR, Firmino H, et al: Financial and testamentary capacity evaluations: procedures and assessment instruments underneath a functional approach. Int Psychogeriatr 26(2):217–228, 2014 24229806

Swanson JW, Swartz MS, Elbogen EB, et al: Facilitated psychiatric advance directives: a randomized trial of an intervention to foster advance treatment planning among persons with severe mental illness. Am J Psychiatry 163(11):1943–1951, 2006 17074946

Uniform Adult Guardianship and Protective Proceedings Jurisdiction Act § 102(5) (2007)

Uniform Guardianship, Conservatorship, and Other Protective Arrangements Act §301(a) (Uniform Law Commission) 2017

Uniform Probate Code § 5–102(4) (2010)

Driving

"My Husband Can Be Absent-Minded When He's Driving, That's All"

Christopher O'Connell, M.D.
Aazaz U. Haq, M.D.

CHAPTER 22

Clinical Presentation

Chief Complaint

"My husband can be absent-minded when he's driving, that's all."

Vignette

Mr. W is a 68-year-old man with a past medical history of coronary artery disease, diabetes, hypertension, and anxiety. He is referred to you by his primary care provider to assist with anxiety management. He has been requiring escalating dosages of diazepam to manage "anxiety attacks." His other medications include metoprolol, simvastatin, and metformin. During your comprehensive mental health evaluation, you diagnose him with generalized anxiety disorder. You notice that during the interview he dozes off frequently, and he admits to being more forgetful. He reports that he fell asleep "briefly" at the stop sign last week.

Discussion

Situations such as Mr. W's are not uncommon in clinical practice and will likely become more common in coming decades.

- There are more than 40 million licensed older adult drivers in the United States (a 33% increase in the past 10 years) (National Highway Traffic Safety Administration National Center for Statistics and Analysis 2017).
- The population of adults older than age 65 years is expected to nearly double, to 98 million, by 2060 (U.S. Census Bureau 2017).
- Motor vehicle collisions (MVCs) are a leading cause of death from unintentional injury in those older than 65 years (Kochanek et al. 2016).
- Adults older than 65 years accounted for 18% of all traffic fatalities and 10% of traffic-related injuries in 2015 (National Highway Traffic Safety Administration National Center for Statistics and Analysis 2017).
- Among older adults, the traffic fatality rate in 2015 was highest for the 85-and-older age group (National Highway Traffic Safety Administration National Center for Statistics and Analysis 2017).
- Medical conditions, including major neurocognitive disorder (NCD), have significant implications for older drivers.

Driving requires a dynamic integration of multiple high-level cognitive skills, and health care providers play a crucial role in the driving safety of the older adult (Betz et al. 2015). Yet many providers may be inadequately trained to assess and counsel older patients about driving (Betz et al. 2015). In this chapter, we aim to review the conditions facing older adults that health care practitioners must keep in mind, including medical, mental, and cognitive impairments, and hope to offer some guidance in approaching these clinical challenges.

Aging and Medical Conditions

Aging can affect vision, proprioception, attention and processing speed, and reaction times, all of which may have implications for driving abilities (Canadian Medical Association 2017). The increased risk of MVCs is just as likely to be related to the cumulative impact of medical conditions (and their associated pharmacological remedies) as it is to aging itself (Rizzo 2011). Beyond normal aging, several chronic medical con-

TABLE 22–1. **Medical conditions associated with increased crash risk[a]**

Epilepsy	Heart disease
Sleep apnea	Stroke
Cataracts	Possibly cancer; diabetes; certain musculoskeletal, endocrine, renal, and respiratory diseases[b]; and decompensated psychiatric illness[c]

[a]Charlton et al. 2010; McGwin et al. 2000.
[b]Jones et al. 2012; Rizzo 2011.
[c]Canadian Medical Association 2017; Pomidor 2015.

ditions have been associated with increased crash risk compared to relevant controls (see Table 22–1).

The treatment of some of these conditions may mitigate this risk, such as continuous positive airway pressure therapy in obstructive sleep apnea, or could potentially raise the risk, such as the use of benzodiazepines in psychiatric disorders (Charlton et al. 2010). For a review of chronic medical conditions and their risk in driving, see *CMA Driver's Guide: Determining Medical Fitness to Operate Motor Vehicles,* 9th Edition (Canadian Medical Association 2017) and Charlton et al. 2010 and Rizzo 2011.

Clinical aids, such as the CanDRIVE fitness-to-drive assessment mnemonic, can assist clinicians in evaluating older drivers with medical illnesses (Molnar and Simpson 2010). It has been noted that older adults' driving experience, as well as the implementation of defensive driving strategies and planning for when and where to drive, can help seniors keep the roads and themselves safe (Canadian Medical Association 2017).

Medications and Substances

Several medications (Table 22–2) may compromise driving and therefore should raise clinicians' concerns. These medications include several central nervous system (CNS)–acting medications that mental health professionals prescribe. Such medications may affect drivers' attention and reaction time or their ability to drive at safe speeds, maintain lane position, and follow traffic signals (Dischinger et al. 2011).

Medications with sedative properties such as antispasmodics, benzodiazepines, muscle relaxants, narcotics, barbiturates, and certain antidepressants have been associated with impaired driving, and their avoidance, dosage reduction, and discontinuation serve as important interventions that may lower driving risks in older drivers (Barco et al. 2015; Carr and

TABLE 22-2. Medications that may affect driving-related abilities[a]

Medication class	Potential adverse effects
Benzodiazepines[b] (especially long-acting)	Slow reaction time, sedation
Anticholinergics (tricyclic antidepressants, antispasmodics, some antipsychotics)	Confusion/sedation, blurred vision
Longer-acting hypnotics (zolpidem, eszopiclone)	Slow reaction time, increased sedation
Opioid analgesics[c]	Sedation, slowed reaction time
Antihistamines	Sedation, dizziness

[a]Canadian Medical Association 2017; LeRoy and Morse 2008; Pomidor 2015; Snyder 2005.
[b]Meuleners et al. 2011 Orriols et al. 2009; Smink et al. 2010; Verster et al. 2004.
[c]Kress and Kraft 2005.

Ott 2010). A retrospective review of medical records (and associated police reports) of all MVC-related admissions to a Baltimore trauma center revealed that the accumulation of psychotropic (CNS-acting) medications increased the crash culpability of older drivers (age >45 years) (odds ration [OR]=1.28 for one agent; OR=4.23 for two agents; OR=7.99 for more than two agents), whereas crash culpability was not significantly increased in drivers younger than age 45 (Dischinger et al. 2011).

The timing of sedative-hypnotic administration may also be important, as illustrated in Verster et al.'s (2014) review examining the effect of "middle of the night" dosing of nonbenzodiazepine hypnotics (so-called Z drugs) on a standardized on-the-road driving test the following morning. Zolpidem and zopiclone significantly impaired next-morning driving; however, this effect was not evident with low-dose zolpidem (3.5 mg) or the shorter-acting agent zaleplon at 10 mg or 20 mg. If there are no alternatives to target insomnia, using a low evening dose of a short-acting nonbenzodiazepine hypnotic may be reasonable (Hetland and Carr 2014; LeRoy and Morse 2008).

Data regarding antidepressants' effects on driving risk are mixed. Some data regarding selective serotonin reuptake inhibitors (SSRIs) and serotonin-norepinephrine reuptake inhibitors point toward an increased collision risk (Hetland et al. 2014). In a time-to-event analysis, Rapoport et al. (2011) found older drivers had a modest but statistically significant increased risk (OR=1.63; 95% confidence interval [CI], 1.57–1.69; χ^2=627.31; *df*=1; *P*<0.0001) of MVCs with second-generation antidepressants (SSRIs and other newer agents) when potentially impairing medications (benzodiazepines, strongly anticholinergic medications) were coprescribed. This risk returned to baseline 3–4 months following drug commencement. Trazodone and mirtazapine have been shown in some studies to elevate risk; the latter appears to have lower risk at high dosages, perhaps due to its theorized inverse dose-dependent sedation. Bupropion is thought to be less risky for drivers (Hetland and Carr 2014). Tricyclic antidepressants' anticholinergic and orthostatic side effects are cited as potential contributors to driving risk, and patients should be counseled to avoid driving during dosage increases and in the first days of initiating the medication (Hetland and Carr 2014).

In their case-crossover study of individuals with dementia who experienced an MVC, Rapoport et al. (2008) discovered that the use of psychotropic medications was associated with an increased risk (OR=1.54; 95% CI, 1.35–1.74) of an MVC. In a retrospective study of 225 older drivers (mean age=68 years) referred to an occupational therapy driving evaluation clinic, Hetland et al. (2014) reported that after controlling for medical impairments, drivers who routinely used potentially driver-impairing medications, based on LeRoy and Morse's (2008) list, demonstrated higher mean Epworth Sleepiness Scale scores (a measure of daytime sleepiness) than control subjects; these higher scores have been linked to risk of MVC (LeRoy and Morse 2008).

Data are similarly mixed for antiepileptic drugs, with some evidence suggesting a nearly twofold increased probability of an accident, and a large multicenter study reporting higher collision rates in nonadherent patients (Hetland and Carr 2014). Antipsychotics may increase crash risk as well, although, again, data are mixed (LeRoy and Morse 2008). Providers must counsel their patients regarding the potential risks of medications with driving, with particular attention given to polypharmacy and drug-drug interactions, and then document these conversations.

Vignette *(continued)*

You discuss a plan to target Mr. W's anxiety symptoms with psychotherapy, as well as the initiation of sertraline. With his consent, you contact his wife to drive him home from the clinic. You counsel both the patient and his wife that he should not drive until the diazepam has been tapered off, given its association with sedation. You taper the patient off of his long-acting benzodiazepine over several weeks. Three months later, Mr. W is off of diazepam and is noticeably more alert and interactive, scoring a 30/30 on his Montreal Cognitive Assessment (MoCA; Nasreddine et al. 2005). His anxiety is also now well controlled. After one more visit, you refer him back to his primary care provider.

Psychiatric Illness

The American Geriatric Society's *Clinician's Guide to Assessing and Counseling Older Drivers,* 3rd Edition (Pomidor 2015), advises that clinicians should recommend that patients cease driving during acute phases of severe depression with suicidal thinking, mania, psychosis, or severe anxiety. The guide also states that patients may resume driving when these conditions are stable. The guide also reminds physicians and other providers to review patients' psychotropic medications and counsel them regarding any potential risks. Lastly, it recommends that patients with severe personality disorders (significant erratic, violent, aggressive, or irresponsible behaviors) with a history of violations be counseled to abstain from driving. Similarly, the *CMA Driver's Guide: Determining Medical Fitness to Operate Motor Vehicles,* 9th Edition (Canadian Medical Association 2017), finds that acute decompensations of psychiatric disorders, including "relapses sufficient to impair perceptions, mood, or thinking," are contraindications to driving.

Alcohol and substance use disorders can also interfere with safe driving, and experts believe patients should abstain from driving until they are sober. Driving under the influence significantly increases risk of MVCs, and clinicians should familiarize themselves with local laws regarding responsibilities for detaining intoxicated individuals who have driven to the clinic or hospital (Pomidor 2015). Older patients are more sensitive to alcohol's effects because of age-related changes in body fat and lean muscle mass compilation, which may be augmented by the addition of CNS-acting medications. Therefore, guidelines recommend clinicians warn older patients against combining alcohol and their CNS-active medications in addition to avoiding drinking and driving (Pomidor 2015).

Many clinicians counsel older patients to abstain from driving while receiving electroconvulsive therapy (ECT). The postictal period, as well as the days surrounding an acute course of ECT, can be wrought with cognitive impairments that may preclude driving (Canadian Medical Association 2017). Expert opinion and guidelines recommend that patients receiving an acute series (e.g., multiple treatments per week) of ECT should not drive, and those receiving outpatient ECT should be discharged to the care of a loved one. However, specific recommendations regarding when patients can resume driving post–ECT treatment are left to the discretion of the provider (Office of Mental Health New York State 2003). Johns Hopkins recommends a 24-hour period of abstaining from driving after outpatient ECT (Johns Hopkins Medicine 2017), while the Mayo Clinic suggests patients cease driving for 1–2 weeks after the last ECT treatment in a series (Mayo Clinic Staff 2017). Other experts recommend that drivers be counseled not to operate motor vehicles for at least 24 hours after general anesthesia, although they do not make specific recommendations regarding ECT (Pomidor 2015). Repetitive transcranial magnetic stimulation has not garnered similar recommendations on driving (Canadian Medical Association 2017).

Major Neurocognitive Disorder (Dementia)

Although many experts, as well as the Alzheimer's Association, recognize that neurodegenerative diseases in and of themselves are insufficient reason to revoke driving privileges, moderate to severe major NCD accompanied by impairments in performing instrumental activities of daily living or activities of daily living precludes driving (Alzheimer's Association 2011; Canadian Medical Association 2017). Up to half of individuals diagnosed with Alzheimer's disease drive an additional 3 years after receiving their diagnosis (Snyder 2005), and pooled data from two longitudinal studies revealed formal on-the-road test pass rates of 88% and 69% for drivers with very mild dementia (clinical dementia rating [CDR]=0.5) and mild dementia (CDR=1.0), respectively (Carr and Ott 2010). Ultimately, the majority of individuals with major NCD will need to retire from driving to protect the safety of themselves and the public (Carmody et al. 2014), because they are at increased risk of automobile collisions (Breen et al. 2007; Carmody et al. 2012; Duchek et al. 2003).

Perhaps more difficult than broaching the topic of driving retirement is the challenge in determining at what point during the illness drivers should retire, because the medical literature offers marginal guidance (Alzheimer's Association 2011). Complicating matters further is inconsistent legislation across state and international lines (Rapoport et al. 2007), as well as the fact that deficits related to the specific etiology of major NCD may significantly alter driver safety (Berger and Rosner 2000). Although experts, consensus statements, and guidelines consistently recommend that individuals with moderate to severe major NCD *not* drive, patients struggling with minor cognitive impairment or mild NCD present a clinical and ethical challenge to all providers who must balance patient autonomy with safety (Carmody et al. 2014). Perhaps most challenging to health care providers is deciding when a patient with questionable or very mild cognitive impairment should retire from driving, because the patient may be able to drive safely for a few years after the diagnosis (Ott et al. 2008), particularly early in the disease. However, a recent study suggests that crash rates may be higher prior to receiving the major NCD diagnosis or earlier in the disease (Meuleners et al. 2016). The authors pointed out, though, that the latter phenomenon may reflect the fact that index hospitalizations for major NCD may lead to driving cessation and therefore lower crash rates (Meuleners et al. 2016). Of note, recommendations for driving retirement may affect patients' ability to access loved ones and services (Chacko et al. 2015).

Vignette *(continued)*

Approximately 10 years later, Mr. W returns to the clinic, again referred by his primary care doctor, for apathy, irritability, and symptoms of depression. Although a review of his history reveals no previous history of depression, on close examination you notice word-finding challenges and short-term memory trouble. He scores a 21 on his MoCA. He is quite irritable and downcast during the examination and states that "everything is fine" when you inquire about his memory and activities of daily living. He will not consent to a referral for neuropsychological testing. His wife joins him and states that he has occasionally rolled through stop signs over the past 6 months, and she has concerns regarding his "absent-mindedness" while driving. She also states that he has been missing doses of his medications; however, he is resistant to help. You counsel the patient and his wife that he should not drive pending further evaluation; however, he declines referral for occupational therapy driving assessment. You explain your concerns regarding his safety and the public's safety and discuss your mandated role in California to prepare a confidential report to the county health department. He is quite angry and storms out of the office. His wife follows, stating, "How could you?! My husband can be absent-minded when he's driving, that's all."

When to Refer and Testing

Deciding Whether to Refer

When to formally assess older drivers' ability to operate automobiles remains a topic of debate (Allison and Lane 2017). Age-based renewal procedures vary by state, with differing intervals between license renewal, and with some states offering restricted licenses with night driving and distance restrictions (Thomas et al. 2013). Many providers do not feel competent in their ability to determine their patient's capacity to operate motor vehicles (Rapoport et al. 2007). In-office cognitive tests and neuropsychological testing are likely insufficient to determine collision risk, and on-the-road driving evaluation remains the "gold

TABLE 22–3. Questions to ask caregivers or family in assessment of older adult driver safety

Any accidents or "near misses"?

Are there scratches or dents on the car?

Any recent citations or tickets? Has the patient been pulled over?

Has the patient gotten lost while driving?

Does the patient veer into other lanes?

Do other drivers honk at the patient?

Has the patient run stop signs or traffic lights?

Has the patient avoided driving or started driving less?

Is the patient watchful and aware of other vehicles and pedestrians?

Would you feel safe being a passenger or having a child be a passenger while the patient drives?

Source. Carr and Ott 2010; Molnar and Simpson 2010.

standard" to assess driving safety (Bixby et al. 2015; Carmody et al. 2012; Chee et al. 2017; Rapoport et al. 2007). A recent study from the Netherlands suggested that a comprehensive approach of clinical interview, neuropsychological testing, and driving simulators may help to predict performance in on-the-road testing (Piersma et al. 2016).

Experienced clinicians may be somewhat more accurate at predicting driving risks compared with family members (Bixby et al. 2015). Many clinicians recognize the role of collateral information from family and caregivers regarding driving safety; however, clinicians must remember that these reports can be compromised because of complicated relationship dynamics and biases (Adler et al. 1996). Questions for family and caregivers that may provide some insight into an older driver's safety behind the wheel are listed in Table 22–3.

Rapoport et al. (2007) argued that "borderline cases" of drivers with mild cognitive disorder are best referred to specialized driving experts for on-road testing. Certified driving specialists and highly trained assessors of driving safety in various populations, including the elderly, can assist in making recommendations about how to drive more safely or help discover alternative means of transportation for impaired drivers (Allison and Lane 2017). Their assessments and recommendations derive from expert consensus (Association for Driver Rehabilitation Specialists 2016). However, the availability of trained occupational therapists to perform on-the-road testing may be limited in certain areas or economically out of reach for patients who may have to pay "out of pocket" for such assessments (Rapoport et al. 2007).

In 2010, the American Academy of Neurology published practice parameters using data from a systematic review to aid clinicians in identifying drivers who may be at increased risk. Having a CDR scale score greater than 0.5–1 and elevated caregiver concern regarding the patient's unsafe driving had the highest evidence for identifying unsafe drivers; having Mini-Mental State Examination (MMSE; Folstein et al. 1975) scores less than 24 and a history of citations, prior MVCs, changes in driving behavior (fewer miles driven or avoiding driving), and impulsive or aggressive personality traits were somewhat less helpful (Iverson et al. 2010). Iverson et al. (2010) recognized that a CDR of 2 or more (moderate to severe major NCD) precluded driving. Of note, the patient's self-report of driving ability was not found to be reliable, and while the CDR remains helpful in informing risk (Chee et al. 2017), it may be less practical for most clinicians because it requires training and time to administer (Canadian Medical Association 2017).

Rapoport et al. (2014) developed a consensus statement and algorithm to aid clinicians when deciding whether to refer older drivers with mild NCD (mild neurocognitive impairment) and major NCD of mild severity (mild dementia) for on-the-road testing and/or reporting to transportation authorities. It may be helpful to note that Rapoport and colleagues are writing from the perspective of a mandatory reporting region. The consensus recommends that the combination of caregiver concern and either abnormalities on the Clock Drawing Test or low scores on MoCA should trigger a report to transportation authorities, while difficulties with Part B of the Trail Making Test should cause clinicians to consider such a report. Other authors have suggested that MMSE scores less than 24 should prompt a driving evaluation and that driving evaluations should be repeated at least every 6 months, or sooner if there are notable changes in cognitive status (Adler et al. 2005).

Health care providers should recommend referral for a functional driving assessment with occupational therapy or the Department of Motor Vehicles/licensing authority if there is uncertainty regarding driving safety in mild cognitive impairment or mild dementia, and those deemed fit to drive should be reevaluated every 6–12 months (Canadian Medical Association 2017).

Broaching the Topic and Referring

Berger and Rosner (2000) recommended that providers counsel older patients and their families about the possible impairments major NCD can bring. It is recommended that providers discuss the topic of driving retirement early in the course of a dementing illness to allow the individual to participate in decision making as much as possible and to allow for loved ones to plan appropriate alternative transportation (Alzheimer's Association 2011; Snyder 2005). Older patients appear to desire that these frequently emotion-laden conversations occur over time and to maintain some degree of agency in this process (Betz et al. 2016b). Carmody et al. (2014) developed a decision aid to help drivers with major NCD facilitate planning for driving retirement, which lowered conflicts surrounding the decision to retire from driving. Some insurance companies have guides to help individuals with major NCD and their families communicate about and plan for driving cessation (Snyder 2005).

Despite clinician aids such as the *CMA Driver's Guide* and the *Clinician's Guide to Assessing and Counseling Older Drivers,* many providers find it difficult to broach the topic of driving retirement. Some call for incorporation of more traffic medicine curriculum in medical education (O'Neill 2017). There are concerns that patients may not be honest or follow the clinician's recommendation to retire from driving (Sokol 2017). In fact, the Alzheimer's Association recognized that despite clinicians' efforts, and even after having licensing revoked by state authorities, some individuals will continue driving (Alzheimer's Association 2011). Therefore, techniques to achieve driving retirement should be employed. The Alzheimer's Association, American Geriatrics Society, and other authors offer approaches (Alzheimer's Association 2011; Pomidor 2015) and recognize that families may resort to filing down or confiscating keys, disabling the automobile, or removing the car from the premises to keep impaired drivers from taking to the road (Alzheimer's Association 2011; Snyder 2005). Carr and Ott (2010) also provide helpful techniques families can try to ensure that at-risk older adults cease driving.

Clinicians caring for older adults are obliged to counsel their patients about potentially impairing medications and diagnoses that raise their patients' collision risk, and to advise driving retirement and report as necessary in compliance with local laws, while minimizing breaching confidentiality. All of these conversations should be documented well (Pomidor 2015).

Vignette *(continued)*

Mr. W and his wife failed to keep the next scheduled follow-up appointment. You call and they hang up immediately, after reporting that they wish to terminate the treatment relationship and are contacting their family attorney regarding a breach of confidentiality.

Ethical and Legal Considerations

Many ethical principles arise for clinicians caring for patients who are older drivers. For many older adults, driving retirement is a challenging and life-changing event (O'Connell et al. 2017; Snyder 2005). Physicians and other health care providers have ethical obligations to honor confidentiality and autonomy while protecting both patient and public safety (Barco et al. 2015; Berger and Rosner 2000). Providers must also keep in mind that while recommending driving retirement or filing a report to the Department of Motor Vehicles may be pursued in good faith to protect the patient and the public, there can nevertheless be significant ethical and legal consequences. Navigating these complex ethical waters may strain the therapeutic alliance (Rapoport et al. 2007), and clinicians may be hesitant to address driving for fear of damaging the patient-provider relationship (Adler and Rottunda 2011).

While many providers are uncertain of their local legal reporting policies regarding drivers with major NCD (or other potentially unsafe drivers) (Barco et al. 2015), ignorance of the law is not a legal defense. Providers can be held liable for not counseling patients about the risks of potentially impairing medications and certain at-risk diseases, such as major NCD. Case law reflects that clinicians may be liable for damages to third parties that their patients injure if they fail to counsel (and document such conversations) or if they fail to notify local licensing authorities of at-risk drivers (Pomidor 2015). Some states, such as California, require providers to notify state licensing authorities/Department of Motor Vehicles (or local health departments) of their patients with specific medical conditions, including major NCD, whereas others mandate that only "unsafe" drivers be reported, at times requesting objective data to explain how the driver poses a risk (Pomidor 2015). The majority of U.S. states do not mandate such reporting. Among the states with voluntary reporting laws, several do not have specific legislation granting immunity from liability for civil damages for privacy violation (Pomidor 2015), and providers must obtain consent to release medical information (Pomidor 2015).

Some have argued that physicians should be immune from liability for reporting to licensing officials if they are operating from a stance of good faith (Bacon et al. 2007); health care providers may have some solace in knowing that several states grant immunity to clinicians who report drivers in good faith (Pomidor 2015). Experts recommend providers disclose to their patients that they will be filing a report to the licensing agency and the legal (and ethical) reasons for doing so, regardless of whether the state or province in question allows anonymous reporting (Barco et al. 2015), and to assure them that only the minimum information required will be released. It is important for health care providers to document conversations regarding these topics (Pomidor 2015); interestingly, in an observational, retrospective chart review of primary care clinics, providers documented less than one-quarter of cases (Betz et al. 2016a).

Clinicians must also attempt to anticipate potential negative health outcomes associated with driving cessation (Alzheimer's Association 2011). Some patients have described the loss of driving privileges as significant as losing the ability to walk (Freedman and Freedman 1996). Driving cessation has been associated with depression (Carmody et al. 2014), including a nearly doubled risk of depressive symptoms (Chihuri et al. 2016). Being an older nondriver has been found to be an independent risk factor for placement into a long-term care facility (Breen et al. 2007; Freeman et al. 2006). Driving retirement may also affect mobility and independence, leading to high morbidity and mortality (Betz et al. 2015).

A qualitative study in New Zealand found that driving retirement had a negative impact on both patients and their caregivers (Chacko et al. 2015). Losing driving privileges contributes to significant stress on the individual as well as on the family, because some view driving retirement as an affront to their independence, and the practicality of finding alternative means of transportation can be quite challenging (Alzheimer's Association 2011). Caregivers and patients are challenged to find reliable, affordable alternative transportation (Taylor and Tripodes 2001), and often licensed close contacts need to take leave from employment in order to drive older adults with revoked driving privileges (Taylor and Tripodes 2001). As the population of older adults grows, it will become increasingly more important to reconsider public policies and infrastructure to accommodate the aging population's transportation needs (Bacon et al. 2007; Berger and Rosner 2000; Hogan et al. 2014; Rapoport et al. 2007; Taylor and Tripodes 2001).

Berger and Rosner, as well as the American Geriatrics Society and the Alzheimer's Association, provide excellent reviews of ethical concerns on the subject (Alzheimer's Association 2011; Berger and Rosner 2000; Pomidor 2015). In addition, the American Medical Association/National Highway Traffic Safety Administration guide covers medicolegal information clinicians may reference (Pomidor 2015).

Conclusion

Older adults are more susceptible to medical and cognitive disorders that may compromise driving. An accumulating pharmacological burden may further impair older drivers. Despite these concerns, many older patients may continue to drive safely. Unfortunately, there remains a dearth of standardized, evidence-based guidelines to aid physicians in determining fitness to drive (Rapoport et al. 2007), and determining a patient's capacity to drive must be assessed carefully using in-office evaluation, objective cognitive examination, collateral information from loved ones, and, if necessary, referral to occupational therapists or other trained driving specialists to aid in this determination. Clinicians should employ an inclusive approach that adopts the values of their patients as much as possible (Carmody et al. 2014). Figure 22–1 offers a potential approach to evaluating older drivers in the clinic.

KEY POINTS

- Many older adults drive safely.
- Major neurocognitive disorders, among other medical and psychiatric conditions, may increase collision risk in older adults.
- Medication lists require scrutiny because some medications may pose a risk to older drivers (e.g., sedative-hypnotics, anticholinergics).
- Providers must familiarize themselves with local laws regarding driving in older adults.
- Driving retirement can impact the psychosocial wellness of patients, and special attention must be paid to clinicians' ethical responsibilities in addressing these topics.

Resources

Resources for Health Care Providers

Organizations

Alzheimer's Association: 225 N. Michigan Ave., Floor 17, Chicago, IL 60601; (800) 272-3900; www.alz.org

Publications

Canadian Medical Association: CMA Driver's Guide: Determining Medical Fitness to Operate Motor Vehicles, 9th Edition. Ottawa, ON, Canadian Medical Association, 2017

Pomidor A: Clinician's Guide to Assessing and Counseling Older Drivers, 3rd Edition. New York, American Geriatrics Society, 2015

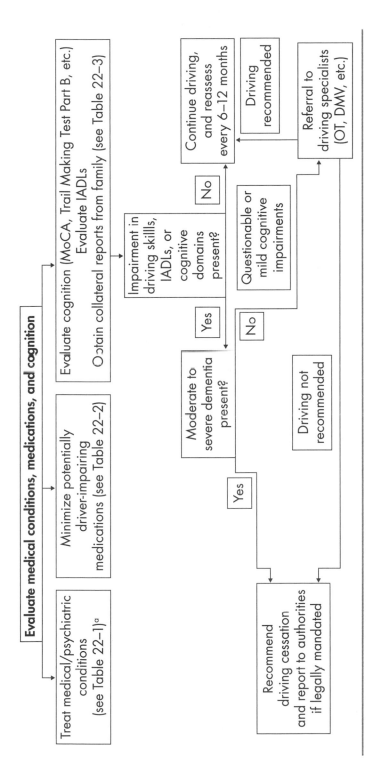

FIGURE 22–1. Approach to evaluating older drivers.

[a]Clinicians should familiarize themselves with local reporting mandates for certain medical conditions. Clinicians should also frequently reassess if treatment of said conditions (or removal of potentially driver-impairing medications) truly mitigates driving risk; if high risk remains, then driving retirement may be recommended.

Note. DMV=department of motor vehicles; IADLs=instrumental activities of daily living; MoCA=Montreal Cognitive Assessment; OT=occupational therapy.

Source. Adapted from Carr and Ott 2010.

Resources for Patients and Families

Alzheimer's Association: 225 N. Michigan Ave., Floor 17, Chicago, IL
60601; (800) 272-3900; www.alz.org

Hartford Center for Mature Market Excellence: www.thehartford.com/
resources/mature-market-excellence/publications-on-aging (Offers several downloadable publications on driving and dementia)

National Highway Traffic Safety Administration: Older Drivers. Available at: https://www.nhtsa.gov/road-safety/older-drivers

National Institute on Aging: Alzheimer's Caregiving: Driving Safety and
Alzheimer's Disease. Bethesda, MD, National Institutes of Health, n.d.
Available at: www.nia.nih.gov/health/driving-safety-and-alzheimers-
disease

References

Adler G, Rottunda SJ: The driver with dementia: a survey of physician attitudes,
knowledge, and practice. Am J Alzheimers Dis Other Demen 26(1):58–64,
2011 21282279

Adler G, Rottunda SJ, Dysken MW: The driver with dementia: a review of the
literature. Am J Geriatr Psychiatry 4(2):110–120, 1996 28531002

Adler G, Rottunda S, Dysken M: The older driver with dementia: an updated literature review. J Safety Res 36(4):399–407, 2005 16226768

Allison CD, Lane A: Risk of motor vehicle collision and driving impairment with
dementia: clinical implications. Am J Geriatr Psychiatry 25(12):1391–1392,
2017 28729140

Alzheimer's Association: Dementia and Driving. Chicago, IL, Alzheimer Association, 2011. Available at: https://www.alz.org/national/documents/
statements_driving.pdf. Accessed November 5, 2017.

Association for Driver Rehabilitation Specialists: Best Practice Guidelines for
the Delivery of Driver Rehabilitation Services. Hickory, NC, Association for
Driver Rehabilitation Specialists, 2016

Bacon D, Fisher RS, Morris JC, et al: American Academy of Neurology position
statement on physician reporting of medical conditions that may affect
driving competence. Neurology 68(15):1174–1177, 2007 17420399

Barco PP, Baum CM, Ott BR, et al: Driving errors in persons with dementia. J
Am Geriatr Soc 63(7):1373–1380, 2015 26140521

Berger JT, Rosner F: Ethical challenges posed by dementia and driving. J Clin
Ethics 11(4):304–308, 2000 11252911

Betz ME, Jones J, Carr DB: System facilitators and barriers to discussing older
driver safety in primary care settings. Inj Prev 21(4):231–237, 2015
25617342

Betz ME, Kanani H, Juarez-Colunga E, et al: Discussions about driving between
older adults and primary care providers. J Am Geriatr Soc 64(6):1318–
1323, 2016a 27321612

Betz ME, Scott K, Jones J, et al: "Are you still driving?" Metasynthesis of patient preferences for communication with health care providers. Traffic Inj Prev 17(4):367–373, 2016b 26507251

Bixby K, Davis JD, Ott BR: Comparing caregiver and clinician predictions of fitness to drive in people with Alzheimer's disease. Am J Occup Ther 69(3):1–7, 2015 25871601

Breen DA, Breen DP, Moore JW, et al: Driving and dementia. BMJ 334(7608): 1365–1369, 2007 17600026

Canadian Medical Association: CMA Driver's Guide: Determining Medical Fitness to Operate Motor Vehicles, 9th Edition. Ottawa, ON, Canadian Medical Association, 2017

Carmody J, Traynor V, Iverson D: Dementia and driving—an approach for general practice. Aust Fam Physician 41(4):230–233, 2012 22472686

Carmody J, Potter J, Lewis K, et al: Development and pilot testing of a decision aid for drivers with dementia. BMC Med Inform Decis Mak 14:19, 2014 24642051

Carr DB, Ott BR: The older adult driver with cognitive impairment: "It's a very frustrating life." JAMA 303(16):1632–1641, 2010 20424254

Chacko EE, Wright WM, Worrall RC, et al: Reactions to driving cessation: a qualitative study of people with dementia and their families. Australas Psychiatry 23(5):496–499, 2015 26104777

Charlton JL, Koppel S, Odell M, et al: Influence of Chronic Illness on Crash Involvement of Motor Vehicle Drivers, 2nd Edition. Victoria, Australia, Monash University Accident Research Centre, 2010

Chee JN, Rapoport MJ, Molnar F, et al: Update on the risk of motor vehicle collision or driving impairment with dementia: a collaborative international systematic review and meta-analysis. Am J Geriatr Psychiatry 25(12):1376–1390, 2017 28917504

Chihuri S, Mielenz TJ, DiMaggio CJ, et al: Driving cessation and health outcomes in older adults. J Am Geriatr Soc 64(2):332–341, 2016 26780879

Dischinger P, Li J, Smith GS, et al: Prescription medication usage and crash culpability in a population of injured drivers. Ann Adv Automot Med 55:207–216, 2011 22105397

Duchek JM, Carr DB, Hunt L, et al: Longitudinal driving performance in early stage dementia of the Alzheimer type. J Am Geriatr Soc 51(10):1342–1347, 2003 14511152

Folstein MF, Folstein SE, McHugh PR: "Mini-mental state." A practical method for grading the cognitive state of patients for the clinician. J Psychiatr Res 12(3):189–198, 1975 1202204

Freedman ML, Freedman DL: Should Alzheimer's disease patients be allowed to drive? A medical, legal, and ethical dilemma. J Am Geriatr Soc 44(7):876–877, 1996 8675943

Freeman EE, Gange SJ, Muñoz B, et al: Driving status and risk of entry into long-term care in older adults. Am J Public Health 96(7):1254–1259, 2006 16735633

Hetland A, Carr DB: Medications and impaired driving. Ann Pharmacother 48(4):494–506, 2014 24473486

Hetland AJ, Carr DB, Wallendorf MJ, et al: Potentially driver-impairing (PDI) medication use in medically impaired adults referred for driving evaluation. Ann Pharmacother 48(4):476–482, 2014 24473491

Hogan DB, Scialfa CT, Caird JK: Consensus statements on the assessment of older drivers. Can Geriatr J 17(2):76–81, 2014 24883166

Iverson DJ, Gronseth GS, Reger MA, et al: Practice parameter update: evaluation and management of driving risk in dementia: report of the Quality Standards Subcommittee of the American Academy of Neurology. Neurology 74(16):1316–1324, 2010 20385882

Johns Hopkins Medicine: Frequently Asked Questions About ECT (website). Baltimore, MD, Johns Hopkins Medicine, 2017. Available at: https://www.hopkinsmedicine.org/psychiatry/specialty_areas/brain_stimulation/ect/faq_ect.html. Accessed November 5, 2017.

Jones K, Rouse-Watson S, Beveridge A, et al: Fitness to drive: GP perspectives of assessing older and functionally impaired patients. Aust Fam Physician 41(4):235–239, 2012 22472687

Kochanek KD, Murphy SL, Xu J, et al: Deaths: Final Data for 2014. Natl Vital Stat Rep 65(4):1–122, 2016 27378572

Kress HG, Kraft B: Opioid medication and driving ability. Eur J Pain 9(2):141–144, 2005 15737803

LeRoy AA, Morse ML: Multiple Medications and Vehicle Crashes: Analysis of Databases. Washington, DC, National Highway Traffic Safety Administration, 2008

Mayo Clinic Staff: Electroconvulsive Therapy (ECT) (website). Rochester, MN, Mayo Clinic, 2017. Available at: https://www.mayoclinic.org/tests-procedures/electroconvulsive-therapy/basics/what-you-can-expect/prc-20014161. Accessed November 5, 2017.

McGwin G Jr, Sims RV, Pulley L, et al: Relations among chronic medical conditions, medications, and automobile crashes in the elderly: a population-based case-control study. Am J Epidemiol 152(5):424–431, 2000 10981455

Meuleners LB, Duke J, Lee AH, et al: Psychoactive medications and crash involvement requiring hospitalization for older drivers: a population-based study. J Am Geriatr Soc 59(9):1575–1580, 2011 21883110

Meuleners LB, Ng J, Chow K, et al: Motor vehicle crashes and dementia: a population-based study. J Am Geriatr Soc 64(5):1039–1045, 2016 27171906

Molnar FJ, Simpson CS: Approach to assessing fitness to drive in patients with cardiac and cognitive conditions. Can Fam Physician 56(11):1123–1129, 2010 21075991

Nasreddine ZS, Phillips NA, Bédirian V, et al: The Montreal Cognitive Assessment, MoCA: a brief screening tool for mild cognitive impairment. J Am Geriatr Soc 53(4):695–699, 2005 15817019

National Highway Traffic Safety Administration National Center for Statistics and Analysis: Traffic Safety Facts (2015 Data, Older Population). Washington, DC, National Highway Traffic Safety Administration, February 2017. Available at: https://www.nhtsa.gov/sites/nhtsa.dot.gov/files/documents/2015_traffic_safety_fact_sheet_older_population.pdf. Accessed May 20, 2019.

O'Connell C, Sommer BR, Dunn LB: Ethical challenges in geriatric psychiatry. Focus 15(1):59–64, 2017

Office of Mental Health New York State: Electroconvulsive Therapy Review Guidelines. Albany, NY, Office of Mental Health, 2003. Available at: https://www.omh.ny.gov/omhweb/ect/guidelines.htm. Accessed November 5, 2017.

O'Neill D: Mandatory reporting of fitness to drive doesn't work. BMJ 357:j2085, 2017 28455346

Orriols L, Salmi LR, Philip P, et al: The impact of medicinal drugs on traffic safety: a systematic review of epidemiological studies. Pharmacoepidemiol Drug Saf 18(8):647–658, 2009 19418468

Ott BR, Heindel WC, Papandonatos GD, et al: A longitudinal study of drivers with Alzheimer disease. Neurology 70(14):1171–1178, 2008 18216302

Piersma D, Fuermaier AB, de Waard D, et al: Prediction of fitness to drive in patients with Alzheimer's dementia. PLoS One 11(2):e0149566, 2016 26910535

Pomidor A (ed): Clinician's Guide to Assessing and Counseling Older Drivers, 3rd Edition. New York, American Geriatrics Society, 2015

Rapoport MJ, Herrmann N, Molnar FJ, et al: Sharing the responsibility for assessing the risk of the driver with dementia. CMAJ 177(6):599–601, 2007 17846442

Rapoport MJ, Herrmann N, Molnar F, et al: Psychotropic medications and motor vehicle collisions in patients with dementia. J Am Geriatr Soc 56(10):1968–1970, 2008 19054208

Rapoport MJ, Zagorski B, Seitz D, et al: At-fault motor vehicle crash risk in elderly patients treated with antidepressants. Am J Geriatr Psychiatry 19(12):998–1006, 2011 22123273

Rapoport MJ, Naglie G, Herrmann N, et al: Developing physician consensus on the reporting of patients with mild cognitive impairment and mild dementia to transportation authorities in a region with mandatory reporting legislation. Am J Geriatr Psychiatry 22(12):1530–1543, 2014 24406250

Rizzo M: Impaired driving from medical conditions: a 70-year-old man trying to decide if he should continue driving. JAMA 305(10):1018–1026, 2011 21364126

Smink BE, Egberts AC, Lusthof KJ, et al: The relationship between benzodiazepine use and traffic accidents: A systematic literature review. CNS Drugs 24(8):639–653, 2010 20658797

Snyder CH: Dementia and driving: autonomy versus safety. J Am Acad Nurse Pract 17(10):393–402, 2005 16181261

Sokol D: Should healthcare professionals breach confidentiality when a patient is unfit to drive? BMJ 356:j1505, 2017

Taylor BD, Tripodes S: The effects of driving cessation on the elderly with dementia and their caregivers. Accid Anal Prev 33(4):519–528, 2001 11426682

Thomas FD III, Blomberg RD, Knodler M, et al: Licensing Procedures for Older Drivers. Washington, DC, National Highway Traffic Safety Administration, 2013

U.S. Census Bureau: Older Americans month: May 2017. Facts for Features, April 10, 2017. Available at: https://www.census.gov/newsroom/facts-for-features/2017/cb17-ff08.html. Accessed November 13, 2017.

Verster JC, Veldhuijzen DS, Volkerts ER: Residual effects of sleep medication on driving ability. Sleep Med Rev 8(4):309–325, 2004 15233958

Verster JC, van de Loo AJ, Moline ML, et al: Middle-of-the-night administration of sleep medication: a critical review of the effects on next morning driving ability. Curr Drug Saf 9(3):205–211, 2014 24909576

LGBT Issues

"I've Been a Woman My Whole Life"

Kevin K. Johnson, M.D.

Clinical Presentation

Chief Complaint

"I've been a woman my whole life."

Vignette

Ms. Z is a 69-year-old white transgender navy veteran who was assigned male sex at birth but now identifies as a woman and uses feminine pronouns (she/her). While the electronic medical record states the veteran's name as "Charles," the veteran prefers to be called "Stacey." She presents seeking medical and surgical interventions for gender dysphoria.

"I've been a woman my whole life," says Ms. Z. She has known she was a girl since grade school but didn't know what transgender was at the time. As a child, she had envied her older sister, who was able to wear dresses and play with dolls while Stacey had to wear her hair short and play with toy trucks. She joined the navy after finishing high school in order to "make a man out of myself" and spent 3 years in Vietnam before being honorably discharged.

She got married at age 23 to a woman she had grown up with and has two adult children, a son and a daughter. She lived as a man throughout the marriage. Her wife passed away 7 years ago after a brief battle with breast cancer. After her wife's death, Ms. Z started experimenting with wearing women's clothing, and "I felt more like my true self." Five years ago, she started doing online research and learned "what transgender was." After reading the definition, she knew instantly that it applied to her. She read more about the transition process. She chose the name Stacey, started growing out her hair, experimented with makeup, and started wearing women's clothing in public on limited occasions in areas where no one would recognize her. At the time, she wanted to come out after she retired to avoid discrimination at work. She retired last year. She came out to her children soon after. Her son, Charles Jr., was supportive of Stacey and easily started using she/her pronouns and referred to Stacey as his mother instead of father. Her daughter, Joan, had a harder time accepting Stacey's identity. Joan expressed concern about the impact it may have on her two young children, who are still unaware of Stacey's transgender identity. Joan continues to use he/him pronouns and has forbidden Stacey to wear women's clothing around them. Stacey expresses concern during the session that Joan may cut off contact with her grandchildren. Aside from a few online friends, no one else knows about her trans identity, and she still navigates the world as "Charles."

Stacey currently smokes one and a half packs of cigarettes daily and drinks 1–2 days per week. When she does drink, she often has one or two glasses of wine with dinner. Her medical history includes diagnoses of diabetes, high blood pressure, high cholesterol for which she takes metformin, a beta-blocker, and a statin. She is followed closely by her primary care physician. She has never been hospitalized medically or psychiatrically. She has never seen a mental health professional but reports intermittent periods of depression and anxiety over the course of her life. She also reports having a history of excessive drinking in her 30s and 40s. She denies a history of substance abuse in the past.

On the mental status examination, the clinician notices that Stacey has shoulder-length hair that has been slicked back into a ponytail, but otherwise she is wearing male clothing (a denim jacket, cargo shorts, and sneakers) and is not wearing makeup. She has some stubble on her face. She is overweight. She is pleasant and makes good eye contact but also appears nervous.

Discussion

Ms. Z is one of nearly 2.4 million people over the age of 50 who identify as lesbian, gay, bisexual, and/or transgender (LGBT) (Choi and Meyer 2016; Fredriksen-Goldsen et al. 2011). This number is expected to double by 2030 (Choi and Meyer 2016; Fredriksen-Goldsen et al. 2011). People who identify as LGBT compose a diverse population that is often neglected in clinical research (Carroll 2017; Choi and Meyer 2016; Fredriksen-Goldsen et al. 2011; Johnson et al. 2018; Yarns et al. 2016), yet they have unique health care needs.

TABLE 23-1. Important terminology

Term	Definition
Sexual orientation	An identity that one uses to describe whom one is attracted to either sexually, romantically, or emotionally. Examples include straight, lesbian, gay, bisexual, queer, pansexual, or a number of other sexual orientations.
Gender identity	One's inner sense of being male, female, both, or neither.
Gender expression or gender role	How one expresses one's *gender identity*. This includes how one dresses, acts, or functions within one's culture or society.
Sex	Generally based on anatomical or biological characteristics, such as genitals, chromosomes, or hormones. This is separate from gender.
Assigned sex at birth, or natal sex	The sex that one is assigned after being born. This is usually based on genitalia.
Transgender	An umbrella term that covers the diversity of those who have a gender identity that does not match their *assigned sex at birth* or *natal sex*.
Cisgender	Refers to those whose *gender identity* matches their *sex assigned at birth*.
Genderqueer, gender nonconforming, gender fluid, nonbinary, or agender	Terms that may be used by the growing number of people who are defining their gender identity outside the limitations of a binary social construct of gender (i.e., either male or female).

Many terms attempt to capture the vast diversity of the LGBT community. Becoming familiar with these terms can assist clinicians in understanding and in working with LGBT patients (Johnson et al. 2018; Yarns et al. 2016). Table 23–1 defines many of these terms. For example, Ms. Z was *assigned male sex at birth* because of her genitals; however, she currently describes her *gender identity* as either female or transfemale (using she/her pronouns for herself), and she has been experimenting with having a feminine *gender expression* in private (i.e., experimenting with makeup, wearing women's clothing, and growing out her hair). In public, she mostly sticks to a masculine gender expression.

Historical Context

When working with LGBT older adults, it is important to consider the impact of culture, politics, and social norms (Fredriksen-Goldsen 2014; Fredriksen-Goldsen et al. 2011; Yarns et al. 2016). For example, those born before 1945 came of age in an environment where same-sex attraction was highly stigmatized and illegal in many places. Homosexuality also was considered a mental illness, and countless individuals underwent numerous "reparative" treatments to "cure" themselves of their sexual orientation. These included involuntary commitments to mental institutions, electroshock therapy, genital mutilation, and castration. Views on homosexuality started to change with the civil rights movement and sexual revolution of the 1960s. The Stonewall Inn riots of 1969 led to the growth and expansion of the gay liberation movement in the early 1970s. In 1973, the American Psychiatric Association (APA) removed homosexuality from DSM—proclaiming that homosexuality is a variant of normal human behavior. However, the historical stigmatization of same-sex attraction as a mental illness has led to a lasting distrust and fear of health care providers among lesbian, gay, and bisexual elders (Fredriksen-Goldsen et al. 2011; Joint Commission 2011; Yarns et al. 2016). Changing attitudes toward lesbian, gay, and bisexual people led to the legalization of same-sex marriage in the United States through landmark decisions in the U.S. Supreme Court in 2013 (United States v. Windsor 2013) and 2015 (Obergefell v. Hodges 2015) (Yarns et al. 2016).

Transgender and gender-nonconforming elders have also reported distrust of health care providers—particularly mental health professionals, who have historically been placed in the position of "gatekeepers" to medical and surgical treatments to aid in the transition process (Carroll 2017; Elder 2016). Shortly after homosexuality was removed from DSM, the APA added diagnoses relating to transgender identity to DSM, starting with transsexualism in DSM-III in 1980 (American Psychiatric Association 1980). This was replaced with gender identity disorder in DSM-IV in 1994 (American Psychiatric Association 1994). These diagnoses were considerably controversial. Many considered the existence of a diagnosis to be pathologizing of normal human behavior. However, many argue that a diagnosis is necessary to encourage insurance companies to cover medical and surgical interventions. Gender identity disorder was changed to gender dysphoria in DSM-5 in 2013 (American Psychiatric Association 2013; Box 23–1) in order to place greater emphasis on the psychological distress that accompanies having a biological sex that differs from one's gender identity. Despite the change, the feeling of stigma from health care providers persists (Carroll 2017).

Box 23–1. Diagnostic Criteria for Gender Dysphoria in Adolescents and Adults

---

A. A marked incongruence between one's experienced/expressed gender and assigned gender, of at least 6 months' duration, as manifested by at least two of the following:

1. A marked incongruence between one's experienced/expressed gender and primary and/or secondary sex characteristics (or in young adolescents, the anticipated secondary sex characteristics).
2. A strong desire to be rid of one's primary and/or secondary sex characteristics because of a marked incongruence with one's experienced/expressed gender (or in young adolescents, a desire to prevent the development of the anticipated secondary sex characteristics).
3. A strong desire for the primary and/or secondary sex characteristics of the other gender.
4. A strong desire to be of the other gender (or some alternative gender different from one's assigned gender).
5. A strong desire to be treated as the other gender (or some alternative gender different from one's assigned gender).
6. A strong conviction that one has the typical feelings and reactions of the other gender (or some alternative gender different from one's assigned gender).

B. The condition is associated with clinically significant distress or impairment in social, occupational, or other important areas of functioning.

Source.   Reprinted from American Psychiatric Association: *Diagnostic and Statistical Manual of Mental Disorders,* 5th Edition. Arlington, VA, 2013, p. 452. Copyright © 2013 American Psychiatric Association. Used with permission.

Aging While LGBT

The data on LGBT aging show vast disparities in mental health, medical comorbidities, and psychosocial issues (Fredriksen-Goldsen et al. 2011). In 2016, the Williams Institute released a comprehensive review of numerous studies covering the known concerns that affect LGBT aging communities (Choi and Meyer 2016). Compared with their heterosexual or cisgender counterparts, LGBT elders are more likely to live alone and less likely to be married or have children (Choi and Meyer 2016).

Because of higher rates of legal and economic discrimination, LGBT older adults are less able to build savings or have consistent benefits (Choi and Meyer 2016); hence, they are less likely to have sufficient financial resources to care for themselves or obtain formal health care (Choi and Meyer 2016).

LGBT adults report higher levels of disability and poorer mental and physical health (Choi and Meyer 2016). For example, LGBT elders have reported rates of depression two to three times higher than those in the general aging population (Fredriksen-Goldsen et al. 2011). The rates are even higher among transgender elders (Fredriksen-Goldsen et al. 2011), with one study noting that 71% of transgender elders reported suicidal ideation (Fredriksen-Goldsen et al. 2011). Lesbian and bisexual older women have a higher risk of developing cardiovascular disease and a lower likelihood of obtaining a routine mammogram compared to heterosexual older women (Fredriksen-Goldsen et al. 2011). Gay and bisexual older men have higher rates of asthma and hypertension (Choi and Meyer 2016).

"Minority stress theory" attempts to conceptualize these higher health risks by suggesting that higher levels of discrimination, social stigma, and victimization lead to a greater risk of adverse health effects (Choi and Meyer 2016; Erickson-Schroth 2014). In the Caring and Aging with Pride project, 82% of LGBT elders have reported at least one lifetime episode of victimization because of actual or perceived sexual orientation or gender identity (Fredriksen-Goldsen et al. 2011). This includes reports of being hassled or ignored by the police (27%), being the target of physical violence (19%), and being threatened with a weapon (14%) (Fredriksen-Goldsen et al. 2011). Fear of discrimination and prejudice can be exacerbated as aging LGBT individuals require long-term care or extended care (Choi and Meyer 2016). Numerous studies report individuals delaying or avoiding entering residential care (Choi and Meyer 2016). In one study, 34% of elderly LGBT respondents believed they would need to conceal their sexual orientation in order to live in a facility (Johnson et al. 2005). One study found a higher proportion of LGBT adults preferring home hospice care compared with heterosexual adults (Choi and Meyer 2016). Another study of gay and lesbian older adults found stronger support for physician-assisted suicide and palliative end-of-life care compared with heterosexual respondents (Stein and Bonuck 2001). In one qualitative study, transgender elders reported favoring ending their lives over entering extended-care facilities (Witten 2014). Hence, it is important for health care providers to keep this in mind when discussing goals of care or long-term medical needs.

Assessment and Diagnosis of Gender Dysphoria

Regarding Ms. Z, the clinician should continue to sensitively gather more information about her gender history to explore how gender has impacted her throughout her life. For example, it is clear that Ms. Z has had feelings of being a girl from a young age. It would be important to explore whether these feelings shifted after the onset of puberty and in what way. She joined the military to "make a man" of herself; however, why did she feel the need to do this? How did she view her gender identity throughout her adult life? It would also be important to explore how Ms. Z perceives her body and what features have triggered dysphoric feelings (i.e., genitals, Adam's apple, facial hair). The assessment would also be a good opportunity to jointly explore the diversity of gender (Elder 2016; Johnson et al. 2018). While Ms. Z may identify with being a woman, she may not be aware of the diversity of genders—including nonbinary gender, as mentioned in Table 23–1. Regarding transition, it would be important to assess her needs and expectations. From there, it would be helpful to develop a set of goals. What would hormones or surgery accomplish? Keep in mind, not every transgender person wants hormones and/or surgery.

During the assessment, it would be helpful to clinically distinguish gender dysphoria (Box 23–1) from mental health conditions that have similar features, such as body dysmorphic disorder, schizophrenia, or another psychotic disorder (Johnson et al. 2018). In addition to this, the clinician should screen Ms. Z for other mental health concerns, such as substance use disorders, mood disorders, anxiety disorders, or trauma-related disorders (Johnson et al. 2018). Transgender geriatric individuals have a higher incidence of mental illness (James et al. 2016). Although having a psychiatric diagnosis is not a contraindication to starting hormone treatment, it can negatively impact the transition process if left untreated. Before transition, Ms. Z may benefit from mental health treatment, such as psychotherapy, psychotropic medication, trauma-focused therapy, or relapse prevention. It would be helpful to explore where she is in the process of coming out and whether there are any barriers in addition to her daughter's resistance. More than half of transgender adults older than 55 years have reported losing friends because of their gender identity (Grant et al. 2011). Hence, it is also important to assess the level of available social support to help Ms. Z endure the physical and emotional changes that accompany hormone therapy and social transition.

Taking a good medical history that includes a sexual history is important to screen for potential medical and social complications associated with starting medical and social transition. Although age is not a contraindication for hormone therapy or gender-affirming surgery (GAS), tobacco use or having numerous medical comorbidities (e.g., heart disease, hyperlipidemia) could increase the risk of medical complications. For example, estrogen can increase the risk of blood clots in smokers (Hembree et al. 2017).

Gender-Related Medical and Surgical Transition

Some (but not all) transgender and gender-nonconforming individuals may want to pursue the process of *transitioning* (Tables 23–2 and 23–3). This refers to the process by which individuals alter their gender expression or other characteristics, such as external anatomy, to more closely reflect their gender identity (Johnson et al. 2018). The person may transition socially, legally, medically, and/or surgically. The World Professional Association for Transgender Health (WPATH; 2016), in its standards of care, recommends transitioning for those who desire it and consider it to be medically necessary. Transgender elders often wait to start the transition process until they are financially or socially able to do so (Carroll 2017; Grant et al. 2011). For many, this may be in retirement, when there is a reduced risk of job discrimination.

Medical transition often includes the initiation of hormone replacement therapy (HRT) to assist the body with developing secondary sexual characteristics that more closely match the person's gender identity. Table 23–3 summarizes the effects and risks/side effects of masculinizing and feminizing hormones used in transitioning. Neither the WPATH's standards of care nor the Endocrine Society's clinical practice guideline lists advanced age as a contraindication to medical or surgical transition (Hembree et al. 2017; World Professional Association for Transgender Health 2011). However, there is very little research on the long-term effects of HRT or its association with age-related illnesses such as neurocognitive disorders, osteoporosis, or heart disease (Mahan et al. 2016). Transition goals for older adults may differ from those of younger adults because menses and menopause have already occurred (Mahan et al. 2016). Fertility preservation is also likely to be less of a concern. Cisgender older men and women already have low levels of testosterone due to aging (Mahan et al. 2016), and it is important for clinicians to keep this in mind when monitoring hormone levels in trans patients. Hence, tak-

TABLE 23–2. Gender-related surgical interventions

Reconstructive chest surgery: Removal of breast tissue (mastectomy) followed by surgical construction of a male chest contour.

Vaginoplasty: Inversion of penile skin tissue that would lead to the creation of a neovagina. This is often followed by a labioplasty and clitoroplasty, which would surgically create a vulva.

Metoidioplasty: Reconstruction of clitoral tissue (often enlarged after testosterone therapy) into a penis. This is often followed by scrotoplasty, which involves the construction of a scrotal sac that would include testicular prostheses.

Phalloplasty: The construction of a phallus from grafted tissue from other sites.

Reduction thyroid chondroplasty: Reduction of Adam's apple.

Facial feminization surgery: Numerous surgeries that assist in body feminization, which may include a facelift, rhinoplasty, and/or blepharoplasty (rejuvenation of the eyelid).

ing an individualized approach in consideration of individual goals is essential.

Numerous terms have been used to describe surgical transition, such as gender-confirming surgery (GCS), GAS, or sex reassignment surgery (Erickson-Schroth 2014; Johnson et al. 2018). The existing research on surgical transition in aging populations is limited to a few case studies and news reports—one of them showing an 81-year-old transwoman who successfully underwent GCS (Duffy 2014). WPATH recommends at least one referral letter from a mental health provider for top surgeries and two letters for bottom surgeries; however, every surgeon has his or her own requirements for what a referral letter should include (World Professional Association for Transgender Health 2011). Both medical and surgical transitions require the person's ability to provide informed consent, which may be a challenge if cognitive abilities diminish (Carroll 2017).

Vignette *(continued)*

Ms. Z was diagnosed with major depressive disorder, which improved with psychotherapy and the initiation of a selective serotonin reuptake inhibitor. She was also diagnosed with gender dysphoria, and on further exploration, she decided to pursue feminizing hormone therapy and GAS. On the urging of her primary care physician, she has quit smoking and has started exercising in order to lower her risk of blood clots. Be-

TABLE 23–3. Medications used for medical transition

	Feminizing medications[a]	Masculinizing medications[b]
Examples	Estrogen, progesterone, androgen blockers (e.g., spironolactone)	Testosterone, dihydrotestosterone (DHT)
Effects	Development of breasts Reduction in body hair Redistribution of body fat—more feminine shape Softening of skin/decreased oiliness	Growth of facial hair and increased body hair Increase in physical energy/strength and sex drive Increase in muscle mass Increase in size of clitoris (typically about half an inch to a little more than an inch) and discontinuation of menstrual periods Deepening of voice
Risks/side effects	Reduction in muscle mass and upper body strength Shrinkage of testicles (if present) and reduction in ability to produce mature sperm Flaccidity of penis (if present); may not get hard enough for penetrative sex Increased risk of blood clots (significantly increased by smoking), breast cancer, prolactinomas	May cause liver damage Increase in abdominal fat—redistributed to a male shape Weight gain Swelling of hands, feet, and legs Vaginal dryness and thinning of vaginal walls Increased risk of heart disease and worsening of cholesterol profile Increased risk of diabetes

Note. Mood changes can occur with both hormones. Taking a higher dose of hormones will not make changes happen more quickly or more significantly.

[a]Estrogen should be discontinued 2 weeks before any surgery (because of increased risk of clots). It is important to screen for family history of blood clots, heart disease, stroke, or breast cancer. Transgender women should conduct regular breast exams and mammograms according to the same guidelines as natal females.

[b]Effects on fertility unknown; testosterone should not be considered a form of contraception. Will not affect breast size. Can start male pattern baldness in those who are genetically predisposed.

cause of her age, her primary care physician is monitoring her estrogen level to match postmenopausal levels (Mahan et al. 2016).

She reports having very few social supports. Most of her friends have either passed away or maintained limited contact with her after she came out as transgender. She did manage to find a religious community that has been affirming of her identity, and she has a few friends who also identify as transgender, whom she met online through the Transgender Aging Network. She has also found a few local events sponsored by SAGE, a national organization dedicated to improving the lives of LGBT older adults. Her son continues to be supportive, and since her daughter, Joan, accepted Ms. Z's invitation to a session with her therapist, her daughter has started to use she/her pronouns. Joan intends to tell her children about Ms. Z's trans identity.

Because of her age, she admits to struggling with feelings of regret of not transitioning at a younger age. Pondering her own mortality, she fears "not having enough time to be myself." She hopes to continue exploring these feelings in psychotherapy.

Sexuality

Taking a sexual history is important in all geriatric populations, but it can be particularly helpful in LGBT geriatric populations. For many, healthy sexuality has long been suppressed because of discrimination, isolation, and/or internalized homophobia or transphobia (Sherman et al. 2014). Some providers may assume that older adults are no longer sexual, so this topic is often avoided (Milspaw et al. 2016). However, this topic should not be neglected; for some LGBT patients, it is the perfect opportunity to come out to their clinician.

It is important for clinicians to raise the topic of healthy sexuality instead of relying on the patient or partner. There are many age-related changes in sexual function to consider, such as hormonal changes, grief and relationship loss, effects of prescription drugs, and medical comorbidities (Milspaw et al. 2016). When a sexual history is being taken, it is important to build rapport with the patient and introduce the topic by putting it into context (Milspaw et al. 2016). The clinician should start with neutral, open-ended questions such as "Have you experienced any changes in your sexual life?" When asking questions, clinicians should avoid using gendered terms at first. It is acceptable to use the gender-neutral word "partners" instead of "men" or "women." Clinicians should ask patients how they identify their sexual orientation. However, it should not be assumed that because a patient identifies as straight that the individual has not had sexual contact with someone of the same sex. A 2006 survey of heterosexual-identified men in New York City revealed 9.4% had had sexual intercourse with at least one man in the past 12 months (Pathela et al. 2006).

Talking about sexuality and sexual health can be particularly stressful for transgender individuals. They may feel uncomfortable referring to their body parts with gendered terms and prefer more gender-neutral terminology, like chest (instead of breasts); "man-hole" or "front-hole" (instead of vagina); and "dicklet" (instead of clitoris) (Erickson-Schroth 2014). Instead of applying labels to gendered body parts, providers must allow patients to take the lead on how they want to describe themselves. Providers should never hesitate to nonjudgmentally ask for clarification.

Vignette *(continued)*

When asked about sexuality, Ms. Z notes not dating or being sexually active since her wife died. She is sexually and romantically interested in women. She hadn't thought about how she describes her sexual orientation, but thinks she identifies as a lesbian. She is not interested in pursuing any long-term romantic relationships until after she starts medically transitioning but has been considering seeking sexual relationships. Currently, she feels uncomfortable with how her genitals appear (and prefers to avoid using the word "penis") and avoids masturbating. She would prefer them not to be touched by anyone during a sexual encounter.

Addressing Sexual Orientation or Gender Identity

Discussing sexual orientation or gender identity can be a way to enhance care, build trust, and improve provider-patient communication (Coren et al. 2011). Despite these benefits, many people may be afraid to come out to their health care provider, fearing negative consequences and lack of confidentiality, or viewing disclosure as unimportant (Eliason and Schope 2001). For example, LGBT veterans have expressed concerns about disclosure and its potential negative consequences when engaging with the Veterans Administration health care system (Sherman et al. 2014). Because of these fears and negative perceptions, it is important to create a safe and welcoming environment that facilitates disclosure. A patient-centered, LGBT-friendly approach requires specific knowledge, skills, attitudes, and behaviors. It is important that health care providers inquire about the sexual orientation and gender identity of all patients as a routine part of the clinical encounter. Many studies have shown that this benefits patients and helps avoid alienating them (Coren et al. 2011). For LGBT communities, acknowledgment of sexual orientation or gender identity facilitates essential screening for suicide, mental health, violence, tobacco and substance use disorders, infectious diseases, and certain cancers for which LGBT populations are at higher risk.

Developing a nonjudgmental method for obtaining this information is essential. Clinical questions should be inclusive and avoid making assumptions about the patient's sexual behavior or relationships (Coren et al. 2011). Not every LGBT patient—even when asked—will disclose sexual orientation or gender identity. Therefore, care must be taken to avoid pressuring patients to discuss orientation or gender concerns. In addition, to avoid the perception of intrusion or curiosity, clinical questions should be restricted to those necessary to address the issue, with explanations on why the information is needed.

Creating a Safe Environment

Clinicians and their entire staff will need to work together to create a safe and welcoming environment for LGBT elders. The following will help achieve this goal:

- Educate ancillary staff, such as nurses, medical assistants, scheduling staff, and security staff, on LGBT issues and cultural sensitivity. Patients' interactions with them often set the tone for the patient experience (Coren et al. 2011). The National LGBT Health Education Center offers online trainings. Training should include topics such as using appropriate language, recognizing and addressing important LGBT health issues, understanding office nondiscrimination policies, and identifying and dealing with any internalized discriminatory beliefs.
- Ensure that intake forms and medical history forms incorporate a diverse range of sexual orientations and gender identities instead of just male and female (Coren et al. 2011).
- Learn pronouns that patients use (masculine/feminine/gender neutral). If not sure about the appropriate pronoun, politely inquire and apologize if the wrong one is accidentally used.
- When interacting with patients, do not assume patients are heterosexual or cisgender. Clinical questions should be inclusive and avoid making such assumptions. For example, when asking about relationship status, avoid assuming the patient has a "husband" or "wife" without clarifying this first. Among lesbian, gay, and bisexual patients affected by cancer, 58% admitted bringing up their sexual orientation as a way to correct a mistaken (often heterosexual) assumption (Margolies and Scout 2013).
- Place objects in the waiting room or office that indicate a safe, supportive space (e.g., rainbow stickers, pride posters, or LGBT-related reading materials or brochures). Some clinicians wear rainbow caduceus pins or lanyards to show solidarity with the LGBT community. One study revealed that 85% of lesbian, gay, and bisexual patients scan the clinical environment for such clues (Eliason and

Schope 2001). In addition, offer gender-neutral or all-gender bathrooms for patients.

- Clinicians should become aware of their institution's nondiscrimination policies and whether they include sexual orientation, gender identity, and gender expression. Develop zero-tolerance policies on issues such as homophobic or transphobic behaviors.

KEY POINTS

- Keep in mind the historical context of the clinical encounter. Older lesbian, gay, bisexual, and/or transgender (LGBT) adults have consistently reported feeling skeptical of health care professionals and reluctant to rely on a system that has discriminated against them (Choi and Meyer 2016; Coren et al. 2011; Elder 2016). It may take some additional effort to gain their trust.
- Remember that not every LGBT patient—even when asked—will disclose their sexual orientation or gender identity (Eliason and Schope 2001).
- When discussing sexual orientation and/or gender identity, remain aware that patients' racial/ethnic identity, religion, dis/ability status, and/or socioeconomic status may play a major role in how they interact with the world.
- Educate yourself on the health needs of the aging LGBT population and familiarize yourself with the concept of gender diversity. Many LGBT elders report frustration with having to educate their clinicians on basic terminology.
- Encourage LGBT elders—especially transgender elders—to complete a living will or power of attorney. Fewer than half of lesbian, gay, or bisexual baby boomers have completed wills or living wills to protect their end-of-life wishes. Among transgender elders this number drops to 5% (Witten 2014).
- It is important for clinicians and their entire staff to create a safe and welcoming environment for LGBT elders.
- When working with LGBT patients, be aware of your own biases and levels of comfort working with this population (Coren et al. 2011). In a 2002 survey, 6% of physicians admitted feeling "uncomfortable" treating a gay or lesbian patient (Kaiser Family Foundation 2002). If you find yourself uncomfortable working with LGBT patients for personal or religious reasons, you can consider seeking guidance from LGBT-oriented health organizations such as those mentioned in the following section, "Resources." However, because it is important to

recognize your limitations in this context, it may also be appropriate to refer the patient to a different clinician (Coren et al. 2011).

Resources

American Society on Aging, LGBT Aging Issues Network (LAIN): www.asaging.org/lain
LGBT Aging Project: http://fenwayhealth.org/the-fenway-institute/lgbt-aging-project
LGBT Elder Initiative: http://lgbtelderinitiative.org
National Resource Center on LGBT Aging: www.lgbtagingcenter.org
SAGE: Advocacy & Services for LGBT Elders: www.sageusa.org
Transgender Aging Network (TAN): http://forge-forward.org/aging

References

American Psychiatric Association: Diagnostic and Statistical Manual of Mental Disorders, 3rd Edition. Washington, DC, American Psychiatric Association, 1980

American Psychiatric Association: Diagnostic and Statistical Manual of Mental Disorders, 4th Edition. Washington, DC, American Psychiatric Association, 1994

American Psychiatric Association: Diagnostic and Statistical Manual of Mental Disorders, 5th Edition. Arlington, VA, American Psychiatric Association, 2013

Carroll L: Therapeutic issues with transgender elders. Psychiatr Clin North Am 40(1):127–140, 2017 28159139

Choi SK, Meyer IH: LGBT Aging: A Review of Research Findings, Needs, and Policy Implications. Los Angeles, CA, The Williams Institute, 2016. Available at: https://williamsinstitute.law.ucla.edu/wp-content/uploads/LGBT-Aging-A-Review.pdf. Accessed December 7, 2017.

Coren JS, Coren CM, Pagliaro SN, et al: Assessing your office for care of lesbian, gay, bisexual, and transgender patients. Health Care Manag (Frederick) 30(1):66–70, 2011 21248551

Duffy N: 81-year-old woman becomes oldest person to have gender reassignment surgery. PinkNews, October 13, 2014. Available at: http://www.pinknews.co.uk/2014/10/13/81-year-old-woman-becomes-oldest-person-to-have-gender-reassignment-surgery. Accessed December 7, 2017.

Elder A: Experiences of older transgender and gender nonconforming adults in psychotherapy: a qualitative study. Psychol Sex Orientat Gend Divers 3(2):180–186, 2016

Eliason MJ, Schope R: Does "Don't ask don't tell" apply to health care? Lesbian, gay, and bisexual people's disclosure to health care providers. J Gay Lesbian Med Assoc 5(4):125–134, 2001

Erickson-Schroth L: Trans Bodies, Trans Selves: A Resource for the Transgender Community. Oxford, UK, Oxford University Press, 2014

Fredriksen-Goldsen KI: Despite disparities, most LGBT elders are aging well. Aging Today 35(3), 2014 25431529

Fredriksen-Goldsen KI, Muraco A: Aging and sexual orientation: a 25-year review of the literature. Res Aging 32(3):372–413, 2010 24098063

Fredriksen-Goldsen KI, Kim HJ, Emlet CA, et al: The Aging and Health Report: Disparities and Resilience Among Lesbian, Gay, Bisexual, and Transgender Older Adults. Seattle, WA, Aging With Pride, 2011. Available at: http:// depts.washington.edu/agepride/wordpress/wp-content/uploads/2012/ 10/Full-report10-25-12.pdf. Accessed December 7, 2017.

Grant JM, Mottet L, Tanis J, et al: Injustice at Every Turn: A Report of the National Transgender Discrimination Survey. Washington, DC, National Center for Transgender Equality and National Gay and Lesbian Task Force, 2011

Hembree WC, Cohen-Kettenis PT, Gooren L, et al: Endocrine treatment of gender-dysphoric/gender-incongruent persons: an Endocrine Society clinical practice guideline. J Clin Endocrinol Metab 102(11):3869–3903, 2017 28945902

James SE, Herman JL, Rankin S, et al: The Report of the 2015 U.S. Transgender Survey. Washington, DC, National Center for Transgender Equality, 2016

Johnson K, Yarns BC, Abrams JM, et al: Gay and gray session: an interdisciplinary approach to transgender aging. Am J Geriatr Psychiatry 26(7):719–738, 2018 29699765

Johnson MJ, Jackson NC, Arnette JK, et al: Gay and lesbian perceptions of discrimination in retirement care facilities. J Homosex 49(2):83–102, 2005 16048895

The Joint Commission: Advancing Effective Communication, Cultural Competence, and Patient- and Family-Centered Care for the Lesbian, Gay, Bisexual, and Transgender (LGBT) Community: A Field Guide. Oakbrook Terrace, IL, The Joint Commission, 2011

Kaiser Family Foundation: National Survey of Physicians, Part I: Doctors on Disparities in Medical Care. San Francisco, CA, Kaiser Family Foundation, 2002. Available at: https://www.kff.org/uninsured/national-survey-of-physicians-part-i-doctors/. Accessed December 7, 2017.

Mahan RJ, Bailey TA, Bibb TJ, et al: Drug therapy for gender transitions and health screenings in transgender older adults. J Am Geriatr Soc 64(12):2554–2559, 2016 27996106

Margolies L, Scout NFN: LGBT Patient-Centered Outcomes: Cancer Survivors Teach Us How to Improve Care for All. New York, National LGBT Cancer Network, April 2013. Available at: https://cancer-network.org/wp-content/uploads/2017/02/lgbt-patient-centered-outcomes.pdf. Accessed December 7, 2017.

Milspaw A, Brandon K, Sher T: Including sexual function in patient evaluation in the rehabilitation setting. Top Geriatr Rehabil 32(3):221–228, 2016

Obergefell v. Hodges, 576 U.S. (2015)

Pathela P, Hajat A, Schillinger J, et al: Discordance between sexual behavior and self-reported sexual identity: a population-based survey of New York City men. Ann Intern Med 145(6):416–425, 2006 16983129

Sherman MD, Kauth MR, Shipherd JC, et al: Communication between VA providers and sexual and gender minority veterans: a pilot study. Psychol Serv 11(2):235–242, 2014 24588107

Stein GL, Bonuck KA: Attitudes on end-of-life care and advance care planning in the lesbian and gay community. J Palliat Med 4(2):173–190, 2001 11441626

United States v. Windsor, 570 U.S. 744 (2013)

Witten TM: It's not all darkness: robustness, resilience, and successful transgender aging. LGBT Health 1(1):24–33, 2014 26789507

World Professional Association for Transgender Health: Standards of Care for the Health of Transsexual, Transgender, and Gender Nonconforming People. Minneapolis, MN, World Professional Association for Transgender Health, 2011

World Professional Association for Transgender Health: Position Statement on Medical Necessity of Treatment, Sex Reassignment, and Insurance Coverage in the U.S.A. Minneapolis, MN, World Professional Association for Transgender Health, 2016. Available at: https://s3.amazonaws.com/amo_hub_content/Association140/files/WPATH-Position-on-Medical-Necessity-12-21-2016.pdf. Accessed December 7, 2017.

Yarns BC, Abrams JM, Meeks TW, et al: The mental health of older LGBT adults. Curr Psychiatry Rep 18(6):60, 2016 27142205

Practical Strategies for Approaching Grief

"When You Don't Know What to Do, Just Be Human"

Alana Iglewicz, M.D.

CHAPTER 24

> *Give sorrow words; the grief that does not speak whispers the o'er-fraught heart and bids it break.*
>
> *William Shakespeare*

This chapter focuses on providing clinical pearls about grief for the primary care provider. When the term *grief* is used in this chapter, it refers to the response to the death of a loved one. This response is composed of emotional, social, cognitive, physical, and spiritual components (Zisook et al. 2014). Through exploring three case vignettes of grief, the reader will learn about how to approach acute and integrated grief, complicated grief, and physician grief. Each case relates to the death of the same person, Mr. Y, who died of a myocardial infarction 10 years ago at the age of 77.

Envision that you had been the primary care provider to Mr. Y, his wife, and their son, John, for the 10 years before Mr. Y's death. You continue to be the primary care provider to Mrs. Y and John, now 10 years after Mr. Y died. You savored providing care to Mr. and Mrs. Y because you found them to be a charming couple who each exuded warmth, humor, and love. They were high school sweethearts who referred to each other as soul mates. They had both retired and divided their time among traveling the world, being engaged in the community, and spending time with their grandchildren. Mr. Y never failed to make you laugh during appointments with his joke of the day, which he prepared just for you.

Vignette 1: Acute and Integrated Grief

Ten years ago, John scheduled a visit to see you after he injured his right knee running. During that visit, John shared with you that his father, Mr. Y, had died of a myocardial infarction 3 weeks earlier while traveling with Mrs. Y in Europe. John was very close with his father. At first John was shocked by the news of his father's death. He had difficulty sleeping for the first 3 nights, at times crying himself to sleep and surprising himself at his emotionality. Shortly after learning of his father's death, he processed it with his wife and reached out to siblings and friends who knew his father well. They recollected funny and touching stories. John shared a sentimental and humor-filled eulogy at his father's funeral. He returned to work within 1 week of his father's death and found he had difficulty concentrating at work for the first 2 weeks.

You saw John for follow-up of his knee injury 1 month later. At that appointment, you learned that within a month of his father's death, John felt integrated back into the flow of his normal life. Although he continued to miss his father, he did not feel consumed by the loss. Now, 10 years after his father's death, John finds that the symptoms of his grief return around times of stress, when he wishes he could ask his father for advice, and during the holidays. He is simultaneously filled with gratitude that he had his father in his life for as long as he did. He does indicate that his mother is having a much harder time adjusting to his father's death than he is.

Discussion: Acute and Integrated Grief

Understanding Acute and Integrated Grief

In this case, John is experiencing grief over the loss of his father. Grief is a near-universal, natural, adaptive, and instinctual human experience (Zisook et al. 2014). Many conceptualize that grief is the price we pay for love and that love is worth this price. If someone were to ask John, he would likely indicate that having his father in his life, their loving relationship, and his cherished memories were well worth the price of the pain he experienced after his father died. Grief can be subcategorized as 1) *acute grief*—the initial painful response; and 2) *integrated grief*—the mitigated and lasting adaptation to the death of a loved one.

At John's initial visit, he was experiencing acute grief. The acute manifestations of grief can range considerably. The intensity spans from mild discomfort or dysfunction to being one of the most—if not the most—painful and debilitating experiences that people will have in their lifetime. John's experience was closer to the mild end of the range. Feeling shocked, as John felt, or struggling to comprehend and accept the finality of the death after learning of a loved one's death, is common in acute grief. Feelings of sadness and yearning often come in waves, as did John's at nighttime. These are often called the "pangs of grief," and with time, they become less intense and frequent. Sleep disturbance is also common, as John experienced. Notably, the pain and sadness that compose acute grief are accompanied by positive feelings and memories (Bonanno et al. 2005). This is highlighted in John's case by his sharing tender and funny stories about his father with loved ones after his father's death. For many, acute grief can be a consuming process, making it difficult to concentrate on other aspects of life (Zisook and Shuchter 1993). We saw this with John, who was initially having difficulty concentrating at work.

When John presented 1 month later, he was experiencing what we refer to as "integrated grief." His grief transformed from preoccupying his mind to finding a resting place in his heart and memories. He became increasingly able to shift his attention from the death of his father to the world around him and his future. For John, as is the case for most people, transitioning from acute grief to integrated grief was an instinctive process. As he comprehended the permanence of his loss, his sadness and yearning lessened and his acute grief resolved. He reengaged fully in his life. Importantly, John, was not "cured" of grief, nor is anyone. Symptoms of acute grief often resurface during important, meaningful times of the year and during periods of stress. For John, the holidays were particularly evocative, as were times of stress when he would normally seek his father's guidance, as he did during his father's lifetime. Yet despite these times and possibly in light of these times, John remained reintegrated and engaged in his life. Integrated grief continues to evolve with time and is conceptualized to be lifelong (Shear 2010, 2015). Although there is no strict timeline by which people transition from the acute stages of grief to integrated grief, most experience a lessening of their acute grief by weeks to months after their initial loss. Studies indicate that the transformation to integrated grief is usually occurring by 6 months (Zisook et al. 2010), and John's was well within that time frame.

Determining How to Approach Grief in the Primary Care Setting

If you were the primary care physician seeing John in Vignette 1, you would need to determine how you would best inquire about and support John in his grief. For some readers, this may come naturally to you. For others, this can be an uncomfortable, if not overwhelming, clinical encounter. In life, there is no recipe book for how to support those who are grieving. Nor is there is a recipe book for how to grieve. Although nothing is written in stone and support always needs to be contextualized and individualized, some basic principles can help guide physicians in providing optimal support for their grieving patients. Similarly, some approaches can be countertherapeutic and thus should be avoided. Optimal approaches that can be integrated easily into the primary care provider's repertoire and countertherapeutic approaches that should be avoided are reviewed in this section and summarized in Table 24–1.

What to Say and Do

There is an adage in medicine that "when you don't know what to do, just be human." This adage can be used as a guide for how physicians should approach grief with their patients. In the spirit of this adage, there are five main things that primary care physicians can say and do in the primary care setting to optimally approach grief: 1) express genuine empathy, 2) ask about the deceased person's name, 3) ask about the relationship, 4) ask about the patient's current support system, and 5) inquire about how the patient is doing. Each of these is described and expanded on in this section.

Several nuances exist for how to "express genuine empathy." These include, but are not limited to, tone of voice, use of pauses in speech, and body language. The words that the physician chooses are often less important than the way in which the words are shared. A physician saying "I'm sorry to hear that" can come across as expressing the opposite of genuine empathy if delivered with a voice stripped of emotion, sounding overly rehearsed and robotic, or—even worse—with undertones of impatience or condescension. This experience would be heightened if there is no eye contact, especially if the physician's back is to the patient and the

TABLE 24–1. Approaching grief: do's and don'ts

What to say and do	What *not* to say and do
Express empathy	Avoid talking about grief
Ask about name of deceased	Avoid eye contact
Ask about relationship with deceased	Type/write in medical record while
Ask about social support	discussing grief
Inquire how patient is doing	Try to "fix the problem"
	Say "I completely understand"

physician is focused on typing in the electronic medical record. However, when primary care providers make eye contact, they should ensure their body language communicates being fully present for the patient, pause after hearing the patient share his or her loss, and in a kind, genuine voice say the name of the patient followed by "I'm sorry to hear this news," followed by another pause—all while maintaining eye contact—the message communicated is one of empathy. In John's case, you as the provider could turn to John after he shares that his father died, make eye contact, and say, "Oh, John," pause, "I'm terribly sorry to hear this," followed by another pause. There are many words the physician can use that are a variation of "I'm so sorry to hear about your loss," but the key is that the words are communicated in a kind, thoughtful manner with adequate pauses and optimal nonverbal communication (Shear et al. 2017).

The next thing a primary care physician can inquire about is the name of the loved one who died. There is an impactful difference between asking about "your husband," "your wife," "your daughter," "your son," "your partner," "your mother," "your father," or "your best friend" and asking about the deceased loved one using his or her actual name. By asking about, and then using, the deceased loved one's name, you are in turn shifting from objectifying the experience of loss to humanizing the experience. By asking about and using the person's name, you are helping to communicate to the patient that you are comfortable leaving the sterile aspects of medicine aside and entering the realm of human relationships, love, and death. In addition, you are communicating that you care. It is helpful to write the loved one's name down in the medical record so that you can review this before the next appointment and return to inquiring about the grief experience using the actual loved one's name. This is especially important if you are not gifted with names. This small touch will communicate volumes.

Another helpful thing to do after learning of a patient's grief is to inquire more about the relationship the patient shared with the deceased.

It is important not to make assumptions about the relationship because the more conflicted the relationship was, the more conflicted the grief can be. Questions that can be posed to someone who lost his or her spouse or significant other include "Tell me about your husband/wife/life partner" (but ideally using the loved one's name); "How long were you married/together?"; "When did you first meet?"; "How did you meet?"; "How was your marriage/relationship?"; and "What sorts of things did you do together?" If you had a long-standing relationship with the patient, you may already know the answers to these questions and thus would not need to ask them. If so, you may choose to share what you recall from past conversations. Relatedly, it is important to get a sense of the kind of death, whether the death was sudden or expected, how long the person was ill (if at all), the degree to which the patient was involved in caregiving, whether or not the patient was present for the death, and details about the funeral/life celebration.

There is one particular kind of death that warrants special attention—the death of a loved one by suicide. Stigma shrouds suicide loss, and the suicide bereaved commonly experience prominent symptoms of anger, shame, confusion, and overwhelming guilt (Tal Young et al. 2012). For these reasons, it is pivotal that physicians listen empathically and nonjudgmentally to the grief experiences of patients whose loved one died by suicide. See the "Resources" section for helpful websites and books for the suicide bereaved.

The next subject to focus on is the patient's support system. It is useful to know who else is in your patient's life. Does your patient have friends, family, colleagues, neighbors, spiritual leaders, or a religious community? If so, do these individuals know about the death? If yes, has the patient opened up to them about his or her grief? Just because patients have people in their life does not at all mean that they are emotionally supported. It is also helpful to find out if a patient is aware of or has participated in a bereavement support group.

After learning the answers to the above discussed questions (in this section "What to Say and Do"), it is optimal to inquire how the patient is currently doing and has been doing since the death. The focus on how someone is doing should be holistic, including at least the physical and emotional components of well-being. Physically, it is helpful to inquire about sleep, appetite, and energy. Simply asking "how have you been doing since your loved one's death?" addresses emotional needs. By asking how someone is and has been doing since the loved one's death, the physician communicates both caring and an openness to helping the patient process his or her grief. If there is enough time, the physician can also learn more about the patient's prior experiences with grief.

These experiences will inform and shape the patient's current grief experience.

Although there is often not enough time in a primary care visit to obtain all of this information, if time is especially limited, the physician should at the very least express genuine empathy, inquire about the name of the deceased loved one (an act that takes very little time and yet communicates much to the patient), and ask the patient how he or she is doing.

What Not to Say and Do

The most important aspects of "what not to do" were just outlined in the previous section depicting genuine empathy. Your patient's grief may be the most painful experience your patient has had, or will experience, in life. When your patient shares that a loved one has died, this is a cue to you to press pause on the agenda you had, set your agenda aside, and be present for your patient's experience with grief. Your tone of voice and nonverbal communication will be key. When your patient shares that a loved one has died, do not keep your back to your patient. Do not continue typing in the medical record. Do not avoid eye contact. Do not remain standing over your patient while your patient is seated. As noted earlier, the physician should not use a dismissive, robotic, condescending, or overly rehearsed response.

Whenever people learn of someone's loss, they often want to say something to make the grieving person feel better. Relatedly, they often want to say or do something to try to fix the problem. This is especially the case with doctors and their patients. These attempts are well intentioned but often not only miss the mark but also make the patient feel more alone, sad, and even angry (Shear et al. 2017). It is not uncommon for physicians who have had a loss in their own lives to want to make their patients feel as though they are not alone. In these cases, physicians may say something to the effect of "I completely understand." I recommend against saying this, especially if it is followed by "I lost my…" and having your deceased loved one be of a different relationship than the patient's deceased loved one (e.g., after a patient tells you his or her adult daughter died, you say, "I completely understand; my mother died 3 years ago"). Even if the loss is similar in terms of relationship, there are many assumptions inherent in making such a claim. Grieving individuals often perceive that the notion that someone else could "completely understand" their loss and pain is simplistic and false. How could another person completely understand every detail of a relationship, be privy to every memory of their loved one, or comprehend the exact nuances of emotional response that comes after their loved one died? Another common expression people use after someone, especially someone who was older, dies is "At least he/she lived a long life." Such statements, although well intentioned, can trivialize a patient's pain, potentially inducing feelings of anger and being misunderstood—the opposite of helping someone feel "better."

Another misstep to prevent is avoidance of the subject matter altogether. As a primary care physician, you are often pulled in many directions. Your older patients in particular usually present with multiple symptoms, have long medical histories, and are taking multiple medications. As such, most providers like to abide by a more focused agenda. In the case of John, the intended focus of his visit was a knee injury, not his grief. After John shares that his father died, some physicians may be so focused on the chief complaint that they might respond, "Oh. So how is your knee pain?" Of course, they may respond with a kinder variation of this, but the theme is one of sticking with the original focus of the appointment and avoiding discussing the loss and resultant grief. A myriad of reasons may underlie this avoidance. The avoidance of discussing grief may reflect that the physician does not recognize the importance of taking time to address grief, does not feel well prepared to address grief, or finds the topic too anxiety provoking and hence avoids it and sticks with a topic that is more comfortable—the medical symptoms.

Vignette 2: Complicated Grief

Mrs. Y, who is now 86 years old, has had a very different experience with grief than has her son. You saw her several times over the year after her husband's death for evaluations of various bodily ailments that were new for her to experience. These included poor sleep, aches, and pains. She canceled several of these appointments at the last minute, which was very uncharacteristic of her. For the first few months after Mr. Y's death, Mrs. Y could not talk about her husband without breaking into tears and softly sobbing. She asked you many questions about the signs of heart attacks and questioned whether she could have caught her husband's symptoms earlier and brought him in for care before his death.

At first you thought that her reaction was normal, especially considering her deep love for her husband of more than 40 years. However, you are now more worried about her and are not sure how best to help her.

You now understand that since Mr. Y died 10 years ago, she has had a profound sense of emptiness. She feels disconnected and directionless. She is consumed with longing and yearning for him. A previously vibrant woman engaged in all aspects of life—who loved entertaining, attending symphonies, eating at restaurants, traveling the world, and babysitting her grandchildren—she now isolates herself in her bedroom every day, wearing her husband's T-shirt, and lays in bed crying. She has stopped returning loved ones' phone calls. She avoids getting rid of Mr. Y's belongings, and even 10 years after his death, she insists that the spare bedroom that Mr. Y used as a home office remain exactly as he left it. Every pen, piece of paper, and book is exactly where it was when he died. This would normally be the room the grandchildren would sleep in when visiting, but she becomes irate when anyone even tries to enter the room, fearing that they will move something that belonged to her husband. She avoids going to restaurants where they used to eat together, has stopped traveling, and has not attended a symphony in the past decade. She is still filled with guilt that she missed the symptoms of her husband's myocardial infarction and is filled with anger at the doctors in Europe for not saving her husband's life. She is not actively suicidal, but she wonders why she is still alive and ruminates about joining Mr. Y.

A colleague of yours recently saw her for a visit when you were out of town. In talking with Mrs. Y, your colleague initially thought that her husband must have died in the past 2 months and was shocked to learn that his death was 10 years ago. Your colleague commented to you that it was like she was "frozen in grief."

Discussion: Complicated Grief

Mrs. Y's grief is clearly different from that of her son, John. You are concerned about her, as is your colleague. Unlike John, who presented with typical grief, Mrs. Y has grief that is debilitating, consuming, and causing significant psychological distress, even 10 years after her husband's death. She is presenting with a form of grief called *complicated grief,* also referred to as *traumatic grief* or *prolonged grief disorder* (Prigerson et al. 2009) in the literature and *persistent complex bereavement disorder* in DSM-5 (American Psychiatric Association 2013). Complicated grief occurs when acute grief does not transform into integrated grief. Rather, the grief process derails, and a person becomes "frozen" in the acute phases of grief, as your colleague astutely observed with Mrs. Y. As summarized in Table 24–2, common symptoms of complicated grief include intense yearning for the deceased loved one; inability to accept the death; perseverative and intrusive thoughts about the deceased; profound anger and guilt about the death; avoidance of reminders of the loss; social isolation; and loss of meaning in life and often resultant suicidal thoughts (Latham and Prigerson 2004; Shear 2015). Additionally, there can be the opposite of avoidance of reminders, something called "proximity seeking." Mrs. Y's avoidance of getting rid of her husband's belongings, keeping his office exactly as he left it, and wearing and smelling his T-shirt on a daily basis are examples of proximity seeking. In its most extreme presentation, proximity seeking can manifest as wishes to die in order to join the deceased loved one. Mrs. Y's avoidance of reminders of her husband are also profound and include avoiding restaurants, symphonies, and travel. Mrs. Y is preoccupied with the "what ifs," "should haves," and "could haves" surrounding Mr. Y's death, which is characteristic of complicated grief.

Mrs. Y's experience with complicated grief is not an outlier. Complicated grief is actually quite common, especially in older adults. Studies indicate that complicated grief is found in approximately 10% of all bereaved individuals, but it is even more prevalent in certain high-risk populations, such as the elderly (Lundorff et al. 2017). A combination of decreased social connections, increased losses, and poorer physical health places older adults at a higher risk for developing complicated grief (see Table 24–1).

Not only is complicated grief common among older adults, but it is also associated with significant morbidity and mortality. From a mental health perspective, complicated grief is associated with functional impairment and increased rates of psychiatric comorbidities—especially major depressive disorder (MDD) (Monk et al. 2006; Newson et al. 2011; Prigerson et al. 1997). In this case, Mrs. Y likely has MDD concurrent with her complicated grief. The symptoms of other psychiatric illnesses heighten when complicated grief is present. Insomnia is common and persistent (Hardison et al. 2005; Simon et al. 2007). Most importantly, individuals with complicated grief are at much higher risk of having suicidal ideation and suicidal behaviors. Complicated grief has been associated with an 8.2 times greater likelihood of high suicidality, even after MDD, posttraumatic stress disorder (PTSD), gender, race, and social support are controlled for (Latham and Prigerson 2004).

From a medical perspective, individuals with complicated grief have worse physical health outcomes. They tend to participate in riskier health behaviors, including increased use of cigarettes and alcohol (Zisook et al. 1987). People with complicated grief have higher rates of hypertension, cardiac disease, and cancer (Prigerson et al. 1997). Unfortunately, despite increased health problems, they also tend to underutilize health resources. It is important for primary care physicians to be cognizant of the anniversary of the death of a spouse. Widows and widowers with complicated grief have significantly higher rates of developing the flu, cardiac problems, and headaches around the time of the anniversary of their spouse's death (Prigerson et al. 1997). Therefore, it is recommended that physicians document in the medical chart the anniversary of the death of a loved one, especially when complicated grief is present. This allows the physician to provide optimal monitoring and treatment of physical symptoms and illness around this salient and significant time in their patient's lives.

TABLE 24–2. Common symptoms of complicated grief

Intense yearning for deceased loved one

Inability to accept the death

Intrusive thoughts about the death/the deceased

Anger about the death

Guilt about the death

Avoidance of reminders of the loss

Loss of meaning in life

Proximity seeking

Typical grief is a normal, adaptive process; should not be medicalized or pathologized; and does not warrant intervention beyond support. In contrast, in light of its serious associated morbidity and mortality and its tendency to persist indefinitely without intervention, complicated grief necessitates treatment. See Table 24–3 for the distinctions between typical acute grief and complicated grief.

The treatment of complicated grief is beyond the scope of what can be provided in a primary care setting, and a referral to a mental health professional is recommended. The treatment most highly recommended for complicated grief is a kind of therapy called *complicated grief therapy* (Shear et al. 2016). Other therapies can also be considered if complicated grief therapy is not available. These include cognitive-behavioral therapy and interpersonal psychotherapy. A kind of therapy called *restorative retelling* can be especially helpful in cases of violent and unexpected deaths (Saindon et al. 2014). Treatment of comorbid psychiatric illnesses, including MDD and PTSD, should also be prioritized. When Mrs. Y's MDD is treated and she is referred to complicated grief therapy to address her complicated grief, she is capable of finding peace with her grief and fully reengaging back in her life.

Now that you know that complicated grief is common (especially in older adults), has serious medical morbidity and mortality, and is treatable, you are now encouraged to better screen for it and refer for treatment when complicated grief is present. To do this, it is helpful to know who is at higher risk for developing complicated grief. As outlined in Table 24–4, certain types of relationships—such as conceptualizing the deceased loved one as a "soul mate," as did Mrs. Y—and types of deaths place people at higher risk for developing complicated grief.

The Brief Grief Questionnaire is a brief complicated grief screening tool (Shear et al. 2011) that can be easily integrated into the primary

TABLE 24–3. Distinguishing between typical acute grief and complicated grief

	Typical acute grief	Complicated grief
Time course	Lessens within 6–12 months or less in most cases	Persists indefinitely without treatment
Transitions to integrated grief	Yes, instinctively	No, not without treatment
Common feelings	Sadness intermixed with happy emotions when recollecting pleasant memories of deceased loved one	Sadness, anger, and guilt
Suicidal thoughts	Less common unless comorbid major depression is present	Often present, with wish to join the deceased loved one
Functional impairment	Intermittent, lasts days to weeks	Pervasive, often lasts months to years
Warrants treatment	No	Yes

TABLE 24–4. Risk factors for developing complicated grief

Type of relationship with the deceased

A child

A dependent child for whom the bereaved was the mother

A chronically ill loved one for whom the bereaved was the caretaker

A "soul mate"

Type of death

Suicide

Murder

Sudden or unexpected death

Traumatic death

Source.   Shear et al. 2011.

care setting when appropriate. It poses five questions that ask how much trouble the person is having about accepting the death, how much grief interferes with the person's life, if there are troublesome of preoccupying images or thoughts about the deceased loved one, whether there are things that person used to do that are now avoided, and whether the person is feeling cut off or distant from others since the death. Ratings for each question range from 0 to 2 (0 = not at all; 1 = somewhat; 2 = a lot), and a positive screen results from a score ≥ 4.

Vignette 3: Physician Grief

As mentioned earlier in this chapter, you really enjoyed working with Mr. Y. You looked forward to each of his visits. In fact, whenever you saw his name listed on your clinic schedule for the day, it would brighten your day. You savored his jokes. With his humor, kindness, and wisdom about life, he reminded you of your own father, who died 5 years before Mr. Y did, as well as a mentor from medical school who died 7 years before Mr. Y did. Providing care to Mr. Y and his family was also a reminder to you of what you enjoyed most about being a primary care provider: meaningful and longitudinal relationships with patients and their family members.

When John, Mr. Y's son, informed you of Mr. Y's death during John's appointment, you were shocked and saddened. You did your best to focus on John, his experience, and his knee injury but had to exert extra effort not to lose your concentration. When John was reflecting on stories about his father, you found your eyes were becoming moist, and you did not know if this was okay. You held back any tears. You were not sure if you should say anything to John about how much you will miss Mr. Y, because you did not want to make the appointment about you. After concluding your visit with John, you had a busy clinic day, and you consciously set aside thoughts about Mr. Y until your clinic was finished. However, on your drive home that evening, you turned on the radio, and a Beethoven symphony was playing. This reminded you of Mr. Y, because you knew how much he and his wife loved classical music and Beethoven in particular. You felt a tightening in your throat and your eyes started to moisten. You found yourself simultaneously smiling, reflecting on how much you enjoyed being Mr. Y's physician over the years. You shared these memories with your spouse over dinner and later that evening shared tender memories not just of Mr. Y but also of your deceased father and your mentor. Ten years after Mr. Y's death, you still think of him every now and then. Whenever someone tells you a good joke, you fondly remember Mr. Y and smile.

Discussion: Physician Grief

This last case was included to remind the reader that physicians are human, often develop meaningful and mutually rewarding "attachments" to their patients, and, as such, may be deeply affected, both cognitively and emotionally, when patients die. Physicians' responses to the deaths of their patients range considerably. It is not uncommon for physicians to cry when learning about a patient death, especially while in training (Sansone and Sansone 2012). It is also not uncommon for a patient death to evoke feelings and memories from a doctor's personal experience of losing a loved one, as was the case with Mr. Y's death. Yet doctors do not typically discuss these emotions. Education on grief in general, and on the emotional lives of physicians more specifically, is deficient in most health care education and training curricula (Ghesquiere et al. 2018; Stroebe et al. 2017; Williams et al. 2005). Most medical schools and residencies do not teach trainees how to optimally counsel grieving families after patient deaths. On the whole, even less focus is placed on teaching trainees how physicians can cope with grief themselves. This "conspiracy of silence toward emotions" can contribute to the development of physician burnout (Redinbaugh et al. 2003). This is especially the case when a physician whose medical error contributes to an adverse event of a patient becomes "the second victim" (Scott et al. 2010). It is thus important for physicians, especially primary care physicians, to allow themselves to grieve their patients' deaths with the support of colleagues and loved ones. Allowing yourself to do this is a reminder that you care and are engaged in your work. This in turn can help prevent physician burnout. *Your* relationship with Mr. Y was a special one. Treating him and reflecting on his life remind you of the meaning of your own work. Reminders of this meaning will reverberate with the care you provide to numerous future patients.

Conclusion

Through exploring three people's experiences with grieving the death of Mr. Y, this chapter reviews the differences between acute, integrated, and complicated grief. Clinical pearls for the primary care physician were highlighted, with the hope that the reader of this chapter will now have more comfort and agility in working with grieving patients. The reader should now know how to provide optimal support for grieving patients in the primary care setting and when to refer grieving patients for mental health treatment. In addition to the death of loved ones, aging is marked by a multitude of other losses. Older adults can experience loss of health, loss of independence, loss of a job, and loss of identity. The approach to grief outlined here can be extended to these other losses, helping physicians optimally support their patients through all life transitions. Finally, it is important for physicians to remind themselves that they are human and thus allowed to grieve. In fact, allowing themselves to feel and to grieve helps physicians to better connect with the meaning of their work, remain engaged and enthused, burn bright instead of out, and provide sophisticated and compassionate care for their patients.

KEY POINTS

- Grief is a near universal, natural, adaptive human experience.
- Typical grief is an instinctive process and does not require formal treatment.
- In typical grief, acute grief naturally transforms into integrated grief.
- Complicated grief, a form of grief that occurs when acute grief does not transform into integrated grief, is associated with considerable morbidity and mortality and requires treatment.
- Common symptoms of complicated grief include intense yearning and sadness, difficulty accepting the death, intrusive thoughts about the death, anger and guilt about the death, and avoidance of reminders of the loss.
- When a patient shares that a loved one died, at a minimum, express genuine empathy, ask the name of the deceased loved one, and inquire how the patient is doing.
- When you do not know what to do or say in regard to a patient's grief, just be human.

Resources

General Resources About Grief

Association for Death Education and Counseling: https://adec.org/
Main/ADEC_Main/Find-Help/ResourcesHome.aspx

Devine M: It's OK That You're Not OK: Meeting Grief and Loss in a Culture That Doesn't Understand. Louisville, CO, Sounds True, 2017

James JW, Friedman R: The Grief Recovery Handbook, 20th Anniversary Expanded Edition: The Action Program for Moving Beyond Death, Divorce, and Other Losses including Health, Career, and Faith. New York, William Morrow, 2017

Westberg GE: Good Grief: 50th Anniversary Edition. Minneapolis, MN, Fortress Press, 2010

Whitmore Hickman M: Healing After Loss: Daily Meditations for Working Through Grief. New York, William Morrow, 1994

Resources for Death of a Spouse/Significant Other

Didion J: The Year of Magical Thinking. New York, Knopf, 2005

Lewis CS: A Grief Observed. London, Faber & Faber, 1960

Resources for Suicide Loss

American Foundation for Suicide Prevention: I've Lost Someone—After a Suicide: https://afsp.org/find-support/ive-lost-someone

Cobain B, Larch J: Dying to Be Free: A Healing Guide for Families After a Suicide. Center City, MN, Hazelden, 2005

Jordan J, Baugher B: After Suicide Loss: Coping with Your Grief, 2nd Edition. Newcastle. WA, Caring People Press, 2016

Myers MF, Fine C: Touched by Suicide: Hope and Healing After Loss. New York, Avery, 2006

Survivors of Suicide Loss: www.soslsd.org

Resources Regarding Death of a Child

The Compassionate Friends: Supporting Family After a Child Dies: www.compassionatefriends.org

Resources About Complicated Grief

The Center for Complicated Grief: https://complicatedgrief.columbia.edu

References

American Psychiatric Association: Diagnostic and Statistical Manual of Mental Disorders. Arlington, VA, American Psychiatric Association, 2013

Bonanno GA, Moskowitz JT, Papa A, et al: Resilience to loss in bereaved spouses, bereaved parents, and bereaved gay men. J Pers Soc Psychol 88(5):827–843, 2005 15898878

Ghesquiere A, Martinez J, Jalali C, et al: Training residents in depression and grief. Clin Teach 15(2):114–119, 2018 28387049

Hardison HG, Neimeyer RA, Lichstein KL: Insomnia and complicated grief symptoms in bereaved college students. Behav Sleep Med 3(2):99–111, 2005 15802260

Latham AE, Prigerson HG: Suicidality and bereavement: complicated grief as psychiatric disorder presenting greatest risk for suicidality. Suicide Life Threat Behav 34(4):350–362, 2004 15585457

Lundorff M, Holmgren H, Zachariae R, et al: Prevalence of prolonged grief disorder in adult bereavement: A systematic review and meta-analysis. J Affect Disord 212:138–149, 2017 28167398

Monk TH, Houck PR, Shear MK: The daily life of complicated grief patients—what gets missed, what gets added? Death Stud 30(1):77–85, 2006 16296562

Newson RS, Boelen PA, Hek K, et al: The prevalence and characteristics of complicated grief in older adults. J Affect Disord 132(1–2):231–238, 2011 21397336

Prigerson HG, Bierhals AJ, Kasl SV, et al: Traumatic grief as a risk factor for mental and physical morbidity. Am J Psychiatry 154(5):616–623, 1997 9137115

Prigerson HG, Horowitz MJ, Jacobs SC, et al: Prolonged grief disorder: psychometric validation of criteria proposed for DSM-V and ICD-11. PLoS Med 6(8):e1000121, 2009 19652695

Redinbaugh EM, Sullivan AM, Block SD, et al: Doctors' emotional reactions to recent death of a patient: cross sectional study of hospital doctors. BMJ 327(7408):185, 2003 12881257

Saindon C, Rheingold AA, Baddeley J, et al: Restorative retelling for violent loss: an open clinical trial. Death Stud 38(1–5):251–258, 2014 24524588

Sansone RA, Sansone LA: Physician grief with patient death. Innov Clin Neurosci 9(4):22–26, 2012 22666638

Scott SD, Hirschinger LE, Cox KR, et al: Caring for our own: deploying a systemwide second victim rapid response team. Jt Comm J Qual Patient Saf 36(5):233–240, 2010 20480757

Shear KM, Jackson CT, Essock SM, et al: Screening for complicated grief among Project Liberty service recipients 18 months after September 11, 2001. Psychiatr Serv 57(9):1291–1297, 2006 16968758

Shear MK: Complicated grief treatment: the theory, practice and outcomes. Bereave Care 29(3):10–14, 2010 21852889

Shear MK: Clinical practice. Complicated grief. N Engl J Med 372(2):153–160, 2015 25564898

Shear MK, Simon N, Wall M, et al: Complicated grief and related bereavement issues for DSM-5. Depress Anxiety 28(2):103–117, 2011 21284063

Shear MK, Reynolds CF III, Simon NM, et al: Optimizing treatment of complicated grief: a randomized clinical trial. JAMA Psychiatry 73(7):685–694, 2016 27276373

Shear MK, Muldberg S, Periyakoil V: Supporting patients who are bereaved. BMJ 358:j2854, 2017 28684392

Simon NM, Shear KM, Thompson EH, et al: The prevalence and correlates of psychiatric comorbidity in individuals with complicated grief. Compr Psychiatry 48(5):395–399, 2007 17707245

Stroebe M, Stroebe W, Schut H, et al: Grief is not a disease but bereavement merits medical awareness. Lancet 389(10067):347–349, 2017 28137681

Tal Young I, Iglewicz A, Glorioso D, et al: Suicide bereavement and complicated grief. Dialogues Clin Neurosci 14(2):177–186, 2012 22754290

Williams CM, Wilson CC, Olsen CH: Dying, death, and medical education: student voices. J Palliat Med 8(2):372–381, 2005 15890048

Zisook S, Shuchter SR: Uncomplicated bereavement. J Clin Psychiatry 54(10):365–372, 1993 8262878

Zisook S, Shuchter SR, Lyons LE: Predictors of psychological reactions during the early stages of widowhood. Psychiatr Clin North Am 10(3):355–368, 1987 3684745

Zisook S, Simon NM, Reynolds CF III, et al: Bereavement, complicated grief, and DSM, part 2: complicated grief. J Clin Psychiatry 71(8):1097–1098, 2010 20797383

Zisook S, Iglewicz A, Avanzino J, et al: Bereavement: course, consequences, and care. Curr Psychiatry Rep 16(10):482, 2014 25135781

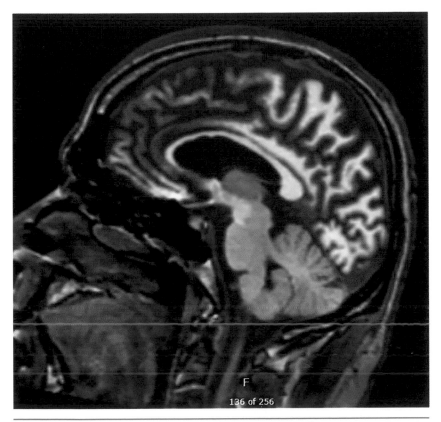

PLATE 1. *(Figure 20–1)* **Sagittal magnetic resonance imaging (MRI) scan of a patient with frontotemporal dementia.**

This MRI scan shows evidence of frontal atrophy in a patient with symptoms of behavioral variant frontotemporal dementia.

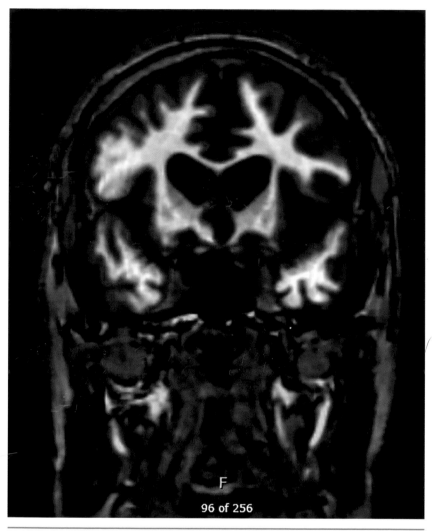

96 of 256

PLATE 2. *(Figure 20–2)* **Coronal magnetic resonance imaging (MRI) scan of a patient with frontotemporal dementia.**

This is a coronal slice of the same MRI scan from Figure 20–1, which shows additional evidence of frontal and temporal atrophy in a patient with symptoms of behavioral variant frontotemporal dementia.

Index

Page numbers printed in **boldface** type refer to tables or figures.

Procainamide, **175**
Processing speed, and cognitive
domains, 256, **257**
Progesterone, **434**
Prolonged grief disorder, 451
PROMIS Depression, 97
PROMIS Emotional Distress-Anxiety
Short Form, **57**
Proximity seeking, and complicated
grief, 451–452
Proxy directives, and powers of
attorney, 393
Psychiatric advance directive (PAD),
392
Psychiatric disorders, and psychiatric
history. *See also* Bipolar
disorder; Comorbidity;
Depression; Generalized anxiety
disorder; Mental health care;
Posttraumatic stress disorder;
Psychotic disorders
driving and, 410–411
post–intensive care syndrome
and, **327**, 334
posttraumatic stress disorder and,
194
Psychiatric symptoms, and cognitive
impairment, 256, **257**
Psychodynamic psychotherapy, for
posttraumatic stress disorder,
205
Psychoeducation. *See also* Education
on BPSD, 273
on generalized anxiety disorder,
52, 58
on mild cognitive impairment,
244
on posttraumatic stress disorder,
199
Psychogeriatric Dependency Rating
Scale (PGDRS), **272**
Psychological distress
chronic pain and, 100, 104–105,
109
somatic symptoms and, 86

Psychosis, and psychotic symptoms.
See also Psychotic depression;
Psychotic disorders
delirium and, 290
frontotemporal dementia and,
377, 378
management of BPSD and, 273–
278
Psychosocial treatments, for somatic
symptoms and anxiety, 88
Psychotherapy. *See also* Cognitive-
behavioral therapy
for bipolar disorder, 182
for depression, 4, **5**, 6–9, 279
for generalized anxiety disorder,
61–62
mild to moderate dementia and,
279
for posttraumatic stress disorder,
200, 203–206
Psychotic depression, 18–19, 25
Psychotic disorders, and differential
diagnosis of posttraumatic stress
disorder, 199. *See also*
Psychosis; Schizophrenia
PTSD Brief Screen, 192
PTSD Checklist, 192

Quetiapine
bipolar disorder and, **178,** 180,
181
BPSD and, 275, **276, 277**
delirium and, 296

Ramelteon, 159, 296–297
Rash, as side effect of lamotrigine,
180
Rating scales
for bipolar disorder, 170
for BPSD, **270–272**
for delirium, 293
for depression in caregivers, 33–
34
for depression in older adults, 2–
3, 16–17